KU-862-686

Empowerment

Madras

Empowerment in community care

Published by Chapman & Hall, 2–6 Boundary Row,
London SE1 8HN, UK

Chapman & Hall, 2–6 Boundary Row, London SE1 8HN, UK

Blackie Academic & Professional, Wester Cleddens Road,
Bishopbriggs, Glasgow G64 2NZ, UK

Chapman & Hall GmbH, Pappelallee 3, 69469 Weinheim, Germany

Chapman & Hall USA, 115 Fifth Avenue, New York, NY 10003, USA

Chapman & Hall Japan, ITP-Japan, Kyowa Building, 3F, 2–2–1
Hirakawacho, Chiyoda-ku, Tokyo 102, Japan

Chapman & Hall Australia, 102 Dodds Street, South Melbourne,
Victoria 3205, Australia

Chapman & Hall India, R. Seshadri, 32 Second Main Road, CIT East,
Madras 600 035, India

Distributed in the USA and Canada by Singular Publishing Group Inc.,
4284 41st Street, San Diego, California 92105

First edition 1995

© 1995 Chapman & Hall

Typeset in 10/12 pt Palatino by Cambrian Typesetters, Frimley, Surrey

Printed in Great Britain by St Edmundsbury Press, Bury St Edmunds,
Suffolk

ISBN 0 412 59880 9   1 56593 421 0 (USA)

A catalogue record for this book is available from the British Library

Library of Congress Catalog Card Number: 94–69064

∞ Printed on permanent acid-free text paper, manufactured in accordance
with ANSI/NISO Z39.48-1992 and ANSI/NISO Z39.48-1984 (Permanence
of Paper).

Contents

List of contributors   v
Introduction   1
Raymond Jack

Part One Empowerment – Meanings and Motives

1 Empowerment in community care   11
   Raymond Jack

2 Defining participative practice in health and welfare   43
   David and Yvonne Shemmings

3 Whose empowerment? Equalizing the competing
   discourses in community care   59
   Suzy Croft and Peter Beresford

**Part Two Empowerment – Practical Experiences in
Self-help and Mutual Aid**

4 Self-help groups as a route to empowerment   77
   Judy Wilson

5 Self-help organizations in Germany: possibilities
   and constraints   96
   Andrea Koch and Monika Reichert

6 Peer support and advocacy – international
   comparisons and developments   108
   David Brandon

7 The third age: a consideration of groups and their
   activities   134
   Tony Chiva

8 Not too 'grey' power   145
   Jack Thain

9 Pensioners' forums – a voice for older people   157
   Tony Carter and Caroline Nash

10 Gaining confidence – speaking out   170
   Zelda Curtis

11 Practical projects for empowering people in health
   and social welfare   184
   Vera Ivers

12 Power and rights: the psychiatric system survivor movement   203
   Vivien Lindow

13 Citizen advocacy and people with learning disabilities
   in Wales   222
   Paul Ramcharan

**Part Three Empowerment – Professional Practice: Challenges
and Opportunities**

14 Effective support for self-help: some lessons from
   the experience of the Self-Help Alliance   243
   *Eric Miller, Fiddy Abraham, Dione Hills, Elizabeth Sommerlad,
   Elliot Stern and Barbara Webb*

15 User first – implications for management   258
   Mervyn Eastman

16 From 'elder protection' to 'adult empowerment':
   critical reflections on a UK campaign   269
   Phil Slater

17 Professional fantasies, consumer realities: a carer's
   view of empowerment   289
   Gillian Hughes

Index   308

Contributors

Peter Beresford and **Suzy Croft**
The Open Services Project, an independent agency promoting the involvement and empowerment of service users. Peter is also senior lecturer in Social Policy, Brunel University College, and a member of Survivors Speak Out. Suzy is also a social worker at St John's Hospice, London

David Brandon
Reader in Social Work, Anglia Polytechnic University, Cambridge, UK

Tony Carter and **Caroline Nash**
Research Institute for the Study of Mid and Later Life, University of Surrey, Guildford, Surrey, UK

Tony Chiva
The Pre-Retirement Association of Great Britain and Northen Ireland and the University of Surrey, Guildford, Surrey, UK

Zelda Curtis
Association of Greater London Older Women
AGLOW is committed to promoting the self-confidence of older women and their full participation in campaigning in all issues which affect their lives.

Mervyn Eastman
Acting Director of Social Services, London Borough of Enfield

Gillian Hughes
Senior lecturer in Social Work, Anglia Polytechnic University, Cambridge, UK

Vera Ivers
The Beth Johnson Foundation, Staffordshire, UK
The Foundation is a charitable trust which promotes innovative ways of working with and improving the quality of life of older people

Raymond Jack
Senior lecturer in Social Work, Anglia Polytechnic University, Cambridge, UK

Andrea Koch and **Monika Reichert**
Lecturers and researchers, Institute of Gerontology, University of Dortmund, Germany

Vivien Lindow
Independent researcher, author and member of various organizations promoting the empowerment of service users and survivors of psychiatric services

Eric Miller, Fiddy Abraham, Dione Hills, Elizabeth Sommerlad, Elliot Stern and **Barbara Webb**
The Tavistock Institute of Human Relations, London, UK

Paul Ramcharan
Research Fellow, Centre for Social Policy Research and Development, University of Wales, Bangor, Gwynedd, UK

Yvonne and **David Shemmings**
Yvonne is Principal Officer, Services for Older People, Essex Social Services Department
David is Director of the Post Graduate Diploma in Community Care, School of Social Work, University of East Anglia, Norwich, UK

Phil Slater
Principal lecturer in social work, School of Social Work and Health Sciences, Middlesex University, and Head of the Student Unit, Social Services Department, London Borough of Enfield

Jack Thain
General Secretary of the National Pensioners' Convention
    The NPC is an umbrella group for pensioners' movements in the UK, the aim of which is to campaign for equality in the basic living standards of all European elderly people.

Judy Wilson
Team Leader and Research Director, The Self-Help Team, Nottingham
    The Self-Help Team provides information and help to people setting up and running self-help groups.

Introduction

Raymond Jack

This book is about people working to gain control over their own lives – trying to empower themselves, and about the way health and welfare professionals working in community care can either help or hinder them. Its diverse readings will interest, challenge and inform service users, providers and managers, and those involved or thinking of getting involved in self-help and mutual aid activity. Students will find here theoretical debate about and practical examples of issues which are fundamental in the development of western societies' health and welfare provision into the 21st century.

Many of the authors have personal experience of overcoming major difficulties in their own lives through self-help and mutual aid, others have spent their professional lives trying to ensure that their practice and their organizations enable this process of empowerment rather than contribute to the disempowerment of the already disadvantaged. Some of the authors have experience from both perspectives: personal and professional. All who contributed did so in the hope that the book will reach a wide and diverse readership of people involved or wanting to get involved in this movement – whatever their role or perspective – and that it will make a very practical contribution to it. Through its exploration of the different ways in which people have successfully empowered themselves in their everyday lives the book begins to redefine not only what empowerment means but what community care can mean when professionals, service users and their carers share common goals rather than being separated by conflicting aspirations.

The choice of title for the book was a deliberate combination of two concepts which, in the measure of their general acceptance as 'good ideas', exemplify a consensus unparalleled in this era frequently characterized as one of the breakdown of consensus over the welfare state. Professionals and politicians of every persuasion are eager to bathe in the 'feel good factor' carried in full measure by notions of both empowerment and community care. Careers have been built on ostentatious allegiance to an apparently common ideology. But, the seeming consensus is only skin deep. Frequently being no more enduring than the expediencies of professional or political aspiration dictate, consensus all too often crumbles in the face of professional rivalry or economic *real politik*, leaving the empty husks of once powerful visions behind, blown away in the vapour trails as professional and political careers take off.

The decision to put together this book of readings was determined by my belief that it is not too late to salvage these visionary conceptions of how health and welfare could be in an age increasingly both aware of and disillusioned by the tokenism of so much of the rhetoric and practice of health and welfare professionals and their political paymasters. This belief that a book about empowerment in community care could still mean something was founded on my own slowly growing (and very belated) knowledge of the immense amount of work being undertaken by disadvantaged people to empower themselves in their communities – helping themselves and others to make their own communities caring. Far from employing the rhetoric and tokenism which threatens to dull these visions, those involved in this work of making these visions real frequently do not characterize it as empowerment or even think of themselves as part of 'community care'. Nonetheless the work of those committed to self-help and mutual aid, rooted as it is in peoples' everyday struggles to master their own lives, is a beacon for those concerned to find the way back to meaningful policy and practice in the human services.

People engaged in self-help and mutual aid will find much that is familiar in these pages and hopefully something new and informative. It is indeed part of the purpose of the book to contribute to the information network which is characteristic of and fundamental to the continued growth of this movement which is burgeoning in all western countries. In those chapters written by health and welfare professionals some insights may be found into practices which have angered and puzzled many service users and their carers and which have sometimes led in reaction to the establishment of self-help groups.

Professionals and politicians with a genuine interest in ensuring that their own practice is about empowerment in community care will find both challenge and opportunity in these pages. It is not the purpose of this book to finally define the word 'empowerment' but to reappraise its meaning and explore its connection with real lives. It is here that challenges will be found. Too much professional practice has become divorced from the real lives of people and their real problems as they experience them, especially those traditionally less favoured by professionals: elderly people, people with physical disabilities and those with learning difficulties. There are harsh words here and severe judgements but those who wish to do so will find not only invective but invitation – a combination exemplified in the words of one writer on disability issues: 'The professionals must decide whose side they're on – they must either join us or get out of the way'.

This has been a punishing period for professionals in health and welfare and some may feel that this is a 'challenge too far' but it is timely nonetheless, for 'empowerment' has become a badge worn by those eager to establish their credibility in a professional environment beset from within by self-doubt and from without by scepticism and popular distrust. There is a danger that this badge is becoming merely another token of good intent, rather than a sign of practical purpose. It seems a good time therefore to reconsider meaning and method.

The notion of the profession has been subject to a sustained critique over the past two decades originally from within the elite ranks of academic sociologists but more recently from a wider constituency including government, the media and a multitude of campaigning pressure groups. In particular those occupations commonly referred to as the 'caring professions' – health, social work and related occupations – have been the subject of criticism perhaps more vitriolic than that received by others in reaction to the suspicion of moral superiority associated with occupations whose often unwelcome task is to enforce standards of conduct.

The critique of professionalism has been broadbased including challenge to the alleged specialist knowledge possessed – or controlled – by the professional; denial of the professional's claim to put the client's interests above their own political and pecuniary advantage; disclosure of the elitist nature of professional education and training. In short, a reinterpretation of professionalism as political tactic rather than principled practice. In Great Britain this critique has been afforded added potency by the suspicion of successive right-wing Conservative administrations of the welfare state apparatus within which most of the caring professions have operated since the Second World War. The demand from government for business-like efficiency and financial accountability in the public service has not only challenged traditional notions of professional autonomy. It has added to the conviction of the radical critique and popular distrust, for as the professions have responded to government demands by becoming more budget driven and entrepreneurial they are seen to be less committed to the interests of their clients – or customers. Any claims still made to moral integrity based on professional vocation and the primacy of the client's interests are seen to be increasingly suspect as the differences between the caring professions and other businesses become less and less apparent.

It is against this background that the notion of empowerment has emerged and become a focus for the continuing revision of the roles and practices of the caring professions in our society. Having said this, however, it is important to recognize immediately that empowerment is not essentially or even primarily about the caring professions. One of the signs of the complacency alluded to at the start of this introduction is the assumption that somehow the empowerment debate begins and ends with its relevance for the caring professions. A major purpose of this book is to challenge this complacency and the assumptions on which it is based – to reappraise the meaning of the badge of empowerment worn so readily by those in the caring professions. This reappraisal is particularly needed in the social care field for two reasons. The critique of the professional has been most severe and sustained in social care and the consequent concern for popular redemption through the notion of client empowerment most pronounced among its professionals. Secondly, the enormous growth in the range and number of self-help, user led organizations in social care over the past two decades – partly in response to the popular disillusion with the professions – demands a reappraisal of their potential role in the process of empowerment. The 'professional imperialism' which underlies the complacent assumption that the traditional professions have a role – let alone a leading one – must be challenged. Can these professions make the connections with peoples' real lives that will make their wearing of the empowerment badge more than tokenistic?

Eager to re-establish the legitimacy of its traditional claim as a profession to have the interests of its clients as its prime concern, those in the caring professions have seen in empowerment a vehicle to achieve this end by espousing client empowerment as a primary goal and defining method. But there is a fundamental contradiction here – whilst claiming to empower clients the caring professions are seeking to re-establish the legitimacy of their claim to professional status – and the authority and power this brings. To acknowledge this contradiction is not to deny any role for the caring professions in the empowerment process, and it is this which provides the second major purpose of the book – to explore the nature of this potential contribution to the struggle people have to gain power and control over their own lives.

Thus our book has two major purposes: to explore meanings, and in so doing disclose contradiction, illogicality and sophistry; and to describe experiences, the ways in which these meanings – their interpretations and practical expressions – are connected to peoples' real lives in the pursuit of empowerment.

Before going on to briefly introduce the content of this collection of readings, I would like to share with you something of the process by which it comes before you. An aspect of the process of its publication which I believe illustrates something of relevance in the empowerment debate. Before being accepted for publication books are read in draft form by independent experts in the relevant field who give their opinion as to the quality of the writing, its accuracy and its potential marketability. This book was so read and opinion duly passed and one or two of the remarks made will serve to illustrate some important aspects of the meaning and method of empowerment whilst also introducing some of the characteristics of the chapters you are about to read. One reviewer asked rhetorically – and somewhat querulously one imagined – 'Is this a personal view?' of a chapter which is demonstrably an account of personal experiences on the road to empowerment. Where were the references to back up these assertions? Was the word 'experiment' used correctly? Now these remarks were made in good faith and with the sole intention of assisting the editor – myself – in meeting the standards and conventions required of an academic text – even one about empowerment. Furthermore, within the context of an academic text these remarks were justified – specific, personal anecdote can be unenlightening in pursuit of the general perspective and the absence of supporting evidence for strongly made assertions can undermine their credibility.

But what would be the point of publishing a text on empowerment which disempowered its contributors by insisting on a uniformity of language and style and demanding adherence to conventions governing the communication of ideas? Although approved of by academic custom, these conventions are alien to several of the authors and much of the potential readership. If one of our purposes in publishing the readings is to promote empowerment through the shared experience of those involved in the variety of its processes, we must surely listen to their experience as they express it, not seek to constrain and reinvent it in forms which certain audiences may find more audible or, in a more sinister interpretation, more acceptable. Such action would be akin to that form of empowerment espoused by some in the caring professions who, while insisting that client participation is a good thing, prefer the bureaucratic and social conventions established for the comfort of the professionals to be observed and respected. The 'assessment' forms must be filled in despite the fact that the client knows what they want and how often have we heard the previously democratic and participative practitioner exclaim 'Don't bring that language in here' in response to an irate client expressing their feelings in the way they find most effective and personally satisfying?

Hopefully this particular anecdote will illuminate some of the reasoning which led to the mix of contributions you are about to read.

Some are unashamedly academic in the best sense in that they are, I believe, erudite and analytical and do observe the conventions by avoiding personal anecdote and meticulously referencing their sources and supporting evidence. Others, however, come from a different heritage and seek to convey their authors' own experience in a way which is personal and practical, informal and sometimes anecdotal. The reader can decide into which category each chapter falls, and it would be wrong to assume that all can be so neatly classified.

Another anecdotal point from the reviewers' remarks which illuminates a further aspect of this book is that one questioned the inclusion of the word 'care' in the title saying the book was not about care. But at least half the chapters are about care – in the form of self-help and advocacy. The problem here is that the reviewer, like many others – particularly professionals in formal caring services – did not perceive such activity as 'real' care, perhaps rather as amateurish attempts at it. Any form of care not provided by trained professionals must be suspect. This type of myopia was another reason for the collection of these readings which put together critical discussion of the concept of empowerment with people's real life experience of empowerment through self-help. The inability of many to see self-help as real care stems from the same professional arrogance and myopia which has led to disillusionment with formal services and the creation of a burgeoning sector of self-help and user led services.

There are 17 chapters in this book, which approach the issues of empowerment from a variety of perspectives and within a diversity of contexts. For this reason the book is divided into three sections, which, broadly speaking, reflect the different perspectives and contexts which their authors are describing. The boundaries between sections are intentionally fluid and there is much in each section which informs the others.

The first, called *Empowerment – Meanings and Motives*, explores what is understood as empowerment by those professionals in health and welfare who claim to be promoting it, and by those who use their services. Is there a common understanding describing a shared mission or is only the rhetoric shared while in fact the aspirations conflict? Do participation and involvement 'empower' service users or is their involvement itself potentially disempowering through absorption, colonization or the bureaucratic dissipation of legitimate protest? The readings suggest that if the professionals' claim to a role in empowerment is to be anything more than rhetoric a new understanding of what 'professional' means and what professional relationships entail is essential.

The second section, *Empowerment – Practical Experiences in Self-help and Mutual Aid*, begins with a consideration of how self-help and mutual aid lead to empowerment. It moves through national and international comparisons of developments to detailed accounts of a wide variety of particular organizations and programmes written by those involved in them. Examples range from health promotion programmes to peer-advocacy systems; from local, national and international political campaigning to assertiveness training groups for black and ethnic elder women and to psychiatric survivor groups which not only campaign for and achieve influence in running local psychiatric services, but enable survivors to celebrate their experience though creative writing and its publication.

Many of the readings relate to older people for the simple reason that they not only experience all the difficulties and disabilities encountered by others, but may legitimately claim to be amongst the most disempowered citizens of this country. Disempowered, that is, by poverty, poor housing and inadequate and frequently discriminatory health and social services. It is particularly important at this time to recognize the need for empowerment among older people because the so-called 'elderly' – a diverse population of ten million people aged between 60 and 100 plus – are increasingly being identified by cost-conscious governments, local authorities and service providers as a 'problem' due to their increasing numbers and, allegedly, greater consumption of health and social services. This constitutes a very real threat to the full citizenship of those arbitrarily consigned to this 'group' and all those claiming an interest in empowerment will therefore be concerned particularly with the plight of elderly people.

This plight is, of course, imposed upon and shared with other so-called 'groups' of people – notably those with mental health problems and those with learning difficulties. Sensitive and moving accounts of those who have survived this oppression through individual courage and mutual aid illustrate in this section the breadth and depth of self-help and mutual aid activity. The energy, innovation and success of those involved belie the discriminatory and potentially debilitating stereotypes of 'the elderly', 'the mentally ill' and 'the mentally handicapped' and may pose for some readers the very real question of what's left for the professionals to do.

In fact the majority of these accounts pay tribute to those 'allies' in the formal health and social services who have contributed in some way to the success of self-help and mutual aid – none doubt that there is a place for the sensitive and imaginative practitioner and manager. There is challenge, but there is also opportunity in the frequently tense, but always potentially creative relationship between professionals and the users – and potential users – of the services they provide.

The third section, *Empowerment – Professional Practice: Challenges and Opportunities* addresses from a variety of perspectives what professionals can do and the potential in this relationship. The readings describe supporting and enabling relationships at a political, managerial and practitioner level which promote empowerment through user participation, self-help and mutual aid. There is danger in the very existence of this still immature relationship between professionals, who always wield power in some sense, and those who seek to gain control over their own lives. But these accounts show how relationships can be developed and shared which bring immense opportunities for creative and rewarding professional practice.

The reader will have noted – perhaps with some frustration – that I have studiously avoided offering a definition of empowerment in this introduction. There are two reasons for this: the first is that the purpose of the book is to allow the reader to explore the various meanings of the term and perhaps come to their own understanding of what it involves. The various contributors have each arrived at their own understanding of empowerment and no pressure has been exerted for uniformity of definition or meaning. The second is that it seems unlikely that any single definition could adequately describe the diversity of oppression and tenacity of spirit shown by those trying to escape it, which are the subject matter of this book. To do so would be but another example of the professional arrogance and myopia that threaten to obscure the vision of genuinely new forms of professional relationship, which the self-help and mutual aid movement offers, and to destroy the mission of empowerment in community care that is there to be shared.

Part One

Empowerment – Meanings and Motives

1

Empowerment in community care

Raymond Jack

DEFINITION

The *Concise Oxford Dictionary* defines empowerment as 'authorize, license (a person to do); give power to, make able (person to do)' – this definition of empowerment has two quite distinct meanings: enablement and empowerment. To authorize, license or make able is a process whereby someone uses their power to enable someone else to do something; what that something is – its nature, goals and extent – is controlled by the enabler. Thus the process of enablement is circumscribed by the power of the enabler and does not involve giving power over that process to the enabled. In contrast, empowerment has been described as '. . . the process by which individuals, groups and/or communities become able to take control of their circumstances and achieve their own goals, thereby being able to work towards maximising the quality of their lives' (Adams, 1990 p. 43). Here the emphasis is on power being 'taken' and its use determined by the goals of its possessor.

In the context of community care a professional may involve a user in the assessment process for a service; the worker may thus 'enable' the user to develop self-confidence, self-esteem and negotiation skills through this process. However, the power to purchase that service and to withdraw it is retained by the professional who has given over none of the power to control the process or its outcome. Empowerment of the user would involve having the money and deciding how it should be spent in pursuit of goals the user determined. There are therefore two quite different activities: enablement which, being about the development of another's capabilities, is a professional skill; and empowerment which, being about the struggle for power and control, is essentially a political activity.

Unfortunately, this apparently simple divide is not so clear-cut in the real world, where the extent to which the professional and political are believed to be separate depends on how one views the relationship between the professionals in community care services and the users of them. It is because the empowerment debate is fundamentally about this relationship and its future development in relation to new forms of health and social care that its importance goes beyond the semantic and the philosophical. As the state of welfare changes, so too do perceptions of the meaning of professionalism and the contribution to health and welfare of the professionals and the bureaucratic organizations they control. The apparently inexorable 'community revolution' which has fundamentally changed the basis upon which community care is provided in Britain brings in its wake questions not only about the role of publicly provided health and welfare services but of the professional status of its providers. As public services are reduced to a residual last resort, and as community care is increasingly redefined as the responsibility of informal carers and voluntary and charitable community networks, the necessity for those who provide services to be qualified professionals is questioned. This is particularly so in social care where professional status has been less securely established than in medical and allied occupations, although even here the 'skill mix' process in nursing is interpreted by some as a way of deprofessionalizing at least some nursing tasks.

It may be no coincidence that in 1989, soon after the *Griffiths Report* (1988) laid out the agenda for action on community care, the British Association of Social Workers (BASW) conference on empowerment was warned by Olive Stevenson, an eminent professor of social work, that 'social work is in deep trouble' and that the increasing role of the independent sector threatened to undermine the independence of the profession which would be limited within a reduced public sector to its 'social control functions' and which now needed to defend its professional status (Stevenson, 1989 p. 7). This view has been recently reiterated by Jones and Novak who similarly note the increasing preoccupation of social work with its child protection, resource allocation and other statutory duties and propose:

> For many clients social work now contributes to their problems and difficulties rather than offering respite and help. Sadly there are few signs of organised opposition to this authoritarian drift of the state's welfare system. The occupation is clearly on the defensive, but is weak, demoralised and in retreat, seemingly incapable of offering a vision of social work which is liberatory and committed to social justice. It would appear that until the political climate changes and there is a widespread revulsion against current trends and social inequalities, social work might continue as an occupation but perish as a caring and liberal profession. (Jones and Novak, 1993 p. 210–11.)

In view of this professional uncertainty it is hardly surprising that most of the literature dealing with empowerment in community care has come from social care professionals – much of it claiming a leading role for them in the empowerment process (Stevenson and Parsloe, 1993; Smale *et al.*, 1993). Similarly North, when comparing the implications of the empowerment debate for health and welfare respectively, wonders if the purchaser–provider split and other measures promoted by the NHS and CCA will 'significantly empower service users as opposed to disempowering statutory providers and the medical profession . . .' (North, 1993 p. 129).

A six-month study of health and welfare professionals in Leeds in 1991 found workers doubtful about their future role as a result of the imposition of the NHS and CC Act with one health respondent asserting that: 'We are becoming more like accountants than health professionals' and another that: 'Because of the pressures of work I am getting further and further away from clients – this is not why I came into nursing' (Higgins, 1992 p. 15).

Thus it is important to consider the empowerment debate within its social and political context – it is after all about power and the defence of sectional interests. As such the debate should be seen as part of a wider process in which professionals are involved in defending their own interests and not simply as a debate about a technique which professionals employ in the interests of service users.

So the nature of the relationship between professionals and service users is central to the empowerment debate and Roger Gomm (1993) suggests that there are basically four interpretations of this relationship. The 'oppressive or liberating relationship' exists in a system where health and welfare organizations are seen as part of the wider political system where power and control are at stake. Their role and that of the professional within them is to maintain a minimum level of functioning in people in order that they may continue to work to increase the wealth and control of the powerful. They also serve to disguise the true nature of this domination and its effects by convincing their users that their dependence on these services is due to their own shortcomings rather than the structural disadvantage which is the true source of their dependency. Professionals collude with this system by turning the political into the personal, that is by 'enabling' users to cope with their shortcomings and adapt to their situation. In this sense they oppress the user as does the wider political system. Alternatively they liberate the user by raising their consciousness of the true source of their problems in social disadvantage – they turn the personal into the political. Professionals are, in this view, inevitably engaged in political activity either in support of the *status quo* or in opposition to it. It is in this sense that those professionals who claim to empower users by enabling them to be involved and participate in decision making without having control over the outcomes have merely 'domesticated' the term in the interests of maintaining the *status quo* (Ward and Mullender, 1992 p. 148).

A second, and related, view of the professional/user relationship Gomm describes as the 'disabling relationship'. Here professionals are in well-paid, secure jobs and use their power to protect their own interests by exaggerating the value of their skills and knowledge and restricting access to them. Their power is founded on their alleged expertise in assessing and defining problems and offering solutions which require the special skills only they possess. This prevents users gaining access to the skills, knowledge and resources they need to deal with their problems themselves – not only, therefore, do professionals not empower or even enable users, they actively disable them through the relationship. In this view professionals who claim empowerment as an aspect of their expertise are merely extending their control by 'colonizing' another activity to which they have no legitimate claim.

The third perspective is that of the 'helping relationship' in which it is accepted that professionals do indeed possess expert skills and know-ledge which users do not, but which they call on to help them identify and meet their needs which would otherwise go unmet. Thus the professionals have a legitimate power which is exercised on behalf of users and in their interests. Here professionalism is seen as essentially apolitical and enablement as part of the armoury of effective professional practice. Finally and, in some senses, not dissimilar is the 'brokerage relationship' in which the expertise of the professional is again accepted but it is a different type of expertise. Here the expertise is less about defining the user's needs for them, and more about negotiating on their behalf the resources the users think they need to meet them.

In the literature on empowerment in community care, these meanings and activities are often confused and the term 'empowerment' has been used to cover a wide range of activities ranging from the power of users to choose what care is provided and how, through involvement and participation in service planning and delivery, to user control of public services. Less frequently, empowerment is discussed in terms of self-advocacy and self-help and as a process through which individuals gain mastery not just over public services but over their lives through a greater understanding of 'power and power relationships within their social, political and economic systems' (Evans, 1992 p. 141).

The role given to the professional in relation to empowerment varies according to which of these meanings is adopted, and it has been claimed that professional practice has to be reinvented and a new culture created in health and welfare organizations in order that professionals can more effectively empower service users. The point of this chapter however will be to suggest that professionals in community care cannot empower users of their services as this is a paradoxical proposition and that even if this were not so, there is little or no mandate for such activity from statute, social policy or public demand. Professional practice designed to promote involvement and participation can be enabling for service users and there is some empirical evidence that such practice is likely to be more effective in meeting the mutually identified goals of users. However, involvement and participation are misleadingly described as empowerment in which process professionals have a much more limited role.

Too often in the empowerment literature professionals in public community care services are placed centre stage in what is claimed to be the empowerment process. This might be expected as much of it is written for professionals by them; however this myopia of therapeutic good intention is misleading since most community care is provided by people who are not professionals, for people who are not service users. Six million informal carers provide more care than all the formal care services put together – most with little or no input from such services (Green, 1988). Furthermore, in the developing mixed economy of care many of those who are receiving services do not receive them from public sector providers – most residential care for example now comes from the independent sector. These are facts almost entirely neglected in the empowerment literature.

In view of the conflicting and changing views in society about the nature of professionalism as identified by Gomm, and the evolution of the mixed economy of care as required by social policy, discussion of empowerment in community care might more reasonably be concerned with the relationship between citizens, services and society rather than limited to that between users of public care services and the professionals who provide them. In this discussion the legitimate role of professional care providers in conventional public community care services would be peripheral rather than central and clearly recognized as enablement rather than empowerment.

As Roger Gomm concludes, 'The term "empowerment" designates many excellent practices and some dubious ones, but exactly what they are and who is doing what to whom is hidden by its usage' (Gomm, 1993 p. 137). In view of this, the chapter will conclude with a less familiar but also less paradoxical model of empowerment in community care. This affords a central role to citizens in the self-help movement whose explicit goal is to empower its members to take control of their own lives through their own efforts and to obtain control of the resources they need so to do.

EMPOWERMENT – A PARADOXICAL PROPOSITION

The notion that professional providers of services can empower service users in the sense of giving over power to them is paradoxical. Power cannot be given but only taken, for to give power implies a gift from a position of power. As Evans points out, there is:

> . . . a basic contradiction in the idea of people empowering others because the very institutional structure that puts one group in a position to empower also works to undermine the act of empowerment. (Evans, 1992 p 142.)

The example given earlier of assessment for service illustrates this well in that although the process of assessment may be enabling for the user in a variety of ways, the institutionalized power of the professional precludes any real user control over the outcome. This will continue to be the case until the institutions are changed or the user creates their own service which they control – both of which require political action by citizens rather than therapeutic intervention by professionals.

The current approach of the disability movement in Britain to statutory care services and professionals within them illustrates Evans' contention that power cannot be given, only taken. A major demand of the disability movement is not that professionals in health and social care empower them by giving up control of services. Rather it is demanding changes in the law governing the disbursement of public funds. These funds are presently allocated by social services departments according to the assessment decisions of professionals guided by what has been termed 'therapeutic good intentions' (Oliver, 1992). The disability movement objects to this, asserting that people with disabilities are disabled as much by economic and social factors which exclude them from work and the wider community, and by professional attitudes which label them as dependent, as by their individual conditions. Professional assessment of need for social care is perceived therefore as not only irrelevant but demeaning and damaging.

The economic problems of disabled people are well documented with nearly half living below the poverty line in Great Britain (Berthoud, Lakey and McKay, 1993) and the movement believes that this true source of their disadvantage is obscured by the alleged requirement for social work assessment of their 'needs' (Mullender, 1992–3; Ellis, 1992). Institutional changes in the way financial resources are allocated would give power to people to control the resources they require to manage their own care services, a development which would, as one study has already shown, not only liberate disabled people through independence, choice and control but actually cost less than existing professionally controlled services (Oliver and Zarb, 1993).

In contrast to this liberating experience, a recent study of assessments of disabled people showed that practitioners brought various pre-conceptions to the assessment including the perception of disability as an individual physical condition rather than a social restriction, and a belief in the paramount value of their professional judgement which led to a devaluation of the views of users and carers (Ellis, 1992). Another found that through their inflexibility statutory services created barriers to independent living and that often less experienced, unqualified, non-professional assistants were felt to be more helpful because they had fewer preconceptions and were more able to give an individualized service (Morris, 1993) – findings previously revealed in a paper graphically entitled 'Untrained carers are tops' which similarly disclosed a preference among people with a disability for untrained carers (Vernon, 1986).

There is therefore empirical support for the conviction of members of the disability movement that rather than being empowered by profes-sionals who seek to involve them in the assessment process, people with disabilities are further disempowered by the perpetuation of their enforced dependence within the social care system, and that access to money and the means of earning it would be the true source of genuine empowerment (Oliver, 1989 p. 21). Thus, in Evans' terms, the institutional structure which allows the professionals to 'empower' users through assessments is the same structure which denies the 'users' the control of those economic resources which would truly empower them. This is why disability groups in Britain are calling not so much for control over public services, which they often feel fail them and increase their dependence, but for anti-discrimination legislation and a comprehensive disability income which would empower people with a disability to live independently of the social care system and its professionals as citizens rather than 'users' (George, 1993). In this sense, therefore, power cannot be given, only taken.

A LIMITED MANDATE

Despite the recent literature exhorting professionals to empower users of public services (Smale *et al.*, 1993; Stevenson and Parsloe, 1993; Morris and Lindow, 1993) there is little or no mandate in social policy or statute for such action by public officials. Empowerment is not mentioned in the *Griffiths Report* (Griffiths, 1988), the White Paper *Caring for People* (DoH 1989) based upon it, the NHS and CC Act 1990 nor the *Policy Guidance* (DoH, 1990) for social services departments and health authorities which followed it. When official guidance on empowerment does appear in the *Practice Guidance for Practitioners and for Managers* (SSI/Scottish Office,

1991) it is highly equivocal and confuses enablement and empowerment.
Thus it begins by asserting that:

> The rationale for this reorganisation is the empowerment of users
> and carers. Instead of users and carers being subordinate to the
> wishes of service providers, the roles will be progressively
> adjusted. In this way users and carers will be enabled to exercise
> the same power as consumers of other services. This redressing of
> the balance of power is the best guarantee of a continuing
> improvement in the quality of service. (SSI/Scottish Office, 1991
> p. 9.)

and later:

> . . . care management is about empowering users and carers,
> enabling them not only to make choices about the services they
> receive but also to be more in control of the process through which
> they gain access to services. (SSI, 1991 p. 31.)

However, the suggestion of 'control' when placed in the context of the
whole document lacks substance. This reveals that what is intended is
enablement, in the sense of promoting participation and involvement,
not empowerment, in the sense of professionals giving up their power
and control. In fact, far from giving up any of their power, the
responsibilities and powers of professionals are frequently reiterated
and the need for them to exercise control over assessment and resource
allocation is emphasized. Empowerment is actually only mentioned four
times in the 98-page document, whereas participation, involvement and
partnership are frequently referred to as basic principles in community
care practice, the goal of which is to promote independence of services,
not surrender control over them: 'All users and carers should be
encouraged to participate . . . because a passive role will only reinforce a
sense of dependence' (p. 51).

Control is never really on offer as the responsible and accountable
practitioner must remain the expert in control of problem definition and
resource allocation: 'The practitioner has to judge how the potential user
can be actively involved in the assessment process' (p. 50); '. . . Because
practitioners and their managers control access to resources the
relationship will never be totally equal . . .'. (p. 16); 'it will not be
logistically possible for all users to have their own care manager and
only a small minority of users will be in a position to perform this
function for themselves' (p. 22). And the final limitation: 'Ultimately
however, having weighed the views of all parties . . . the assessing
practitioner is responsible for defining the user's needs' (p. 53).

If anything, these statements suggest that greater power is to be
invested in front line professionals with devolution of budgetary control

and the power 'to define' users' needs and indeed the guidance admits that:

> . . . the devolution of responsibility to allocate resources, changes the nature of the relationship between practitioner and user. Practitioners are less able to act as advocates on users' behalf. (p. 22.)

Not only does the devolution of decision making to the front line professional limit their ability to act as an advocate for service users, it may also further disempower users by leading to restricted access to the more costly services. Kathryn Ellis found in her study of the involvement of disabled people in assessments – which involved observations of 50 assessment visits and detailed discussion of each with all participants – that the closer the individual practitioners were to budgeting decisions, the more conservative was their management of referrals and agency resources. Ellis found that sometimes restrictions were presented as options: people could express preferences but only within the limitations of the services. For example, one home care manager equated 'negotiation' with enabling the user to decide which rooms could be cleaned on which days. A good example of enabling participation in the process but giving no power over the outcome – the amount of service received. In such circumstances it is unsurprising that many people wondered why needs related to disability had to be assessed by professionals in this way in any case (Ellis, 1992).

Thus there is certainly no mandate for empowerment if by this is meant user control of services – a fact sometimes ignored in the literature on empowerment. Thus in guidance from the Users' Group of the Community Care Support Force, 'control' and 'veto' are clearly identified as two elements which define participation in public services – the others being involvement, consultation and campaigning. User participation is said to be 'the currency which will empower those for whom community care services are provided' (Morris and Lindow, 1993 p. 15). Again, and in direct contradiction to the policy guidance quoted above, Smale and his colleagues in their pamphlet on empowerment and assessment assert:

> Any approach to 'giving people choice', short of enabling them to buy the services they require, obtain them as a right or develop them through their personal relationships, runs the risk of maintaining or even increasing people's powerlessness. There has to be a good reason for not allowing people to be their own care manager. (Smale *et al.*, 1993 p. 5.)

Despite these interpretations there is no mandate for empowerment in the sense of giving power to control services. Where there does appear to be a mandate it is for the promotion of the rights of service users as consumers akin to those possessed – albeit tenuously – by consumers of any other service. This social policy mandate is clearly in keeping with the consumerist philosophy underpinning a decade of government reforms in public services. However this does not extend to user control – the ability to choose between brands of cereals in the supermarket does not carry with it the right to a seat on the board of directors of the corn flake company.

EMPOWERMENT AS CONSUMERISM

The goal of the consumer movement is to shift power form the provider to the purchaser. Potter identifies five factors which must be addressed if this goal is to be achieved: access, choice, information, redress and representation (Potter, 1988). These activities have an unequivocal mandate in social policy where the notion of empowerment as consumerism is directly invoked as we saw earlier in this quotation from the *Practice Guidance*: 'In this way users and carers will be enabled to exercise the same power as consumers of other services. This redressing of the balance of power is the best guarantee of a continuing improvement in the quality of service' (SSI/Scottish Office, 1991 p. 9). The White Paper and the NHS and CCA imposed duties on local authorities which directly reflect the five factors of consumerism identified by Potter – the requirements to establish transparent assessment procedures, to promote choice through establishing a mixed economy of care, to publish information, to establish complaints procedures and encourage independent advocacy.

However, there are a number of differences between the market for commodities and that for public services which bring into the question the extent to which the application of consumerist principles can in any real sense empower users of public services. The first is that the consumer of publicly provided services is not necessarily the purchaser. Such services are paid for by tax payers and the professional purchasers of them are accountable, if at all, to the tax payer not the consumer. One of the grounds of accountability is value for money which means that the availability of publicly financed services will reflect not only the choice of the consumer but that of the professional purchaser who must achieve this. This may conflict with freedom of choice for the consumer who may have to accept the cheapest rather than the preferred option. Again, the choices of the professional purchaser must reflect decisions about how public finance can best promote the public good – therefore choice in the public service market reflects competition between consumer groups as well as preferences within them. Finally, the consumer of publicly financed services has often not chosen this option freely but has taken it because they lack the finances to purchase care privately. As we have seen, this is well attested in relation to disabled people and there is similar evidence in relation to older people among whom even the 50% who possess housing capital would have difficulty privately purchasing adequate care (Gibbs, 1993; Oldman, 1991).

In a detailed discussion of the relevance and application of the consumerist philosophy to public services, Jenny Potter concludes that because of these and other problems:

> Consumerism can help authorities to advance from considering individual members of the public as passive clients or recipients of services – who get what they are given for which they must be thankful . . . but it will rarely be enough to turn members of the public into partners, actively involved in shaping public services. For this to take place, the arguments must be shifted into the political arena . . . Consumerism is fine as far as it goes, but it does not go far enough to affect a radical shift in the distribution of power. (Potter, 1988 p. 157.)

In fact the political decision to impose the 'discipline of the market' via the NHS and CC Act may have acted to shift the power of choice further from the consumer. Nancy North suggests the creation of the NHS internal market could lead to GPs being even less likely to be interested in power sharing as a result of GP fundholding. This has encouraged GPs to take more power rather than less in decision making and control of resources, such that 'the structuring of incentives within general practice may disempower patients' encouraging fundholding GPs to avoid certain types of expensive patients or despatch them to cheaper hospitals outside local communities (North, 1993 p. 131). The chairperson of the British Medical Association Council recently wrote that: 'The intolerable two tier service that is now the norm in the acute hospitals' is endangering patients and that the burgeoning bureaucracy required in an attempt to make the internal market work is oppressive. He asserts that 'In many hospitals there is a climate of intimidation, of fear to speak out about such matters' (Macara, 1993 p. 27). The chairman of the joint consultants committee of the BMA and the Medical Royal Colleges, Mr Paddy Ross, has recently been reported as claiming that NHS hospital consultants have yielded to 'moral blackmail from managers to give a quicker service to GP fundholders' patients, even if more seriously ill people have to wait longer for treatment' (Jones, 1993 p. 3). This hardly constitutes evidence for user empowerment through consumerism in health care and neither does the growth of the 'burgeoning bureaucracy' taken to run the internal market of the NHS. A recent investigation by the *Sunday Times* revealed that the number of senior managers has risen from 510 to 13 500 over a six year period and their wage bill from £11m to £251m in the same period. Health service experts claim that 200 000 administrative jobs could be cut within the next five years without harming patients. This does indeed suggest that the only people who have been 'empowered' by these changes are the manager purchasers not the patient consumers of health care (Chittenden and Ramesh, 1993 p. 6).

Similar developments have occurred in response to the Act in social care where previously the direct Department of Social Security (DSS) funding mechanism did not require that care be purchased through health or welfare departments but was a means tested entitlement to benefit. This has been replaced by a cash limited welfare service to which citizens have no specific entitlement, and access to which is only available through professional assessment of 'need'.

Thus, the introduction of the mixed economy of care through the NHS and CC Act and its consumerist mandate has effectively empowered the purchasers but not the consumers of publicly financed services. Far from being empowered as consumers, consumers have been disempowered as citizens by being redefined as clients. This tendency is not only encouraged by the Act but is the unacknowledged corollary of much of the empowerment debate with its emphasis on the centrality of health and welfare professionals in the empowerment process.

THE MYOPIA OF THERAPEUTIC GOOD INTENTION

The discussion of empowerment often confines itself to those services providing 'care' in the community, but mainstream services such as education, housing, transport, leisure and town planning are used far more widely, and though not usually included in discussions of empowerment, could be more influential in promoting it. Such services play a crucial role in determining the quality of peoples' lives in communities and the extent to which they are able to participate in community life, which has been seen as a measure of their citizenship. For example, if architects and town planners were more sensitive to the needs of people with physical disadvantages the extent of their 'disability' would not be so great, and their need to use formal services commensurately less. Often the environment is more disabling than the individual's condition.

It is in this sense that 'therapeutic good intention' when introduced into the empowerment debate diverts attention from real sources of disadvantage and disempowerment to the needs of clients for 'care', rather than the rights of citizens to independence. An example of this myopia of therapeutic good intention is the pamphlet by Stevenson and

Parsloe (1993) *Community Care and Empowerment*. The authors acknowledge that they are employing a narrow focus on the issues of
empowerment and allude to the problems which such an interpretation
brings; however they choose not to amend it in favour of a broader
analysis – they say:

> We realise that for many people and especially for community
> workers, empowerment implies an increase in power in political
> processes. We do not use it in this sense but rather to describe
> work with individuals and families within a relatively circumscribed
> context, that of their need for formal community services. We
> consider their empowerment in relation to the articulation and
> meeting of their needs. (Stevenson and Parsloe, 1993 pp. 6–7.)

The centrality afforded to care services and their professionals in this
version of empowerment could not be more clearly illustrated than in
their conclusion where they assert:

> Empowerment is about processes which permeate organisations
> and professional thought. The challenge is to create a culture in
> which such processes are able to thrive. (Stevenson and Parsloe,
> 1993 p. 58.)

The validity of this interpretation is questioned by the findings of the
Birmingham Community Care Special Action Project which was a series
of initiatives specifically designed to promote user influence and
involvement in services. In their review of the project Wistow and
Barnes (1993) suggest that empowerment may be more about people
gaining control over their lives than over public services. The burden of
such control would, they point out, divert already overstretched
personal and financial resources. Users would rather devote their often
meagre resources to running their own lives independently than to
doing for nothing what others are paid to do – albeit sometimes with
limited effectiveness. Surveys of users' views in Birmingham suggested
that:

> . . . it is dissatisfaction with services which motivates involvement.
> If the services they receive meet their needs in a sensitive way,
> control in itself may not be something they would wish to seek and
> choice may be less significant. (Wistow and Barnes, 1993 p. 293.)

Rejecting the view put forward by Stevenson and Parsloe on the
necessity for a 'new culture', Wistow and Barnes propose that on the
basis of their study:

> The evidence suggests that carers at least may be less concerned
> about cultural change than practical improvements to services such

as ensuring that transport runs on time. It may be that a willingness on the part of providers to give priority to achieving such basic improvements in services quality would in itself be an indication of cultural change. While this [improving service sensitivity] may lead to a sense of empowerment over their own lives, the indications are that the objectives of most [carers] do not extend to user control. (Wistow and Barnes, 1993 p. 296.)

This is a finding supported by Richard Wood who, as Director of the British Council of Organisations of Disabled People, asserted that professionals claiming to be committed to user involvement were really only 'picking the brains' of disabled people who have consequently decided to:

> . . . put whatever resources we've got into disabled peoples' organisations . . . If you want us to participate, you go and find more money and we can get some development workers. (Croft and Beresford, 1992 p. 39.)

Rather than being preoccupied with the alleged role of health and welfare professionals and their care services in empowerment, the debate could more legitimately focus on mainstream services and opportunities in community life too often routinely denied to disabled and otherwise disadvantaged people. Shifting the focus of the debate away from 'care services' and the professionals who control them, Wistow and Barnes create links between the normalization movement and empowerment, describing how the philosophy of normalization promotes the view that people with health and social care needs should live as normal a life as possible and that:

> . . . in stressing the importance of gaining access to 'ordinary' lifestyles, it implies an increasing role for mainstream services at the expense of specialised – and often segregated – residential and day services. (Wistow and Barnes, 1993 p. 283.)

They later suggest that this redefinition of the nature of problems and their solution away from care and therapy towards services and rights could leave medical and social care professionals isolated and redundant as 'experts on disability' as groups of users form alliances:

> . . . between people with disabilities and, for example, architects, planners and engineers who are able to make changes in the physical environment which promote mobility and independence. Services provided by social care agencies may also become redundant as access to mainstream facilities becomes more possible and, for example, leisure and education services supersede traditional day care. (Wistow and Barnes, 1993 p. 284.)

This would lead to empowerment in the sense of people taking power over those aspects of everyday life previously denied to them. Wistow and Barnes conclude, therefore, that empowerment in the sense of giving over control is not something which professionals can readily do, nor is it apparently what many users want. However there remains an important role for professionals if they can rid themselves of the myopia of therapeutic good intention, and adopt new definitions of problems with broader approaches to their resolution.

ENABLEMENT AND THE ROLE OF THE PROFESSIONAL

Although practitioners cannot claim to empower users of public services in any meaningful sense, this does not imply that they can have no role in the empowerment process as it is pursued by citizens on their own behalf. As Evans suggests:

> Workers need not be immobilised in empowering efforts because of these structural inequalities . . . [for although] empowerment is a process capable of being initiated and sustained only by the agent or subject who seeks power or self-determination. Others can aid . . . in this empowerment process by providing a climate, a relationship, resources and procedural means. (Evans, 1992 p. 142.)

A recent discussion document from the National Health Service Management Executive Focus Group on 'Empowering the Patient' clearly identifies both the paradox and the proper role of the professional in resolving it:

> Although empowering the patient may be a useful slogan, there is a danger that it acts as an ill-defined, or even misleading, banner to travel under. Empowering literally means the giving of power, but might more accurately be interpreted as creating opportunities which enable and encourage power to be taken. Patient self-empowerment is therefore a more accurate description than 'empowering patients'. While we cannot empower patients, practices and structures can be changed so that people are no longer disempowered in being unable to exercise existing powers of control or choice – be it through feelings of vulnerability, the power of the professional or the opaqueness of the organisation – and can take further powers. (National Health Service Management Executive, 1992 p. 1.)

Wistow and Barnes refer to these more limited goals of professional practice as 'think big but act small'. They suggest that users can be helped to empower themselves by professionals who provide more effective, more responsive services based on new definitions of problems and their resolution. This involves extending user choice and control of their everyday lives through interpreting community care 'as a corporate or "whole authority" responsibility' rather than the exclusive province of 'care' services. Practical examples of this from the Birmingham project include a special unit formed within the corporation's economic development department involving service providers and employers in promoting better access for people with physical, sensory and learning difficulties to local training and employment opportunities; day centre staff redefined their role to identify opportunities for recreation, training, leisure in mainstream community resources rather than providing traditional centre based activity; a mobility task group was formed within the central executive department involving architects, engineers, transport staff and service users in improving physical access and transport services across the whole community (Wistow and Barnes, 1993 p. 293–4).

There are numerous other practical examples of such new approaches to problem definition and resolution. A recent evaluative study from the School of Advanced Urban Studies at Bristol University describes six community care projects in which professionals have adopted innovatory approaches to the self-empowerment of individuals and groups. These range from a care management project in Cheltenham in which service users assess their own needs and determine priorities in the light of scarce resources on which information is provided by the professionals to a care and repair scheme in Radnor in which frail older people identify what they need and receive help from professionals in obtaining the resources to achieve their goals (School for Advanced Urban Studies, 1993).

Despite being one of the professionals' most severe critics, Michael Oliver proposes that there is an important task for the professionals if they can dispense with their traditional view of disability as individual dysfunction and loss, and the view of their role as helping people to adjust to this. Part of this task will be helping disabled people 'to locate the personal, social economic and community resources to enable them to live life to the full' (Oliver, 1989 p. 21). An example of this approach is described by Morris in her study of the effectiveness of an independent living advocate (ILA) working in the National Spinal Injuries Centre (NSIC) at Stoke Mandeville hospital. Here, an advocate – himself disabled – was appointed under a joint initiative between the user-led Spinal Injuries Association and the NSIC. The task was to act as an advocate on behalf of clients with spinal cord injury and tetraplegia to enable them to organize their own independent living schemes using personal assistance support in pursuit of their own self-defined aims. The ILA was successful in maximizing the benefits derived from rehabilitation programmes within the hospital by engaging users and professionals in shared user-defined goals; in promoting skills of care management in users, thus enabling them to find, employ and manage their personal care assistants, and in creating effective partnership between a statutory organization and a user led one (Morris, 1993).

Even within more traditional professional/service user relationships on an individual and small group level these broader perspectives can inform practice. For example, Smale and his colleagues (1993) describe three models of the process of assessment in community care. The 'procedural' model assumes that service managers who set criteria for service eligibility are the experts, and assessors simply measure service users against these criteria. In this model both the professional and the client are effectively disempowered by having little or no choice about process or outcome. The 'questioning' model assumes that the professional has expertise in the user's problem and having asked questions, decides what is the best course of action. Here the client is the passive beneficiary of the professional's expertise. The 'exchange' model, however, recognizes that both service user and professional possess expertise though in different areas. The user is an expert in their own problem in that they have personal experience of it, the professional has knowledge of services which are available and might contribute to this process. This model interprets assessment as negotiation about who should do what for whom. It avoids the myopia of therapeutic good intention by not assuming that people only exist as clients who bring nothing to the situation other than their 'needs'. It recognizes the expertise and skills they have thus enabling their development in the interests of achieving the goals they have themselves defined. The broader approach to professional community care practice described by Wistow and Barnes, and Oliver is supported in the exchange model which recognizes that:

> . . . assessment involves an understanding of a social situation, of the pattern of relationships in which a persons need's are perceived by somebody as not being met. It is not just the assessment of an individual but of the relationship between them and the people with the resources to support or change the situation. (Smale *et al.*, 1993 p. 43.)

Although this chapter has been critical of Smale and his colleagues' description of this relationship as 'empowerment', it is enabling in that it promotes the development of the skills service users bring to the assessment situation and this form of enablement does allow the professional to contribute to the process of user self-empowerment.

A further detailed account of practice based on similar principles is by Marsh and Fisher (1993) who describe an empirical study carried out over three and a half years in four social services departments. The action research project included training staff in techniques of user involvement and evaluations of outcomes for users and staff. 'Partnership practice' draws on the theories and methods of task-centred work with its emphasis on clearly identified and mutually agreed goals, contracts and frequent review and evaluation. These methods are well established and enjoy empirical support for their claims to effectiveness as well as legitimacy in terms of user involvement.

Ward and Mullender offer a different model of practice based on the skills of group work. They suggest that the consumerist version of empowerment promoted by current social policy is a chimera designed to obscure the true origins of disadvantage and that the role of the professional in the empowerment process is to disclose as public ills what professional practice and ideology too often obscure as private sorrows (Ward and Mullender, 1992 pp. 21–31). This is achieved through 'self-directed groupwork' which they believe offers opportunities for people to become aware that their problems derive not from their own inadequacy but from shared disadvantage. Professionals, whose monopoly of power is minimized in the group setting, enable this process of consciousness raising by encouraging user-led analysis and user-led action whereby:

> Alternative explanations and new options for change and improvement can be opened up. The demoralising isolation of private misfortune reinforced by public disinterest or, worse, moral condemnation and day to day surveillance, can be replaced with a new sense of self-confidence and potency as well as tangible practical gains which individuals on their own could not contemplate. (Ward and Mullender, 1992 p. 29.)

There are other recent studies, too numerous to describe in detail, that have explored various issues and practices in enablement through involvement and participation. These include the involvement of disabled people in assessment (Ellis, 1992); user involvement in community care planning (Bewley and Glendinning, 1992; Deakin, 1992), research (Davis and Fleming, 1992) and policy making (O'Donnell, 1993); and the impact on practice of an organizational commitment to greater user participation (Lupton and Hall, 1993). The effectiveness of client participation on the effectiveness of community social work is described by Itzhaky and York (1991). Though somewhat less developed there is an emerging literature from health on user participation in decision making (Meredith, 1993).

Most of these works share the incrementalism of Wistow and Barnes and explore how professionals within current institutional frameworks can enable user participation and involvement in the interests of service effectiveness or user self-empowerment.

These are enabling processes which are not new to professional practice, for which there is considerable empirical support in terms of their contribution to effective intervention (Marsh and Fisher, 1992 p. 9; Smale *et al.*, 1993 pp. 48–65), and which therefore do not require 'a new culture' – contrary to some of the grandiose claims of empowerment pundits. This contribution does depend, however, on the abandonment of what we have called the myopia of therapeutic good intention and unfortunately there is considerable evidence that this may be an elusive goal.

DISABLEMENT AND PROFESSIONALIZATION

Marsh and Fisher, in their study of partnership practice, assert that 'The principles are not radically new . . . they are widely accepted within social care. However, practice often runs counter to these principles . . .' (Marsh and Fisher, 1992 p. 13). They found a widespread belief that partnership practice – which includes informing and involving users and negotiating action with them – undermined professionalism. Even after training, social workers felt that such practice was only suitable for certain types of practical problems, and that psychological problems required different, and more highly valued, professional skills. The propensity of many social work commentators in the empowerment literature to make rather grandiose and unrealistic claims for their role in the process is illuminated by Marsh and Fisher's finding that:

> . . . they had a professional rating scale for the outcomes of the work . . . The most professional outcome was seen as grand changes in the users' circumstances; to aim for smaller changes was seen as easier and less professional . . . The fact that quite small changes could be of great significance to people on the margins of coping . . . was not the general view. (Marsh and Fisher, 1992 p. 50.)

It seems that many professionals find it difficult to adhere to Wistow and Barnes' exhortation to 'think big, act small' and that this may well be a consequence not only of the threat to the professional status of social work identified by Stevenson, but more fundamentally of the value placed by professionals on the type of psychological interpretations and interventions which Oliver dismisses as disempowering therapeutic good intention.

Further examples of such professional myopia are rife – evidence of the arrogance of simplistic interpretations of professionalism comes from Lupton and Hall whose study of user involvement in a social services department found that workers believed that: 'Choice is limited by what we consider to be good practice: our beliefs can at times be in advance of carers and society at large' (Lupton and Hall, 1993 p. 80). In view of this it is unsurprising to learn that 'social workers are finding the concept of listening to clients very difficult' (Lupton and Hall, 1993 p. 10). A recent year-long consumer survey of 543 disabled users of social services by RADAR found that users' confidence had fallen due to lengthy waiting lists for assessments and assistance, and that there had been unilateral withdrawal of highly valued home help in favour of the provision of personal care, which many disabled people said they did not want. In addition, many users were reluctant to complain for fear of being labelled as troublemakers (RADAR, 1993). The Ellis study referred to earlier suggest that such fears are well founded with its finding that:

> People who were knowledgeable about their entitlements were regarded as 'demanding', those attempting to exercise choice as 'fussy' or a 'nuisance', those who challenged judgements as 'manipulative'. (Joseph Rowntree Foundation, 1993 p. 3.)

Such findings have led Michael Oliver, Professor of Disability Studies at the University of Greenwich, to assert that 'Disabled people are treated as the lowest of the low by Social Services Departments, and for at least ten years they have failed to take on board what disabled people have been telling them they want' (George, 1993 p. 18). In terms of the client group preferences of social workers Oliver's words are supported by a series of studies over two decades which show that among the groups least favoured by social workers are elderly and physically impaired people (Borsay, 1989). There is evidence of similar prejudice and disadvantage in health care where Allen *et al.* (1992) refer to a BMA report in 1986 which found that 'many doctors feel that looking after older people is a second rate speciality' and to a more recent claim that 'nurses and other health-care professionals label older people as "hopeless", "undeserving" or "incurable" solely on the basis of their age and frailty'. It is often the least well qualified and least trained workers who provide services for elderly and disabled people within health and welfare bureaucracies and so, ironically, these people suffer most from the self-serving prejudices of the professionals whilst benefiting least from their alleged expertise.

There seems to be ample evidence of the tendency of the relationship between professionals and service users to fall remorselessly into the oppressive/disabling categories identified earlier by Gomm (1993). Oliver suggests that the denial of control to disabled people of the services they need is due to 'an over-professionalised and bureaucratic system of provision which keeps people dependent' (George, 1993

p. 18) and Ellis illustrates the response among users to such relationships that 'Users tended to limit their demands on services as a result of their valuing self-reliance and privacy. Those turned down felt humiliated, angry or cynical about the claims of community care . . .' (Joseph Rowntree Foundation, 1993 p. 1). The conviction that this is so, that oppression and disablement are indissolubly linked to the professional-ization of caring, has been one of the motivating factors underpinning the massive growth of the self-help movement. So too has the evolving nature of community care services and beliefs about who should provide them – the state or the community. Along with the increasing disenchantment with and distrust of professionals and the health and welfare bureaucracies they control has come a belief among many that self-help is the only path to self-empowerment.

EMPOWERMENT AND SELF-HELP

Whilst recent studies have confirmed users' disillusion with health and welfare bureaucracies and the professionals who control them the origins of the self-help movement go further back and are broader based.

There has been a phenomenal increase in the number of self-help groups in western societies in recent years, in fact some claim it '. . . has developed worldwide into a major social phenomenon' (Hasenfeld and Gidron, 1993 p. 217). In the UK there are no reliable national figures but Wilson illustrates this growth by reference to the city of Nottingham where in 1982 there were 60 recorded groups and 155 in 1992 (Wilson, 1993). Matzat (1993) estimated in 1993 that there were 50 000 self-help groups in what had been the Federal Republic of Germany – according to federally funded research there was one such group to every 1000 people in urban areas and about half this in rural ones. Several factors have been identified as contributing to the growth of the self-help movement (Adams, 1990; Wilson, 1993; Matzat, 1993). At the most general these have included industrialization and technological develop-ment, which have led to depersonalized and dehumanized institutions, and the alienation of people from communities, institutions, each other and themselves. All of which have led people to seek to re-establish greater control over their own lives and recreate community and fellowship in alternative forms. The increasing demand for more local democracy and devolution of previously centralized decision making is evidence of this.

In relation to health and welfare these wider social factors have combined with a disillusion with professional 'therapies' which had begun in the anti-psychiatry movement of the early 1960s. This disclosed the politics of the psychiatric experience, challenging the expertise of the professionals involved in it, and their claim to therapeutic altruism – reinterpreting individual therapy as social control and asylum as incarceration. The anti-institutional literature and the decarceration movement provided professional legitimation for the policy of community care which had become increasingly attractive to governments as the costs of maintaining ageing institutions mounted. Interestingly, however, the anti-psychiatry movement did not demand an end to institutional care in favour of community care – rather it developed the notion of the therapeutic community. The anti-therapy movement was reinforced by the resurgence of the women's movement in the early 1970s with its assertion that 'the personal is the political' which had resonance for many other disadvantaged groups who now sought to reject professional, individual and personal explanations for their problems in favour of other definitions which recognized the social construction of individuals' problems in terms of their social and political disadvantage. Individuals with physical disabilities, mental health problems, and learning difficulties formed themselves into groups and redefined their problems in social terms, identifying the disabling effects of the physical and socio-economic environment – and of professional therapies which located the origin of problems within individuals and sought to 'treat' them or help them 'come to terms with' or 'adapt' to their disadvantage.

In the 1970s and 1980s the social policy responses of government to recurrent economic crises, with the rediscovery of market forces as an instrument of social policy, have undermined the case of public providers to be the primary source of health and welfare and the accompanying constraints on public expenditure have demoralized professional providers within public bureaucracies. Regular highly publicized scandals in health and social care throughout the 1980s have contributed to the demystification of the professional and their claim to expert status, reinforcing a view promoted by government and some academics of the professional as incompetent, secretive, self-serving and altogether too powerful. The health and welfare bureaucracy has thus become part of the problem instead of part of the solution, and the professionals who control it and their therapeutic methods part of the cause of countless ills rather than part of their cure.

Robert Pinker suggests that there are three cultural traditions which have characterized the development of social welfare since the mid 19th century. First came the social administration tradition in which:

> The provision and expansion of social services has been charac-
> terised by the growth of complex bureaucratic and professional
> hierarchies. Along with the steady growth of modern social
> services the pursuit of equity, consistency and efficiency has

turned the conventional informal practices of giving and receiving help into a largely impersonal enterprise. (Pinker, 1992 p. 280).

This tradition saw welfare bureaucracies and the professionals who worked in them as guided by the notion of disinterested public service, characterized by an absence of profit motive, an understanding of human need, and ethical codes reinforced by public accountability. Pinker then proposes that as the mixed economy of welfare develops stimulated by political ideology and economic necessity, divisions between statutory and independent sector providers break down and a new cultural tradition becomes established. 'Entrepreneurial management' has come to permeate the public sector changing the administrative frameworks of public service, but also those of independent welfare agencies which in order to compete for the public funds being managed by the public sector have more closely to conform to the structure and processes of business to ensure survival. Pinker sees this as a potential threat to the historical independence of the voluntary sector and the diversity which it provided. In other words the welfare pluralism which the promotion of the mixed economy is supposed to provide is actually threatened by the way it is funded. The third tradition is what Pinker calls the 'communitarian' or 'populist' tradition which he points out 'affects more people throughout their lives than the other two combined' (p. 281). This is the tradition of informal care and mutual aid epitomized by the self-help movement.

Self-help groups have been defined in the following terms:

. . . made up of people who experience the same problem or life situation, either directly or through their family and friends. They come together for mutual support and to share experiences, information and ways of coping. Groups are run by and for their members. Some self-help groups expand their activities . . . they may provide services for people who face the same problem or life situation; or they may campaign for change. Professionals may sometimes take part in various ways, when asked to by the group. (Wilson, 1993 p. 212).

Matzat (1993) adds several other defining characteristics including the absence of a profit motive, a stress on authenticity, equality and a common language. He proposes three types of self-help groups. The 'anonymous type' the model for which was Alcoholics Anonymous (AA) and which has no formalized membership, no board or committee but which does have a 'programme', in the case of AA the 'Twelve Steps' to recovery, adherence to which guidelines for daily life and confessional ceremony in the event of failures to meet them form the cathartic core of the meetings. The second type Matzat refers to as 'self-help groupings' which include large patient organizations such as the Alzheimer's Disease Society in the UK. These have a formal structure and status, employ full-time staff and function nationwide, they represent the interests of not only their members but any who have the same problem, and only a minority of their members are activists – the majority being consumers of their services, i.e. information bulletins, advice services, campaigns and so on. Thirdly there are 'psychosocial self-help groups'. These are small closed groups with membership:

> clearly defined by self-declaration and mutual agreement . . . and by regular reliable participation and attendance, but not by subscription and fees. [They] meet regularly . . . over a considerable period of time. They have an open discussion on very personal matters . . . try to be as frank and open as possible and to clarify their points of view. (Matzat, 1993 p. 35.)

As the public monopoly of health and welfare provision has been increasingly questioned interest has grown in identifying differences between self-help groups and formal health and welfare organizations. Most commentators agree that formal health and welfare organizations tend to be monolithic, bureaucratic and hierarchical, peopled by career-oriented professionals working within clearly defined roles and statuses, guided by formalized theoretical and procedural knowledge. In contrast self-help groups have an anti-bureaucratic, non-hierarchical ethos within which roles are informal and interchangeable, personal know-ledge and subjective experience guide behaviour and common experi-ence and mutual support are valued as opposed to the professionals' maintenance of distinct client/professional roles (Adams, 1990 pp. 17–18; Hasenfeld and Gidron, 1993 p. 218).

Matzat summarizes the research literature on the benefits of self-help groups which include:

- reduced depression,
- increased self-esteem,
- more personal contact,
- increased skills in conflict management,
- a comparative perspective on one's own problems,
- more selective use of the formal care system.

Matzat proposes that these benefits are the product of particular processes characteristic of self-help groups. These include:

- modelling, whereby members learn from others coping with the same problem successfully;
- the 'helper therapy principle' – mutuality assures that everyone has

the opportunity to enjoy the sense of competence, self-esteem and assurance derived from helping another;
- direct empathy – because others share the problem understanding is virtually assured, which is not so with professionals who may have no personal experience of the problem;
- destigmatization – many of the problems people have are subject to stigma – AIDS for example; within groups of people who share a problem it is the 'norm' and no longer a minority issue;
- the 'combination of potentials' – professionals are trained to assess and search for problems and look to their techniques to resolve them. This undervalues the strengths individuals possess which combined in self-help groups are a potent force for change.

Matzat concludes that 'Most therapies are nothing more than a systematic and elaborated application of certain elements of natural helping behaviour' (Matzat, 1993 pp. 38–39) and as such are possessed in some measure by non-professionals who can employ them in self-help activity (Matzat, 1993 pp. 36–39).

Despite the apparent benefits and evident popularity of self-help groups among people in difficulties there exists a tension in the relationship between self-help groups and human service organizations and the professionals who work in them. This relationship has become a focus for concern as the number and influence of such groups expand and the monopoly of public sector care services declines (Hasenfeld and Gidron, 1993; Wilson, 1993; Adams, 1990 pp. 26–34). Hasenfeld and Gidron propose a model describing the determinants of the relationship between self-help groups and formal human service organizations – the key factors involved are domain and mission, i.e. what problems they are concerned with and why; the extent of their respective dependence on external resources including people and finance; service technology, i.e. theories and methods used to effect change; internal structure whether formal or informal, with fixed or interchangeable roles. They assert that depending on the similarity or difference in these respects the relationship will be basically competitive or co-operative. Competition or conflict exists when the formal and self-help organizations rely on the same source for external resources of people or finance, when their respective missions are opposed, and when their service technologies and internal structures are different. This is especially so when social change is the goal of the self-help group.

The disability movement in the UK provides an example of this, as we have seen, with its rejection of psychological and medical models of disability and the accompanying therapies, its insistence on a social model of disability and its accompanying demand for radical change in the way resources are allocated. In addition its active dissemination of information and recruitment of new members presents a challenge to mainstream services.

Co-operation can range from the mutually beneficial such as exchanging referrals, through co-ordination of policies, coalition in campaigning, to co-option with its attendant danger of colonization of the self-help group by the usually stronger formal organization. Hasenfeld and Gidron warn of dangers to newly emergent self-help groups where, in order to sustain the relationship and the benefits it derives from it, the self-help group may be forced to adopt organizational structures and managerial methods which could 'erode the very unique contribution each can make to the welfare and wellbeing of the people it serves'. They conclude:

> . . . self-help groups whose distinct mission is to challenge human service organisations and to provide alternative service systems will be ill-served by interorganisational relations, especially during their formative phase. Only after they become sufficiently institutionalised and secure can they afford to initiate or accept such relations. (Hasenfeld and Gidron, 1993 p. 234.)

Despite the organizational differences and the dangers of certain forms of co-operation to self-help groups many commentators have been eager to identify the potential role for individual professionals in relation to such groups. Matzat suggests five ways in which professionals can contribute – disseminating the idea of collective self-help as an alternative to or complement to professional services. They include:

- giving information and helping people make decisions about membership;
- helping to get groups started, perhaps by bringing potential members together, providing a room and offering initial guidance on group processes;
- transferring of any personal experience of self-help group membership to the new group;
- offering consultation or supervision whilst remembering that group members can decide what is useful;
- promoting the idea of self-help groups widely among colleagues and helping them with their doubts and concerns about their role in relation to them.

In an earlier, though still relevant, paper Powell reported the views of consumers comparing professional and self-help groups from personal experience and found that many view the two different systems as complementary rather than conflicting. He proposes that the 'insularity, condescension and sometimes outright hostility which characterises relations between these systems is hardly congruent with these findings' (Powell, 1979 p. 564). He proposes that workers in both types of organization can contribute to people's wellbeing by ensuring that service users are able to move freely between both systems deriving maximum benefit from both. Powell also sees benefits to professionals from maintaining close links with self-help groups, suggesting that they '. . . are exemplary models of the qualities associated with therapeutic outcomes in professional programmes' by which he means the qualities of authenticity, supportiveness and caring shown to be associated with effective intervention by Traux and Mitchell (1971) and others since. He asserts that reciprocal relations can provide professionals with information and understanding of subcultures, distinctive problems and special resources that some clients need (Powell, 1979 pp. 564–5). Writing a decade later, Adams reiterates these possibilities, placing them within the British context of the early 1990s and, in particular, emphasizing the possibilities for professionals to learn from self-help groups which will contribute to 'personal and professional growth' (Adams, 1990 p. 74). He asserts that professionals should avoid the danger of perceiving self-help activity as criticism or rejection and the consequent withdrawal into the isolation of what he describes as 'core duties'.

So, despite the very different approach and philosophy underpinning self-help, and the disillusion with professionals that has contributed to its growth, professionals should not feel immobilized in the empowerment process – there remains a valuable contribution. However, it is impossible to avoid the question mark which hangs over the willingness and ability of professionals in health and welfare bureaucracies to make this contribution. Hasenfeld and Gidron are not alone in their scepticism about the benefits of closer co-operation between self-help groups and formal care services.

Thus, Robert Pinker wonders whether the relationship which is being promoted between formal social services and the informal sector will result in the latter being 'colonised or asset stripped'. He suggests that the outcome is unlikely to be beneficial in view of the fact that:

> A growing body of research suggests that the moral and behavioural dynamics of informal care and mutual aid are fundamentally different from those relating to formal social services . . . All past experience, from the origins of the poor law to the household means test, suggest that, when officials who are strangers intrude into these private homes and communities in an attempt to manipulate them, they often cause offence, with resulting damage to the effectiveness of these private systems of mutual aid. Although our understanding of the cultural dynamics of mutual aid is incomplete, there is little reason to assume that benevolent intentions will result in more beneficial outcomes. (Pinker, 1992 p. 282.)

Wilson suggests that this inherent tension has been largely ignored in the UK literature which has emphasized the benefits of co-operation and minimized the dangers. In conclusions reminiscent of our own earlier assertions about the need for professionals to relinquish their myopia of therapeutic good intention she proposes:

> Professionals who seriously want to work with self-help groups will have to reappraise their own roles, accept the strengths and potential strengths of their clients and be prepared to give up some of their power. Without some acknowledgement of these im-balances and of the need to change, conference conclusions on partnership may be mere platitudes. (Wilson, 1993 p. 216.)

SUMMARY AND CONCLUSIONS

This chapter and the empirical evidence on which its analysis is based suggest that health and welfare organizations and the professionals who control them are unwilling or unable to surrender power to their users and thus meaningfully empower them. This is a conclusion reinforced in a recent article by Vivien Lindow and Peter Beresford who have previously campaigned energetically for greater user involvement in formal community care services in the interests of user empowerment. In a recent paper they assert that:

> . . . getting involved with existing providers can feel like a futile struggle with enormous effort resulting in limited improvement, which is only on the surface. Those who use services remain at the bottom of hierarchies . . . People are looking for a more direct way to improve their lives. (Lindow and Beresford, 1993 p. 24.)

Several examples of user-controlled services in the USA and the UK are described which offer 'a model for different more empowering ways to run and manage services' (Lindow and Beresford, 1993 p. 24). These authors are among the most influential contributors to UK literature on user involvement and participation. Both are members of the service users group established by the Department of Health in Britain to promote user participation in public health and welfare organizations and both are members of self-help groups. That they should reach such conclusions seems to support the contention with which this chapter began which was that true empowerment in community care is attainable only through self-help activity and user-led services.

The empowerment debate has been stimulated in the UK by the NHS and CCA despite the limited mandate it offers. There is a question mark over the consumerist mandate it does offer as to the extent to which this empowers the users of health and welfare services as opposed to the purchasers of them. There is considerable evidence that professionals find it difficult to adapt to those practices that have been shown to promote effective service and that people say they want, and which in this chapter are described as enabling – though not empowering. Much of the debate, in its preoccupation with the role of professionals in health and welfare bureaucracies, ignores the fact that if these workers wished to practise in more enabling ways before the Act there was no reason why they should not have done so. The values of participative practice have been claimed as the foundation of the social care professions for decades, but as we have seen professionals still choose not to realize these values in their practice and continue to disempower service users by their actions.

This chapter began by suggesting that the empowerment debate must be seen within the overall context of the changing relationship between citizens, services and the professions. The credibility of the health and welfare professions is currently at a low ebb, whilst the creation of user-controlled alternatives to their services is at its most prolific. The current claims of professionals to a leading role in the empowerment process could be seen as a reflection of this alienation from their constituency and its consequent threat to their autonomy and power. It is hardly surprising, therefore, that against this background the beleaguered professions should welcome with open arms an apparently new opportunity to regain the public confidence upon which their legitimacy as 'experts' depends, and of course the status and power that goes with it. As Roger Gomm proposes, people who claim to be in the business of empowering rarely seem to be giving up their own power, and sometimes may actually be protecting it by appearing to share it with people who might otherwise take it all (Gomm, 1993 p. 137).

Increasingly people are becoming aware that public health and welfare bureaucracies and the professionals who work in them do not hold the monopoly of knowledge, skill and resources and the power these bring. Empowerment will result from people with needs taking control of the means to meet them. This is happening now and if health and welfare professionals are to play any role in this they must provide the effective service people want rather than the treatment the professionals think they need.

REFERENCES

Adams, R. (1990) *Self-Help, Social Work and Empowerment*, Macmillan, Basingstoke.

Allen, I., Hogg, D. and Peace, S. (1992) *Elderly People: Choice Participation and Satisfaction*, Policy Studies Institute, London.

Berthoud, R., Lakey, J. and McKay, S. (1993) *The Economic Problems of Disabled People*, Policy Studies Institute, London.

Bewley, C. and Glendinning, C. (1992) *Involving Disabled People in Community Care Planning*, Manchester University, Dept. of Social Policy and Social Work, Manchester.

Borsay, A. (1989) First child care, second mental health, third the elderly: professional education and the development of social work priorities. *Research, Policy and Planning,* **7** (2), pp. 22–30.

Chittenden, M. and Ramesh, R. (1993) *The Sunday Times,* 3 October, p. 6.

Croft, S. and Beresford, P. (1990) *User Involvement in Social Services,* Open Services Project, London.

Croft, S. and Beresford, P. (1992) The politics of participation. *Critical Social Policy,* issue 35, **12** (2) pp. 20–44.

Davis, A. and Fleming, A. (1992) User-commissioned research – the shape of things to come? *Social Services Research* (1), pp. 50–53.

Deakin, D. (1992) How far can users be involved in the planning of social services? *Social Services Research* (1), pp. 1–8.

Department of Health (1989) *Caring for People,* HMSO, London.

Department of Health (1990) *Community Care in the Next Decade and Beyond – Policy Guidance,* HMSO, London.

Ellis, K. (1992) *Squaring the Circle: User and Carer Participation in Needs Assessment,* Joseph Rowntree Foundation, York.

Evans, E.N. (1992) Liberation theology, empowerment theory and social work practice with the oppressed. *International Social Work,* **35**, pp. 135–147.

George, M. (1993) Unmet rights. *Community Care,* 14 October, pp. 18–19.

Gibbs, I. (1993) Financial resources of older people and paying for care in later life. *Social Policy Research Findings,* July (40), Joseph Rowntree Foundation, York.

Gomm, R. (1993) Issues of power in health and welfare, in *Health, Welfare and Practice – Reflecting on Roles and Relationships,* (eds Walmsley, J., Reynolds, J., Shakespeare, P., Woolfe, R.), Sage Publications, London, pp. 131–138.

Green, H. (1987) *Informal Carers: General Household Survey, 1985*, HMSO, London.

Griffiths, R. (1988) *Community Care: Agenda for Action,* HMSO, London.

Hasenfeld, Y. and Gidron, B. (1993) Self-help groups and human service organisations: an interorganisational perspective. *Social Service Review,* **67** (2), pp. 217–236.

Higgins, R. (1992) Room to consume. *Social Work Today,* 26 March, pp. 14–15.

Itzhaky, H. and York, A.S. (1991) Client participation and the effectiveness of community social work intervention. *Research on Social Work Practice,* **1** (4), pp. 387–398.

Jones, C. and Novak, T. (1993) Social work today. *British Journal of Social Work,* **23**, pp. 195–212.

Jones, J. (1993) The National Health Service market out of control. *The Independent,* 16 September, p. 3.

Joseph Rowntree Foundation (1993) (March) *Social Care Research Findings* (31).

Lindow, V. and Beresford, P. (1993) Taking charge. *Community Care,* 7 October, pp. 24–25.

Lupton, C. and Hall, B. (1993) Beyond the rhetoric: from policy to practice in user involvment. *Research, Policy and Planning,* **10**(2), pp. 6–11.

Macara, S. (1993) *The Independent,* 21 September, p. 27.

Marsh, P. and Fisher, M. (1992) *Good Intentions: Developing Partnership in Social Services,* Joseph Rowntree Foundation York.

Matzat, J. (1993) Away with the experts? Self-help groupwork in Germany. *Groupwork,* **6** (1), pp. 30–42.

Meredith, P. (1993) *Sociology of Health and Illness*, **15**(3), pp. 315–336.

Morris, J. (1993) *The Independent Living Project – Final Evaluation*, Spinal Injuries Association, London.

Morris, J. and Lindow, V. (1993) *User Participation in Community Care Services*, Community Care Support Force, DoH, Leeds.

Mullender, A. (1992–1993) Disabled people find a voice: will it be heard in the move towards community care? *Practice*, **6**(1), pp. 5–15.

National Health Service Management Executive (1992) Corporate Affairs Directorate, October. Unpublished discussion document, Leeds.

North, N. (1993) Empowerment in welfare markets. *Health and Social Care*, **1**(3), pp. 129–137.

O'Donnell, S. (1993) Involving clients in welfare policy-making. *Social Work*, **38** (5), pp. 629–635.

Oldman, C. (1991) *Paying for Care: Personal Sources of Funding Care*, Joseph Rowntree Foundation, York.

Oliver, M. (1989) Social Work with disabled people. *Social Work Today*, 6 April, p. 21.

Oliver, M. (1992) Civil rights and citizenship – a case of disabling welfare, in *Who Owns Welfare? Questions on the Social Services Agenda*, (ed. T. Harding), National Institute for Social Work, London.

Oliver, M. and Zarb, G. (1993) Personal services. *Community Care*, 4 March, pp. 22–23.

Pinker, R. (1992) Making sense of the mixed economy. *Social Policy and Administration*, **26**(4), pp. 273–284.

Potter, J. (1988) Consumerism and the public sector: how well does the coat fit? *Public Administration*, **66**, Summer, pp. 149–164.

Powell, T.J. (1979) Comparisons between self-help groups and professional services. *Social Casework*, November, **60**(9), pp. 561–565.

RADAR (1993) *Disabled People have Rights*, Interim Report, London.

School for Advanced Urban Studies (1993) *Working Together for Better Community Care*, Bristol University.

Smale, G., Tuson, G., with Biehal, N. and Marsh, P. (1993) *Empowerment, Assessment, Care Management and the Skilled Worker*. HMSO, London.

Smith, R. (1993) Helpers in harmony. *Community Care*, 1 April, pp. 25–26.

Social Services Inspectorate and the Scottish Office (1990) *Case Management and Assessment – The Practitioners' Guide*. HMSO, London.

Social Services Inspectorate and the Scottish Office (1990) *Case Management and Assessment – The Managers' Guide*. HMSO, London.

Social Services Inspectorate and the Scottish Office (1991) *Case Management and Assessment, Practice Guidance*, HMSO, London.

Stevenson, O. (1989) *Social Work Today*, 13 April, **20**, p. 7.

Stevenson, O. and Parsloe, P. (1993) *Community Care and Empowerment*, Joseph Rowntree Foundation, York.

Traux, C.B. and Mitchell, K.M. (1971) Research on certain therapist interpersonal skills in relation to process and outcome, in *Handbook of Psychotherapy and Behaviour Change*, (eds A.E. Bergin and L.G. Solomon), John Wiley, New York, pp. 299–344.

Vernon, G. (1986) Untrained carers are tops. *Community Care*, 11 September, (628), pp. 28–29.

Ward, D. and Mullender, A. (1992) Empowerment and oppression: an indissoluble pairing for contemporary social work. *Critical Social Policy*, issue 35, **12** (2), pp. 21–30.

Wilson, J. (1993) Vital yet problematic. Self-help groups and professionals – a review of the literature in the last decade. *Health and Social Care*, **1** (4), July, pp. 211–218.

Wistow, G. and Barnes, M. (1993) User involvement in community care: origins, purposes and applications. *Public Administration*, Autumn, **71**, pp. 279–299.

2

Defining participative practice in health and welfare

David and Yvonne Shemmings

INTRODUCTION

There is little doubt that, in future, the provision of health and welfare services must include more participative practice with the people receiving those services. But at a time when there have been cutbacks in these services, in real terms, it is extraordinary that the term 'empowerment' should be used to describe the way they are to be delivered; within social services departments, even more curious is the notion that parents or carers accused of abusing a child are expected to relate as 'partners' to those investigating the allegation.

People receiving health and welfare services have rarely described their experience with those providing them in language suggestive either of 'empowerment' or 'partnership'. Because community care involves rationing, prioritizing and charging for state intervention, they are even less likely to use such language in the future. This raises questions about why health and welfare professionals have started to do so now, but the possibility should not be overlooked that:

> . . . the received language of care performs an important, conservative illusion in society. It consoles us with the belief that something is being done to relieve distress and oppression. (Rojek *et al.*, 1988 p. 159.)

After discussing the significance of the language used to describe 'empowerment', and 'partnership' (see Department of Health, 1991 p. 21) in community care, we consider the reaction of helping organizations and professions to the changes that have already increased the rights of the 'consumers' of health and welfare services.

We contend that professionals and managers cannot yet claim to be 'empowering' consumers or engaging in 'partnerships' with them.

Finally, by considering the views of those on the receiving end of health and welfare, those with least formal power, the conclusion is reached that participation is not a linear concept but a dynamic one: it will vary depending upon the circumstances, the context, the setting and the people involved. We draw a distinction between participatory practice and participative practice, and depict 'empowerment' and 'partnership' as the higher rungs on a **ladder of participation** (Arnstein, 1969). Reaching the top of this ladder, however, is considered unlikely in most situations within the context of community care because of the structural inequalities existing between those providing services and those receiving them.

'EMPOWERMENT' . . . 'PARTNERSHIP' . . . ? WHAT'S IN A WORD?

Four overlapping and connected sociological, philosophical and socio-linguistic developments each conclude that language is the pivotal concept shaping how humans understand the world and each other.

Firstly, while structuralism and functionalism both assume categories such as 'class' or 'capitalist society' as the architectural foundations responsible for the construction of meaning and experience, post-structuralists see language as having primacy in the social organization of human behaviour (see Sarup, 1988; Norris, 1993). Understanding human social behaviour is about understanding discourse, an aggregation for 'language, knowledge, myths, and assumptions' (Rojek *et al.*, 1988).

Secondly, and as a direct consequence of post-structuralist interpretations of meaning and experience, post-modernists argue that as language is pivotal, there can be no such thing as 'truth' or 'taste'; there is no such thing as objective 'reality', something touchable, 'out there', to measure and control or any other 'meta-narrative' (see Rosenau, 1992 p. 12). Insecure as this may leave us, post-modernism asserts that existence, though not a level playing field, is a transitory, human construct achieved by negotiation through language. 'Truth' is a flexible concept which changes over time. Meaning is manoeuvrable and subject to manipulation by those groups and individuals in society who have the power to set agendas and define social action and interaction. Referring to Law (1986 p. 5) Sibeon reminds us that 'power is emergent; an effect, not a cause, of strategic success achieved in and during social interaction among actors' (Sibeon, 1992 p. 185).

Thirdly, some sociologists are beginning to argue that reductionist constructions such as 'class' or 'men' are 'social aggregates possessing' (for example) 'interests that are "objective" (or "real"), i.e. interests that are structurally determined . . .' (Sibeon, 1992 p. 184). Sibeon presses for an anti-reductionist sociological exposition on the premise that the whole is **not** greater than the sum of the parts because the whole was erroneously invented **by** some of those parts, i.e. human actors. Thus we return to our theme of the centrality of language in the construction of meaning.

Fourthly, recent developments in the field of socio-linguistics have been concerned with a logical consequence of these ideas: if language does not reflect an 'objective reality' but instead builds meaning, then it should be possible to reverse the process and find underlying meaning in language or more specifically, in metaphor (see Ortony, 1988; Lakoff and Johnson, 1980). Embedded in the metaphors hidden in speech and writing are indications of our underlying value system. It is the metaphorical structure of the language selected which is the window to our thought. But more than simply the cognitive basis of thought is revealed: language throws light on the attitudes of actors in social situations. Language is a 'carrier of ideology' (Rees, 1991). Lakoff and Johnson show as an example how different metaphors might be selected to speak about the concept of **argument**. If, for example, **argument** is experienced as a battle or as a war, words and phrases like 'defeat', 'defend' or 'take sides' will be chosen to describe it. It is possible to reverse this analytical process by posing questions such as: if different words and phrases are selected, like 'construct', 'build' or 'lay the foundations of', then what does such language suggest metaphorically about the underlying meaning attached to 'argument'? Lakoff and Johnson suggest this is an 'arguments are buildings' generative metaphor – 'generative', because the metaphor will occur repetitively and routinely in the speech and writing of its owner. The metaphors favoured are neither fixed nor static. Generative metaphors suggesting 'arguments are wars' are used when situations are seen in that way, but 'arguments are buildings' metaphors may have been chosen depending upon the circumstances. Naturally, there are many different metaphors available but Lakoff and Johnson (1980) found that culture affected the repertoire.

The relationship between these ideas and the concept of 'empowerment' in community care exists at two levels. At a fundamental level it is clear from the above discussion that what those with power say significantly defines meaning and experience. But something odd is implied by the language currently being used to describe relationships between the wide range of 'bureau-professionals' and managers in health and welfare organizations who have more formal and structural power, and those who have less. By describing their intention as that of 'empowerment' the former are implying that they are going to 'give' their power to the latter. In one sense this is patronizing but there is another more fundamental question to be considered. At a time when virtually all professional and occupational groups are under extreme pressure, with some feeling their very survival is in doubt, then why, with the possible exception of the medical professions, are such groups talking about giving power to the 'consumer'? While it is true that many nurses and social workers have always felt uneasy about the formal powers they possess – and perhaps would prefer sometimes to rid themselves of the responsibility – it is surprising that they should suddenly decide to offer it to their clients and patients. Are we witnessing the beginnings of professional suicide or merely observing occupational panic? Or are we seeing *la condition post-moderne*?

One way to understand the move toward 'empowerment' is by viewing it as a race for the ownership of language. The key to each professional group's survival is to get to the finishing post before rivals. Each profession is training itself to win, not because those receiving services have demanded 'empowerment', but because each profession is determined to be first past the finishing post. The prize is worth all the effort and its trophies are to be treasured: improved security of employment and the right to determine one's professional future. There are other races too. Nowadays, knowing exactly when to speak and write about 'greater choice', the establishment of a 'total quality management environment' is of greater strategic importance than any accompanying action. It is also less costly.

But the race itself, the 'competition', was not instigated by the professions. It is seen as being created by government, as part of its reversal of Keynesian, demand management economics (see for example Farnham and Horton, 1993 pp. 3–26). It is at the centre of neo-conservative and New Right moves to introduce popular capitalism and to untie significantly individuals from notions of 'society' and, in particular, to uncouple them from expensive attachments to the state. (We are reminded at this point of Prime Minister Thatcher's telling statement 'There is no such thing as society, only individuals and their families.) With specific reference to the concept of 'empowerment' Rees observed:

> Right-wing politicians use it to stress the merits of economic independence at all costs: somewhat ingenuously, they have argued that citizens have a right to fend for themselves. (Rees, 1991 p. 3.)

But to achieve this citizens need to be 'given' something; something to make them believe it is safe, indeed preferable, to live life as an individual rather than as part of society. Looked at in this light it may partly explain why a range of legislation has been enacted, in a very short space of time, giving people more rights as consumers of health and welfare services.

'CONSUMER' RIGHTS IN HEALTH AND WELFARE: CRUMBS FROM THE TABLE OR A GENUINE ATTEMPT AT OPENNESS?

Many of the recent changes in public sector policy are predicated on the belief that the management and delivery of health and welfare services are no different to the management of retail and commercial enterprise. Metaphors abound to support these changes. Clients and patients become 'consumers' or even 'customers'; 'business plans' and 'mission statements' are produced after a series of 'awaydays'; services are 'purchased', often from different sections of the same organization – what Common *et al.* (1993 p. 16.) described recently as 'playing at shops'. 'Nurses' and 'social workers' are unceremoniously replaced by 'care managers'.

But the structural relationship between receivers and providers of health and welfare services is markedly different from commercial relationships for at least three reasons. First of all, most people would prefer not to need health and welfare services at all, in the sense of preferring not to be ill, vulnerable, frail or abused. They are not doing what most people would consider as 'shopping'.

Secondly, and as Smale and his colleagues have recently illustrated so powerfully, commercial organizations do not 'assess need':

> Imagine turning up at the supermarket to be met by an 'assessor', or 'gatekeeper of resources', perhaps called a 'shopping manager' . . . this person explains that their job is to work with you to identify your needs, and to form an opinion of what kind of package of goods you need . . . (Smale *et al.*, 1993 p. 4).

This kind of advice might be given to a customer planning a new kitchen but this is a very different kind of activity from that of assessing need in the context of health and welfare provision.

Thirdly, the aim of commercial enterprise is to increase demand and thus persuade customers that they want more of what is on offer. The task of health and welfare organizations usually resembles the complete opposite. They do not want to increase 'trade': on the contrary, they have to ration and prioritize demand. Unlike health and welfare organizations, supermarkets do not turn their customers away.

So, we argue, to create the myth that clients and patients are 'customers' (and then persuade them of this) they had to be accorded some of the rights enjoyed by 'consumers'. How was this achieved?

Over the past six years a phenomenal change has taken place in the amount, and detail, of legislation giving the new 'customers' rights as 'consumers'. Those receiving health and welfare services can now:

- see information about them held on computer records or manually-produced files (as a result of the Data Protection Act, 1984; the Access to Personal Files Act, 1987; the Access to Medical Reports Act, 1989; and the Access to Health Records Act, 1990).
- attend important meetings in the field of child protection (following the publication of the Department of Health guidance *Working Together* in 1991). Similar arrangements could well be applied to the protection of vulnerable adults in the community.
- make complaints about the services received or not received (as a result of the Children Act, 1989 and the National Health Service and Community Care Act, 1990).
- receive services based upon clearer standards, and more 'assured' levels of 'quality' (following the publication of Citizens' Charters and Patients' Charters).

The most noticeable aspect of these changes was the speed at which they occurred. To use one example as an illustration, in 1988/9 the official view of the British Association of Social Workers (BASW), and of the (then) Department of Health and Social Security (DHSS) was, in effect, that parents of children should not be invited to child protection conferences. After the publication of the most recent guidance by the Department of Health (DoH) in 1991 the position was almost reversed: it must now be assumed that a parent or carer will be invited to **all** conferences about his or her children unless there is a good reason why they should not attend. The public scandals in Cleveland and Rochdale no doubt hastened the speed of this change but a similar urgency is noted with the other developments (see Shemmings, 1991, for example, in respect of access to records legislation).

But are these changes merely 'crumbs from the table'? The answer depends upon whether certain other promises made are honoured, for example in respect of improved access to health and welfare resources or the recent proposals to devolve management to localities for the commissioning and provision of health services. The extent to which 'opportunities' are 'equal', the 'community' really 'cares' and whether or not there is an overall health 'gain' in society will also determine its answer; so will the amount of 'service quality' which is **actually** 'assured'.

Clients of social services departments have welcomed these hard-won rights when they have been put into practice (Raymond, 1989), as have, for example, general practice patients (Bird and Walji, 1986) but, so far, such practice has been sporadic and subject to the enthusiasm of particular teams and individuals (see Øvretveit, 1986; Marsh and Fisher, 1992; Shemmings, 1991).

Referring to the kinds of 'consumer rights' described above Parsloe drew attention to the challenge facing social services departments (which could equally have been issued to health authorities). As yet it is not possible to feel confident that either of these agencies have responded with much commitment. In 1988 she wrote:

> Recent events provide the greatest challenge social services departments have faced since their inception, since they lay bare their value base. They provide an opportunity for departments to achieve the kind of relationship with clients and with the public which Seebohm envisaged, but which has been distorted by the demands flowing from a large organisation. Now there is a second chance. (Parsloe, 1988 p. 90.)

PROFESSIONAL AND ORGANIZATIONAL REACTIONS TO DATE

The reaction of health and welfare organizations and professionals has been one of resistance, and sometimes hostility. There is ample evidence that social services departments have not welcomed the idea of sharing their records with their clients without waiting to be asked for formal access (Doel and Lawson, 1986; Raymond, 1989; Øvretveit, 1986; Shemmings, 1991); that the nursing and medical professionals have also resisted the move to open records (Maquire *et al.*, 1986; Quine and Pahl, 1986); that professionals from the key child protection agencies have been resistant to the idea of parents and carers participating in child protection meetings (McGloin and Turnbull, 1986), despite the evidence that between 80–90% of children on child protection registers **carry on living at home** with their parent or carer.

The views of patients and clients about the extent to which they now have greater choice about the services received are not encouraging, despite the promises made. This example from a recent study on the views of older people by Allen and her colleagues is typical:

> Few, if any, elderly people interviewed had any choice in what went into their package of care and some did not have anything in their package at all. They usually had no choice about the time at which the service was delivered, the person who delivered it or how much they received . . . Choice and participation by elderly people usually took a negative form, with elderly people refusing services . . . (Allen *et al.*, 1992 p. 325.)

Although there is less research evidence to date about the introduction of complaints procedures it is likely to reveal a similar incongruence between words and action. Anecdotally, between us we have experience of working with over 2000 professionals, in a variety of training events on the subject of complaints procedures. The experience has, if anything, been more indicative of professional resistance to the idea of clients and patients complaining than with the other policy developments. An illustration of this is that as soon as it became clear the Department of Health was planning to introduce formal complaints procedures into health and welfare organizations, some immediately sought to control the language by attempting to redefine a complaint as a 'representation' or a 'suggestion'. Seen in this way handling complaints presents no difficulty because clients and patients are not really making a 'complaint'. Again, we are spectators at a race to occupy politico-linguistic space, but this time one of the competitors is the 'consumer'. After numerous role-plays and discussions about complaints procedures the overwhelming impression we are left with is that, far from being a 'partner' or someone about to be 'empowered', clients and patients who have the temerity to complain about their treatment may find they are treated as enemies.

A summary of our argument is that health and welfare organizations do not seem comfortable with many of the changes which have given clients and patients some additional rights as 'service consumers' (albeit with little change in the overall balance of power to allocate resources). But due to a number of social policy directives driven firmly from central government, each aimed at legitimizing the market, and not political systems, as the preferred mechanism of providing health and social services (see Farnham and Horton, 1993 pp. 3–26) they were given little option.

There are no indications that, left to their own devices, health and welfare organizations would have voluntarily introduced greater 'user involvement'. It will surely be an everlasting embarrassment of the profession of social work – and to the welfare bureaucracies that employ most of its members – that almost nothing was done to implement the findings of *Clients are Fellow Citizens'* (BASW, 1980). In this report BASW concluded that to breathe life into social work's stated value system it would need to: show people what is written about them; invite them to decision-making meetings; provide for second opinions; allow people to have a friend or representative present; and provide clients with independent, formal complaints procedures. And when, in 1983, the Department of Health and Social Security Circular LAC (83) (1983) 14 was issued, encouraging departments to prepare their records with access in mind, few departments did anything to introduce open records practice.

Marsh and Fisher came to a similar conclusion, partly evident in the title of their report *Good Intentions* but revealed more particularly in the following short passage:

> At an early stage . . . we were struck by the difference between the language used to describe the practice of staff and the actual work undertaken. For example, the use of 'agreements' was stated to be widespread, clients were described as 'participating' in decision-making meetings, and 'open' records were apparently in regular use. (Marsh and Fisher, 1992 p. 37).

Largely concurring with our own research findings, their conclusions indicated a lack of congruence between the words used by workers to **describe** their actions and what they did in practice. Although the notion of 'written agreements' has been subject to criticism (see Rojek and Collins, 1987) when they were proposed as a way of increasing client participation in social work the reaction of workers in Marsh and Fisher's study was quite different from healthy criticism. The authors describe the reaction as 'rather lukewarm'; and additionally 'it was not evident to practitioners that anything was new. We came to describe this as the DATA effect – we **D**o **A**ll **T**his **A**lready' (Marsh and Fisher, 1992 p. 37). The report concluded, however, that they did not.

We consider it unwise to leave it to managers and professionals in health and welfare bureaucracies to define terms such as 'empowerment' and 'partnership', for they are too apt to do so in ways which suit their own professional interests; or as Hallett put it, 'each is free like Alice's Humpty Dumpty to make the word mean exactly what he or she wishes it to mean' (Hallett, 1986 p. 10). Michael Ignatieff develops this point:

> Words like fraternity, belonging and community are so soaked in nostalgia and utopianism that they are useless as guides to the real possibilities of solidarity in modern society . . . and our language stumbles behind like an overburdened porter with a mountain of cases. (Ignatieff, 1984 p. 138).

THE EXPERIENCE OF THE 'CONSUMERS' OF HEALTH AND WELFARE: PARTNERS OR POOR RELATIONS?

This section considers the views of those on the receiving end of health and welfare. It is unashamedly about the **practice** of community care. It seeks to address the kind of interpersonal relationships valued by them. Why should they be any better than professionals at defining such relationships? This is probably not the best way of looking at the issue. It is not a question of whether they are any better at defining the nature of empowerment or partnership; it is simply right and proper that their views be given an airing and taken seriously. No romantic view that clients and patients 'know best' is offered, but we do share a belief that the insights of the least powerful actors in social behaviour are as important as those of the most powerful. And, if left unchecked, the voices of managers and professionals soon drown those of clients and patients.

A number of research studies have been drawn upon which have sought the views of clients and patients, who at best could be described as reluctant, often more accurately as resistant and sometimes as hostile, to what they felt was an unwelcome intrusion into their lives. Included are the views of family members attending child protection conferences, in particular from research undertaken for the Department of Health (and in which one of us has been directly involved – see Thoburn *et al.*, 1995); we draw upon reactions to the sharing of records in the fields of both health and welfare (see Øvretveit, 1986; Raymond, 1989; Shemmings, 1991); also some of Howe's findings are referred to, from his study of consumer reactions to family therapy (Howe, 1989). Finally Marsh and Fisher's research project is used because it sought the views of carers and family members who were looking after older people experiencing severe confusion (Marsh and Fisher, 1992).

No summaries of these research studies are provided; rather, the implications are presented and discussed which have a direct bearing on clients' and patients' views about the way they were treated by members of the 'helping' professions.

The conclusion is drawn that two necessary, but not sufficient, conditions are required if professionals hope to convince clients and patients that the planning and allocation of community care services are moving in the direction of empowerment and partnership.

As stated earlier, when describing their experiences of health and welfare practice clients and patients rarely use language containing metaphors redolent of empowerment or partnership, but they regularly and routinely speak in metaphorical language suggesting different shades of **participation**.

We argue that participation is a better term than empowerment or partnership. This is why a modification of Arnstein's Ladder of Citizen Participation (Arnstein, 1969) has been designed to conceptualize the notion of participation having different shades or 'levels'. Our everyday metaphorical awareness of a 'ladder' embraces at least two concepts: the possibility of ascendance but accompanied by ever-increasing difficulty. This neatly captures the reality of participation in community care: the higher 'rungs' are harder to reach, so the lower ones are easier and safer. As we can see, as the 'ladder' is climbed the task gets more difficult:

Rung 8: Citizen control
Rung 7: Delegated power
Rung 6: Partnership
Rung 5: Consultation
Rung 4: Involvement
Rung 3: Keeping fully informed
Rung 2: Placation
Rung 1: Manipulation

Although the bottom two rungs are not examples of true participation they are included because they can sometimes masquerade as such. It is possible to invite someone to a meeting, apparently as a participant, only for them to find out they are not allowed to speak. Worse still, they might have been led to believe they are being listened to, but in reality are being ignored because the professionals have already decided what they are going to do. Thus it is axiomatic that Rung 3, keeping fully informed, is the basic step on the way to higher levels of participation.

We also believe it will be more helpful in future to refer to those aspects of services concerned primarily with the relationships between receivers and providers as **participative practice** and those concerned with the involvement of clients and patients in the organization, planning and delivery of those services as **participatory practice**.

Necessary conditions for participative practice

From the research, it seems that two conditions are necessary before those receiving health and welfare services will even think about 'participation'. They need to experience **mutuality** (see Maluccio and Marlow, 1974) with those providing services, and they must experience **trust**. But this 'trust' requires an additional dimension to that originally described by American pioneers and researchers in the field of counselling and psychotherapy in the 1960s and 1970s (Rogers, 1951; Traux and Carkhuff, 1966; Egan, 1990). When the power relationship is structurally unequal, for trust to be experienced, and then sustained, it must be **demonstrated** by professionals at all times. Health and welfare professionals offering help to those who may not have asked for it cannot expect clients and patients to have faith in them: they will regularly need to **prove** themselves to be trustworthy.

Condition 1: The Metaphor of Mutuality

Applied to health and welfare in community care **mutuality** implies that clients and patients have to be treated by professionals in exactly the same way the professionals would wish to be treated, were the roles to be reversed. This 'do unto others' metaphor is present in virtually all research into the perceptions and preferences expressed by clients and patients about the way they were treated – or would have preferred to have been treated – by professionals. Returning to Lakoff and Johnson's (1980) metaphorical analysis of language, the underlying meaning carried by this metaphor is markedly different from everyday notions of empowerment or partnership which, when applied to health, welfare and community care, signpost relationships suggesting promises of freedom and equality rarely possible in practice. Again, this is why they were placed at the top of the 'ladder of participation'.

In interpersonal terms, those receiving services are saying that what they want from health and welfare professionals is different from equality; it is more akin to the notion of **reciprocity**.

What does this mean in practice? In one sense all that is required to answer this question is to consider how we, ourselves, would want to be treated if we ever needed to be 'cared for in the community'. The research findings suggest that two qualities must be present which at first sight may seem contradictory. For clients and patients to experience mutual and reciprocal relationships professionals must behave at one and the same time in a direct and sensitive manner. **Directness** and **sensitivity** are the two essential ingredients of mutuality. One skill may at times eclipse the other, but for mutuality to exist the other must be present, albeit in the background. On a course concerned with the participation of family members in child protection conferences, a health worker made the following observation about the concept of mutuality in practice: 'It's like the ability to give people "bad news" while cuddling them at the same time but without the cuddle masking the "bad news" '.

Her statement reaches the core of the 'mutuality metaphor' as defined by people receiving health and welfare services, so many of whom have used it to describe what they want from those providing them. It is remarkably simple to understand yet enormously difficult to achieve in practice. Most of us can be direct when we need to be; most of us can recognize when people need sensitivity. But combining the two in the right proportion and offering them both at once is not an easy task.

The combination of directness and sensitivity consists of getting to the point without being brusque, coarse or harsh. Health and welfare professionals who demonstrate this skill are found to be unambiguous yet tentative, concrete and compassionate, simultaneously empathic and challenging.

Condition 2: The Metaphor of 'Demonstrable Trust'

Within the helping professions it is axiomatic that, for it to be effective, those receiving 'help' need to experience a trusting rapport with the 'helper'. But, it seems, the literature on counselling and helping relationships has so far ignored an aspect of trust which is of immense importance to those who hope to be on the receiving end of it; yet it is something spoken about regularly by clients and patients in the research studies referred to earlier.

Outside of the world of health and welfare the most typical generative metaphor for 'trust' includes an intangible quality within the relationship which can never be appreciated fully. 'Trusting' involves indeterminate and elusive qualities bestowed by one person on another. Although it contains immensely complex and paradoxical constructions, ultimately it seems to have a lot to do with faith.

But for people receiving health and welfare services, deciding when it it safe to trust professionals cannot be based upon faith alone; or rather, such faith – which still needs to be present – must be constantly proved and demonstrated.

What does 'demonstrable trust' look like? How does practice need to be adjusted to respond to these challenges? To put meat on the bones of this embellished concept a rich seam of ideas is appearing in the literature, and it is based upon the views of the less powerful (see Beihal and Sainsbury, 1991; Marsh and Fisher, 1992 pp. 13–15; Rees, 1991 pp. 86–98; Thoburn *et al.*, 1994 p. 3). It tends not to be found in policy statements emanating from the main statutory health and welfare organizations responsible for providing community care.

For a worker to be seen as trustworthy they will always make it clear who they are, who they work for and why they are involved, especially if there is any reluctance shown on the part of the client or patient. The worker will always offer to share what they write in files with the client or patient and will invite them to any key decision-making meetings. In situations when this cannot be done (for legal reasons) the worker will explain why and then outline the complaints procedure. They will encourage people to have a friend or representative with them during such explanations – and in such situations it may also be appropriate to consider whether to tape-record interviews. Trustworthy professionals are experienced by clients and patients as **even-handed**, which they demonstrate by always fully explaining what they are doing and why. But most important of all, workers must explain how they are thinking, as well as what they are thinking: how assessments are formed, and how decisions are made, are of central importance to clients and patients.

Are we inventing yet another 'received idea' within the helping professions? Rojek and his colleagues are critical of concepts such as 'mutuality' because 'logically it has no basis in experience for it is precisely the absence of mutuality in everyday social work that (Maluccio and Marlow, 1974) are commenting on' (Rojek *et al.*, 1988

p. 9). They rightly place 'mutuality' alongside 'trust', 'respect', 'acceptance', 'self-determination' as 'abstractions' (Rojek *et al.*, 1988 p. 174). As we have attempted to assert, the problem centres on who defines such abstractions. It may be possible to meet these criticisms if terms such as 'mutuality', 'trust' and 'empathy' are **defined in operation** by those on the receiving end. Doing so may mark the beginning of the 'move from a donatory to participatory form of care' (p. 178) which Rojek and his colleagues – and many others – are keen to see.

CONCLUSION

We have raised questions about the meaning of 'empowerment' and 'partnership' as defined by health and welfare organizations for two reasons. Firstly, to prevent clients and patients from having their expectations raised inappropriately; secondly, and as a consequence of the first reason, we remain concerned about the effect such raised expectations could have upon health and welfare practitioners, so many of whom have told us that they are beginning to feel sandwiched between the service user and senior management.

It is our contention that the primary motivation behind the introduction of 'empowerment' and 'participation' into health and welfare organizations is best understood as resulting from the marketization of these services. Thus the attempt to give clients and patients 'consumer' status by introducing empowerment and participation is a predictable consequence of the creation of the illusion that receiving a health or welfare service is no different from purchasing goods at the supermarket. We believe that they are **radically** different.

The other clear aim of the government's health and welfare policy has been to increase competition significantly (see Farnham and Horton, 1993, for example). Here is possibly another reason why the emphasis on empowerment and partnership in health and welfare service provision has achieved such ascendancy.

Although participative practice is well within the range of skills of any competent health or welfare professional we remain both cynical and sceptical about promises to 'give power' to clients and patients at a time when government policy looks set to change the basis of provision towards leaner and meaner, privately-owned, services in which, with a strange twist of Darwinism, only the most fit and socially acceptable will be welcome. The rest look likely to be squeezed into an increasingly resource-starved and marginalized public sector.

Finally, it is almost self-evident that for practitioners to be able to empower others they in turn must feel valued and supported. But with the rise of short-term contracts, redundancies and the ever-present fidgeting which accompanies departmental reorganizations, it is difficult to feel confident about their ability to do so when they feel uncared for. Perhaps this is why, so far, they seem not to have responded to the challenge of particip**ative** practice with much enthusiasm or commitment.

REFERENCES

Allen, I., Peace, S. and Hogg, D. (1992) *Elderly People: Choice, Participation and Satisfaction*, Policy Studies Institute, London.

Arnstein, S.R. (1969) A ladder of participation. *Journal of the American Institute of Planners*, **35** (4), pp. 216–224.

Beihal, N. and Sainsbury, E. (1992) From values to rights in social work. *British Journal of Social Work*, **21**, pp. 245–257.

Bird, A.P. and Walji, M.T.I. (1986) Outpatients have access to their medical records. *British Medical Journal*, 1 March, pp. 595–596.

British Association of Social Workers (BASW) (1980) *Clients are Fellow Citizens*, BASW, Birmingham.

Common, R., Flynn, N. and Mellon, E. (1993) *Managing Public Services: Competition and Decentralisation*, Butterworth-Heinemann, Oxford.

Department of Health (1991) *Working Together under the Children Act 1989.* HMSO, London.

Department of Health LAC (83) (1983) *Disclosure of Personal Information*, HMSO, London.

Doel, M. and Lawson, B. (1986) Open records: the client's right to partnership. *British Journal of Social Work*, **16** (4), pp. 407–430.

Egan, G. (1990) *The Skilled Helper*, 3rd edn., Brooks-Cole, Monterey.

Farnham, D. and Horton, S. (1993) *Managing the New Public Services*, Macmillan, London.

Hallett, C. (1986) In whose best interests? in *Parental Participation in Case Conferences*, (eds T. Brown and J. Waters), Association for the Study and Prevention of Child Abuse and Neglect, pp. 9–26.

Howe, D. (1989) *The Consumer's View of Family Therapy*, Gower, Aldershot.

Ignatieff, M. (1984) *The Needs of Strangers*, Chatto and Windus, London.

Lakoff, G. and Johnson, M. (1980) *Metaphors We Live By*, University of Chicago Press, Chicago.

Law, J. (1986) On power and tactics: a view from the sociology of science. *Sociological Review*, **34** (1), pp. 1–38.

McGloin, P. and Turnbull, A. (1986) *Parent Participation in Child Abuse Review Conferences: A Research Report*, Directorate of Social Services, London Borough of Greenwich.

Maluccio, A.N. and Marlow, D.W. (1974) The case for the contract. *Social Work*, **13** (1).

Maquire, P., Fairburn, S. and Fletcher, C. (1986) Most young doctors are bad at giving information. *British Medical Journal*, 14 June, pp. 1576–78.

Marsh, P. and Fisher, M. (1992) *Good Intentions: Developing Partnerships in Social Services*, Joseph Rowntree Trust, York.

Norris, C. (1993) *What's Wrong With Postmodernism: Critical Theory and the Ends of Philosophy*, Harvester-Wheatsheaf, London.

Ortony, A. (1988) *Metaphor and Thought*, Cambridge University Press, Cambridge.

Øvretveit, J. (1986) *Improving Social Work Records and Practice*, British Association of Social Workers, Birmingham.

Parsloe, P. (1988) Social services: confidentiality, privacy and data protection, in *Personal Data Protection in Health and Social Services*, (eds P. Pearce, *et al.*), Croom Helm, London.

Quine, L. and Pahl, J. (1986) First diagnosis of severe mental handicap: characteristics of unsatisfactory encounters between doctors and patients. *Social Science and Medicine*, **22** (1), pp. 53–62.

Raymond, Y. (1989) Empowerment in practice: users' views on seeing their records. *Practice*, **3** (1), pp. 5–23.

Rees, S. (1991) *Achieving Power*, Harvester-Wheatsheaf, London.

Rogers, C.R. (1951) *Client-Centered Therapy*, Houghton-Mifflin, Boston.

Rojek, C. and Collins, S.A. (1987) Contract or con-trick? *British Journal of Social Work*, **17** (2), pp. 199–121.

Rojek, C., Peacock, G. and Collins, S. (1988) *Social Work and Received Ideas*, Routledge, London.

Rosenau, P.M. (1992) *Postmodernism and the Social Sciences: Insights, Inroads and Intrusions*, Princeton University Press, New York.

Sarup, M. (1988) *An Introduction to Post-structuralism and Post-modernism*, Harvester-Wheatsheaf, London.

Shemmings, D. (1991) *Client Access to Records: Participation in Social Work*, Gower, Aldershot.

Sibeon, R. (1992) Sociological reflections on welfare politics and social work. *Social Work and Social Sciences Review*, **3** (3), pp. 184–203.

Smale, G. and Tuson, G. with Biehal, N. and Marsh, P. (1993) *Empowerment, Assessment, Care Management and the Skilled Worker*. HMSO for the National Institute for Social Work, London.

Thoburn, J., Lewis, A. and Shemmings, D. (1995) *Partnership or Paternalism? Family Participation in Child Protection*. HMSO, London.

Traux, C.B. and Carkhuff, R.R. (1967) *Towards Effective Counselling and Psychotherapy*, Aldine, Chicago.

3

Whose empowerment? Equalizing the competing discourses in community care

Suzy Croft and Peter Beresford

THE EMERGENCE OF EMPOWERMENT

There is now considerable interest in issues of involvement and empowerment in community care. The publication of this book is one more expression of it. Much work is currently being done on the analysis, development, implementation and evaluation of involvement and empowerment. However, much less attention has been paid to the social construction of the debates and developments taking place; to the influences, ideologies, organizations, institutions and interests which affect and shape them. This is what we want to focus on here.

A small industry has developed round empowerment and involvement. Its growing apparatus includes legislation, government guidance, mission statements, charters, literature, participatory projects, committees, working parties, researchers, consultants, trainers, managers, development workers and much more.

While discussions and developments around user involvement and empowerment in community care focus on challenging the traditional relationships and distribution of power between service users and service agencies and authorities, they are also circumscribed and overshadowed by these. As a result the debate is a heavily contested one. Ironically the debate and development about involvement and empowerment are often themselves excluding and disempowering.

It is likely to be helpful to explore this hidden history of involvement and empowerment both to do justice to the experience and difficulties experienced by people struggling to be involved and empowered and also to improve progress in this field.

Our own interest in this issue arises from our experience as service users, our involvement in service user movements and our work in a small independent project, the Open Services Project, seeking to support people's involvement and empowerment. This work has given us the opportunity to explore a wide range of participatory initiatives and to meet many people involved both as service users and providers in progressing participation and empowerment. We have also experienced first hand many of the issues and problems which apply more generally through our own involvement in a number of participatory developments.

TWO COMPETING DISCOURSES

Current discussion about participation in community care mirrors many of the tensions, problems and possibilities of participation itself. There is not so much a debate or dialogue about empowerment and involvement as at least two different discourses (Beresford, 1994a). There is the discourse of politicians, policy makers, service providers and their associated analysts, consultants and spokespersons and then there is the discourse of disabled people, service users, their organizations, movements and allies. This is not to say that there isn't contact and collaboration between the two, but there are also tensions, ambiguities, distrust and uncertainties. At the same time there are overlaps between them. Some people have a foot in both camps. Individuals may be service users and providers. There are also some determined efforts to make links and encourage co-operation and understanding, like the *Building Bridges* initiative (User Centred Services Group, 1993). But there are also real differences and it is helpful to look at some of these.

There are fundamental differences in the nature, concerns and ideology of the two discourses as well as in the language and definitions they use. Let's begin with the form they take. The discourse of people who use services is not predominantly a written one, as is that of service providers. It is much more an oral and interpersonal one, developing through people's shared experience, contacts, networks, collective action, struggles and organizations, with written and other recorded material just the tip of an iceberg of analysis, experience and discussion, much of it local and undocumented. Where it is recorded, connections between the personal and the political tend to be more clearly drawn. People's histories and interests tend to be made more explicit.

SERVICE USERS' DISCOURSE

The importance of non-written discussion among community care service users may be partly due to the different cultures and histories of disabled people and other service users compared with most service providers. They are more likely to have experienced segregated and limited educational opportunities. They tend to have less support to write; less time and money, fewer secretaries and administrative back-up, fewer word processors, training opportunities and chances to meet and exchange information, particularly nationally and internationally, and less access to transport.

Deaf people and non-readers also communicate in different ways. Service users produce material in diverse forms and are also pressing service providers to produce material in non-print forms including audio-cassette, braille, pictures, on disc, video and signed video. While disabled people and other recipients of community care services have been subject to many constraints, their debates are nonetheless sophisticated and have developed rapidly. What characterizes them most is that they are part of a discourse concerned with liberation.

Disabled people and community care service users have created their own broadcast and print media, their own journals and newsletters. Their cultures extend beyond the office and print-based ones of social services to include direct action, poetry, cartoon, illustration, music, comedy, drama, cabaret and song.

The discourses are also concerned with solving different problems. That of service providers and their associates is crucially concerned with their agencies and services; how to make them more efficient, cost-effective, better managed and responsive. That of disabled people and service users is primarily concerned with their lives, rights, choices and opportunities.

COMPETING APPROACHES TO PARTICIPATION

The differences in concerns of the two discourses are also clearly reflected in their approaches to the idea of participation. We have discussed these in more detail elsewhere (Croft and Beresford, 1992a). The terms 'consumer involvement' and 'user involvement' originate from the service system, not from disabled people or other candidates for community care. Many dislike being defined in terms of services which they see as inappropriate and unhelpful. Like many psychiatric system survivors, Viv Lindow objects to the term 'consumer' where people have no choice about the 'service' they receive and are 'damaged' by the product (Lindow, 1990).

The meanings that disabled people and other recipients of community care services attach to user involvement are concerned with having more say and control in their lives and over organizations, services and institutions that affect them. They are concerned with securing people's independence, their civil rights, equal access and opportunities and, in some cases, the achievement of broader social change. Involvement in services is not their primary focus. Instead people's full participation and inclusion in society is. Their concern with services extends beyond dedicated community care provision to how public policy and provision overall relate to their lives and support or restrict their inclusion and independence.

If the approach to user involvement pursued by disabled people, recipients of community care and their allies can be described as a **democratic** one, concerned with people's rights as citizens and their participation in decisions which affect them, that of service providers can best be described as a **consumerist** one. Here the focus is on the individual as user or consumer of community care services under the new arrangements and market ideology of a 'mixed economy of care'. This approach is service-centred. The involvement of service users is through consultation and market research to contribute information and ideas to improve management, economy and effectiveness. Power and control remain with services and their providers and purchasers. People can feed in their views and experience, but agencies still make the decisions.

COMPETING IDEAS OF EMPOWERMENT

This brings us to empowerment. In community care, discussion of empowerment has largely taken place in the context of debates and developments concerned with user involvement. The two terms involvement and empowerment are often used interchangeably. This can be confusing because initiatives for user involvement are often disempowering and empowerment is not only concerned with people's participation. It is important to distinguish between the two and to recognize that the relationship between them is often complex and unclear.

We haven't always done this adequately ourselves. For example, we have also described the democratic model of involvement as an empowerment model, because of its commitment to people having more say and control over their lives (Beresford, 1988). We define empowerment to mean:

> Making it possible for people to exercise power and have more control over their lives. That means having a greater voice in institutions, agencies and situations which affect them. It also means being able to share power or exercise power over someone else, as well as them exercising it over you. (Beresford and Croft, 1993.)

Many people involved in disabled people's and service users' organizations use the term without explicit definition, because they know what it
means for them; it has shared meanings and these meanings are clear
and self-evident. Empowerment means challenging their disempowerment and the discrimination they face, not being subject to service
providers' arbitrary control, achieving their rights, and being able to live
their lives like other people.

Peter Campbell, a founding member of Survivors Speak Out, the
national organization of people with mental distress, says for example:

> What people are looking for with empowerment is a greater degree
> of control and say in what goes on in their lives; to have greater
> freedom and autonomy in services and much more widely. It's an
> objective. (Campbell, 1994.)

But as Raymond Jack showed in Chapter 1, there is no overall agreement
about empowerment. Many different strands can be identified in the
idea's development and usage. There are managerialist, self-help,
liberational, professional and market models of empowerment
(Beresford, 1994b). They are in a complex relationship with each other.
While there are overlaps between them, there are also important
differences. The two approaches most in evidence in community care
are the professional and liberational ones. The first is narrowly
concerned with personal empowerment; people taking increased
responsibility for managing their lives, relationships and circumstances,
to live in conformity with prevailing values and expectations and to
change in accordance with professionally set goals and norms.

Professional interest in empowerment has developed in response to
the new demands of the consumerist care market. It seems to reflect the
increasing uncertainty and insecurity of professions like social work and
nursing. Empowerment offers them a new professional ethos. It
provides professionals who are under attack and in retreat with a relevant
and legitimate philosophy for the new welfare consumerism, as well as
an argument for their own autonomy and consolidation by emphasizing
the prior need for their empowerment if they are to empower service
users (Stevenson and Parsloe, 1993).

By contrast, the liberational model of empowerment developed by the
movements of disabled people, older people and survivors is concerned
with changing their position in society. It doesn't ignore issues of
personal empowerment, but these are framed in terms of ensuring
people have to support, skills and personal resources they need for self-
organization and participation to achieve broader social change.

What can we learn from this empowerment debate? Firstly the shared
interest of service providers and service users in empowerment does not
necessarily represent a cessation of tensions or differences between the

two, but instead may reflect the lines on which struggles between them are currently drawn. While service providers are operating within the parameters of an individualized market model of welfare and the preoccupations of professionalization, movements of disabled people and service users are seeking to transcend these with a commitment to people's needs and to their civil and human rights.

Secondly, debates and developments about empowerment and involvement are a conflict-ridden area of activity. This conflict is not just central to the issues of participation and empowerment, but also to the discourses, structures and processes which have developed around them. This is heavily disputed territory. Roles, relationships, analysis and the distribution of power are all being contested. Just as participation is political – although this reality is often understated or ignored – so are the debates and developments around it.

THE CHEQUERED PROGRESS OF EMPOWERMENT AND INVOLVEMENT

It might be expected that the existence of these different, frequently conflicting interests around empowerment and involvement in community care would have had some bearing on their progress. This progress seems to be limited, patchy and qualified. In 1990, we reported the findings of the first national survey of user involvement in voluntary and statutory social services (Croft and Beresford, 1990). At this time, just under a third of social services departments and nearly half of voluntary organizations surveyed reported that they had formal policies to involve service users in the provision of their services. But there seemed to be few coherent, agency-wide schemes and policies for involvement and empowerment. Very few statutory departments seemed to offer service users a direct say in policy or provision.

In mid 1994, a year on from the full implementation of the community care reforms, the situation does not seem to have improved greatly. The research officer of a major funding organization working in this field told us that her impression from research on user involvement and empowerment, which it was supporting, was that the key issues emerging included tokenism, inadequate resources, low priority and the need for more time. Daphne Statham, Director of the National Institute for Social Work, has argued that participation and empowerment 'are not working that well in many areas' (Statham, 1994). In their study of disabled people and community care planning, Catherine Bewley and Caroline Glendinning found that its purpose was often unclear and that many disabled people, particularly black people and members of ethnic minority groups, were likely to be left out (Bewley and Glendinning, 1994). In a study of user empowerment and social services departments,

Lesley Hoyes and others reported that 'the ideals of choice and control for service users and carers are still a long way off' (Hoyes *et al.*, 1994). All this reflects our own experience in a national project we are currently undertaking, putting together service users' first-hand accounts of community care and participation.

THE FAILURE TO LOCATE THE DEBATE

This uncertainty in the development of user involvement and empowerment in community care reflects a more general hesitancy in their development over a much longer period and in other fields. Perhaps we should not be surprised, with such contentious and politically loaded issues. But there also seem to be two particular difficulties in the area of community care obstructing progress. The first of these has been the frequent failure to **contextualize** involvement and empowerment and the second the continuing conflicts and competition between service users and providers. It is worth looking at both of these more closely, beginning with the contextualizing of involvement and empowerment.

This tendency to abstracted discussion has been a common feature of social policy and social administrative discussions and developments. Some would argue it is one of their defining characteristics. It has certainly been true of the dominant service provider discourse around involvement and empowerment. While service users often face particular difficulties making connections, because of their limited access to information and opportunities for exchange, the exclusion and institutionalized discrimination which they routinely experience and feel has encouraged a search for broader understanding (Barnes, 1991).

The dominant discourse on involvement and empowerment, on the other hand, has not been adequately linked either to broader developments and discussions around participation and democracy or to major current debates about the future of welfare and the welfare state. Both of these have fundamental implications for community care and empowerment. Let's begin with the first.

THE NEED TO MAKE THE BROADER POLITICAL LINK

There has frequently been a failure for participatory policy and practice to build on existing ideas and experience. This has been particularly true in community care, where many of the lessons learned in community development, land use planning and other fields have had to be relearned. Perhaps even more important is the frequent failure to relate the discourse about involvement and empowerment to broader political discussion and political theory; to ideas about the role and nature of the state, democracy, citizenship, rights and power.

The reasons for this are not clear. Perhaps it is felt that more responsive, user-centred services are achievable in isolation. However the lesson of the last 15 years in the UK has been that political and socio-economic structures have a profound bearing on public policy and services. It is even more questionable whether democratization can be pursued at a micro level without reference to broader political structures. Practical issues also arise in relating and reconciling structures for participation and empowerment with existing political arrangements and structures for local and central democracy.

On the other hand, service providers may be reluctant to relate involvement and empowerment to these broader issues because of the far-reaching and constraining implications they have and prefer instead, as we have seen particularly with the idea of empowerment, an individualizing focus.

It remains difficult to see though how discussions about the control people can have over their own life, in relation to other people and over agencies, organizations and services affecting them, can be had in isolation from broader political, social and economic institutions. The suggestion that they can, implicit in much discussion and practice around involvement and empowerment, may explain the suspicion with which many disabled people and service users regard them.

COMMUNITY CARE, EMPOWERMENT AND THE FUTURE OF THE WELFARE STATE

There has been a similar failure to make connections between community care, empowerment and the welfare state more generally. The future of the welfare state is in the melting pot. There is broad political and expert agreement that it must change, but fierce ideological and political differences about the nature of that change (BBC, 1993). While the political left seeks to redefine the welfare state's universalist base, the political right argues for a shift away from it. The left argues for full employment as a pre-condition of a future welfare state; the right argues that this is not a feasible option, and the government continues to pursue economic policies associated with high unemployment. Meanwhile major demographic changes are taking place, particularly an accelerating increase in the number and proportion of very old people in the first half of the 21st century. There is fierce disagreement about the feasibility of resourcing social security for the future at current levels and government is constrained by short-term concerns to limit public expenditure to meet a large-scale budget deficit (Oppenheim, 1994). There has also been a reluctance to involve service users fully in the discussion about the welfare state (Croft and Beresford, 1993a).

Whatever the outcome, changes in the welfare state will have an important bearing on community care, the needs it has to address, its potential for involvement and empowerment and the extent of budgetary constraints. Change will affect both how much funding is made directly available to community care, as well as the level of resourcing for public provision – the context in which community care policy operates. Little attention is being paid to this in the dominant community care discourse, but service users are already being affected in the run-up to change with cuts in benefits and attacks on disabled people as scroungers.

CONFLICT AND INEQUALITY IN THE EMPOWERMENT DEBATE

The second major problem we identified impeding progress on involvement and empowerment is the continuing conflict and competition between the discourses of service users and providers. As we pointed out earlier, the two have significantly different personal, professional, political and organizational concerns. But what is particularly important here is the imbalance of power and resources between them.

Disabled people and other service users have less access to the mainstream, less support, fewer resources and less credibility. Funding is a pivotal issue. The funding of service users' organizations is generally inadequate and insecure. Underfunded projects are often expected to rely on one single and/or part-time workers. They frequently lack the essentials for administration and outreach work, making do with poor premises, second-hand equipment and relying on free photocopying and other support services from sympathetic allies. This is in sharp contrast to conventional academic and research institutions, large charities and statutory organizations.

A pilot research project indicates that user-led groups experience additional obstacles in gaining funding to non-user-led organizations (Barnes and Thompson, 1994). While service users often receive no or low pay for their expertise, consultancy and training, conventional consultants, whose knowledge is largely drawn from service users, command fees as high as £1000 per day (Croft and Beresford, 1992b). People involved in the provider discourse have better access to print and broadcast media and to publishers. Most of the books on involvement and empowerment in community care have been written or edited by people located in the provider discourse. The large research projects have all gone to conventional research organizations, even though service users have sometimes sought to carry them out. The National User Involvement Project, funded by the National Health Service Executive, represents the first major national research and development project led and undertaken by service users.

There is another perhaps more subtle expression of the power imbalance between the two discourses. While, as we have said, there are positive examples of collaboration between service users and providers, there are also many cases of incorporation and co-option, where service providers seek the legitimacy and expertise of service users, but want to keep control and retain their own agendas. The difficulty for service users and their organizations is that they are still often dependent on organizations and individuals involved in the provider discourse for resources, access, training, consultancy, networks and information. Service users can find themselves caught up in a heavily political world which is stressful, confusing, competitive and unfriendly. They can expect to work with agencies which preach empowerment but act in painful and excluding ways. This is frequently divisive and damaging for service users. We have also heard of service workers who have been sidelined and denied promotion because of their activities as allies. This is part of the hidden history of involvement and empowerment, which people involved in service users' organizations know about only too well, but may not be able to talk about publicly if they want to maintain effective working relationships, attract funding and not be marginalized by service providers and their associates.

The heart of the problem is not the differences between the two discourses, but the **inequality** of power between them. It affects both how much progress is made and the direction of developments. It effectively means that service users are continually disadvantaged in their efforts to challenge the definitions and goals of the service provider discourse. In our view this imbalance of power plays a crucial part in obstructing the development of participatory and empowering policy and practice.

It is also especially important because participation and empowerment policies and practice are notoriously contradictory. Their history suggests that they are used as often to disempower as to empower people. This leads us back to the potentially conflicting objectives of the two empowerment discourses. Karen Baistow raises fundamental questions about professional empowerment, posing the issue that it may actually be concerned with extending the professional domain and increasing professional intervention, and have major regulatory as well as liberatory implications (Baistow, 1995). By adding their weight to the service provider discourse, service users may be unintentionally assisting an unhelpful development.

ENCOURAGING EMPOWERMENT

Existing inequalities between the discourses need to be challenged if the debate about empowerment and involvement is to be a progressive one.

So far we have tried to identify some of the problems associated with the discussion about empowerment. Now we want to turn to some ways forward. We want to headline six here. These are:

- the redistribution of resources
- a new emphasis on constructive partnerships
- a changed approach to research
- a twin-track approach to involvement and empowerment
- a greater emphasis on broadbased involvement
- highlighting the personal.

Let's look at each of them briefly in turn.

The redistribution of resources

If policy makers and funders are serious about empowerment and involvement, then they will have to direct the lion's share of resources – for their analysis, dissemination, exchange and development – to user-controlled initiatives. Funders and policy makers are likely to be much closer to the ideology, approaches and world view of service providers than of service users. They generally have closer and longer term links with the former. There is no doubt that many still have doubts about the ability and reliability of service users and their organizations. They must be prepared to review and challenge their traditional allocation of resources, develop anti-discriminatory policies and practice, and set up effective schemes to monitor and evaluate progress. Only by doing this are they likely to develop trust for the future and break down a user-versus-provider culture which continues to block progress.

A new emphasis on constructive partnerships

We have talked about the destructiveness of unequal relationships between service users and providers. Like other service users, we have had our quota of these, where agencies and individuals want to pick your brains, expect you to fit in with their schedules, don't get back to you when they say they will, expect you to do things for nothing and use your work without acknowledgement or agreement. If anything, this emphasizes the importance of constructive partnerships. What distinguishes them is that service providers are prepared to be open and receptive to the views and ideas of service users; collaborate on equal terms; put their contacts, networks, resources and credibility at the disposal of service users and their organizations; acknowledge their mistakes and are flexible enough to learn to work in different ways which are comfortable for service users.

Such relationships are not only important, they are also possible. You don't always know which will blossom and which won't, so service users have to take risks, but the building up of trust is possible. We have our own first-hand experience of such positive and fruitful collaboration with both the Race Equality Unit and the National Institute for Social Work. People can begin to recognize and value their overlaps, instead of having to get behind the barricades of their difference.

A changed approach to research

Disabled people and other community care service users are demanding a different kind of research. This has implications for the kind of questions asked, who asks them and how and why they are asked. Such participatory or emancipatory research is concerned with changing the social relations of research (Oliver, 1992a). Now the subjects of research may also be the researchers. There is already a significant and growing body of such research coming from people with learning difficulties, people with impairments and from psychiatric system survivors (Croft and Beresford, 1993b). Such research clearly has a central role to play in the analysis and evaluation of discussions and developments around user involvement and empowerment. The journal *Disability & Society* has proposed guidelines for undertaking disability research, which are helpful here (Oliver, 1992b). These prioritize the involvement, critiques and equal opportunities of disabled people, and offer a model of broader relevance to community care research funders.

A twin-track approach to involvement and empowerment

Much of the discussion and development around user involvement and empowerment has focused on involving people in services and service agencies and developing participatory forums and structures within them to do so. There has been a mushrooming of participatory planning and working groups, joint planning arrangements and consultative committees. But this approach has its defects. The gains from involvement in such structures are often limited and uncertain. Their connection with the decision-making process is often weak. Service users are generally disadvantaged and outnumbered in such representative structures. As Catherine Bewley and Caroline Glendinning report, such involvement is a drain on the resources of both disabled people's organizations and of individual disabled people (Bewley and Glendinning, 1994). It often works to divert and contain people's demands and requirements.

A 'twin-track' approach is more helpful here, working outside such agency structures, as well as using them to advantage. There are two aspects to this for service users. First it makes use of existing democratic and representative structures, including MPs, local councillors and the law. Second, it places a premium on developing your own self-organization, networking with other user-led organizations and setting up your own services. Effective self-organizations seem to be involved in both collaborative activities from within and campaigning activities from outside.

A greater emphasis on broadbased involvement

Relatively few people get actively involved in political and community life. There isn't a strong tradition of such participation in Britain (Croft and Beresford, 1992a). There are also additional obstacles in the way of disabled people and other community care service users. Progress in developing user involvement and empowerment which involves as wide a range of eligible participants as possible and challanges discrimination on the basis of age, race, disability, gender and sexual orientation has so far been limited. Both service users' organizations and service providers face major difficulties in gaining such involvement, despite the priority it has for them both: service providers so that they can gain the 'representative' involvement which remains one of their key concerns and service users' organizations in order that people can truly 'speak for themselves'. Service providers need to increase both the **access** to their organizations and decision-making and the **support** for service users, which are the basis for broader involvement (Croft and Beresford, 1993c). More work needs to be done to research and develop innovative, accessible and anti-discriminatory ways of involving people.

Highlighting the personal

More attention needs to be paid to the personal issues raised by user involvement and empowerment. So far the focus has been on services, organizations, structures and management. Much less attention has been paid to personal concerns: for example, how people feel about being involved and about efforts to empower them; how they experience them; what they mean for them and why people might want to be involved and empowered. This may help explain why many initiatives for involvement and empowerment are actually experienced as instru-mental, unpleasant and anti-personal. It has largely been left to service users to develop this discussion and explore a more humanistic paradigm which takes account of people's feelings, hopes and goals. This concern with the personal should not be confused with individual-izing models of personal empowerment. Instead it represents a recognition of the need to unify the personal and political if empower-ment and involvement are to be positive and real for people.

CONCLUSION

Two overarching themes emerge from these six pointers for empowerment policy and practice. The themes are **redistribution** and **inclusion**. So long as there are two unequal and competing discourses around empowerment, the outcome will be disempowering. If discussions and developments about empowerment are to avoid mirroring the problems which they are supposed to address, they must treat service users with greater equality, challenge existing distributions of personal, social, economic and political power and break down divisions between service providers and service users. Service users must be fully and equally involved in the conceptualization and formulation of empowerment policy and practice. It is such redistribution and inclusion which lie at the heart of empowerment in community care.

REFERENCES

Baistow, K. (1995) Liberation and regulation: some paradoxes of empowerment. *Critical Social Policy*, **14** (3), Winter pp. 34–46.

Barnes, C. (1991) *Disabled People In Britain And Discrimination: A Case for Anti-discrimination Legislation*, Hurst and Company/University of Calgary.

Barnes, C. and Thompson, G. (1994) *Funding For User Led Initiatives*, User Involvement Group, National Council for Voluntary Organisations.

Beresford, P. (1988) Consumer views: data collection or democracy? in *Hearing The Voice Of The Consumer*, (eds I. White, M. Devenney, R. Bhaduri *et al.*), Policy Studies Institute, pp. 37–52.

Beresford, P. (1994a) Developing the discussion about user involvement, in *User Involvement in Social Services: An Annotated Bibliography, part 2: 1992–1993* (ed. A. Upton), pp. 5–6.

Beresford, P. (1994b) Mental health and empowerment, in *Promotion Of Mental Health*, (eds D.R. Trent and C. Read), Volume 3, 1993, pp. 27–37.

Beresford, P. and Croft, S. (1993) *Citizen Involvement: A Practical Guide for Change*, Macmillan, London.

Bewley, C. and Glendinning, C. (1994) *Involving Disabled People In Community Care Planning*, Joseph Rowntree Foundation and *Community Care* magazine.

British Broadcasting Corporation (1993) *The Future Of The Welfare State*. The Radio 4 Debate, October 27.

Campbell, P. (1994) *A Survivor's Perspective On Mental Health*, Lecture, West London Institute, 24 April.

Croft, S. and Beresford, P. (1990) *From Paternalism To Participation: Involving People in Social Services*, Joseph Rowntree Foundation/Open Services Project.

Croft, S. and Beresford, P. (1992a) The politics of participation. *Critical Social Policy*, (35), Autumn, pp. 20–44.

Croft, S. and Beresford, P. (1992b) User views, changes. *International Journal of Psychology and Psychotherapy*, **10** (3), September, pp. 266–267.

Croft, S. and Beresford, P. (1993a) A poor show. *New Statesman And Society*, 19 March, p. 23.

Croft, S. and Beresford, P. (1993b) User views, changes. *International Journal of Psychology and Psychotherapy*, **11** (2), pp. 179–180.

Croft, S. and Beresford, P. (1993c) *Getting Involved: A Practical Manual*, Open Services Project/Joseph Rowntree Foundation, York.

Hoyes, L., Lart, R., Means, R. and Taylor, M. (1994) *User Empowerment And The Reform Of Community Care, Findings, Social Care Research 50*, Joseph Rowntree Foundation, May.

Lindow, V. (1990) Participation and power. *OPENMIND*, (44), April/May, pp. 10–11.

Oliver, M. (1992a) Changing the social relations of research production? *Disability, Handicap & Society*, **7** (2), pp. 101–114.

Oliver, M. (1992b) Guidelines for funding applications to undertake disability research. *Disability, Handicap & Society*, **7** (3), pp. 279–280.

Oppenheim, C. (1994) *The Welfare State: Putting the Record Straight*, Child Poverty Action Group, London.

Statham, D. (1994) The challenges for social work education, presentation, *Social Work Education And The Community Care Revolution Conference*, National Institute for Social Work and West London Institute, 24 March.

Stevenson, O. and Parsloe, P. (1993) *Empowerment In Community Care*, Joseph Rowntree Foundation/*Community Care* magazine.

User Centred Services Group (1993) *Building Bridges – Between People Who Use and People Who Provide Services*, National Institute for Social Work.

Part Two

Empowerment – Practical Experiences in Self-help and Mutual Aid

4

Self-help groups as a route to empowerment

Judy Wilson

Self-help groups have been described as one of the great voluntary sector success stories in recent years. Yet it is not a co-ordinated development. People are rarely aware either of being part of a movement or of the concepts that underlie this special type of voluntary group when they set out on their self-help journey. This chapter sets out to explore what self-help groups are and do, and their benefits as members see them. Its sources come from the work of the Nottingham Self-Help Team over 12 years, and a recent research project in the Trent Region on self-help groups and professionals. The values and roles of the Team, and the definition it uses are summarized. The challenging nature of self-help and the question of support to self-help groups are discussed. Finally, the constraints which hold back the development of self-help are reviewed before reflecting on the extent to which self-help groups are a route to empowerment.

INTRODUCTION

Members' stories

Sue and Elizabeth, Cath and Chris are all members of self-help groups in Nottingham. Their stories appeared in recent newsletters. Sue is registered blind. She has some sight but suffers from a progressive condition called retinitis pigmentosa.

> I was 27 and just married when this bombshell dropped. At that moment, my life ended and as a human being I felt totally

worthless. A Nottingham group was just starting up and I went along to a meeting. From that day I've never looked back. To say that my life has changed beyond all recognition would be an understatement. As well as being welfare officer for the group, my confidence has grown and blossomed, enabling me to become involved in activities outside the group and my home. These include being a school governor at two local primary schools, one of which recently asked me to take over the role of chair – I felt very honoured and proud. Far from feeling a non-person, I now feel a fulfilled and useful member of society – and all this because I joined a self-help group.

Elizabeth is a social worker, addicted to tranquillizers until she joined a tranx release group.

Not only was I addicted to a powerful drug for nine years, but I was also too frightened of admitting this because I might lose my job. Our job is to help other people through their problems. We are people trained to show strength and stability. Self-help groups had always been for my 'clients', so taking the step to join the group needed me to swallow my pride and to change my attitude. The group has helped me to plan my withdrawal, which my GP was very supportive of. I know I will be able to withdraw totally over the next 18 months. I've come clean with my colleagues at work. I've got a long way to go, but I know with the support around, I'll make it.

'The Graduates' is a group of people who had attended a mental health day centre. Cath and Chris had found there a level of understanding, support and caring which had led them to start their own group when they stopped attending the centre.

Ours was the University of Life, the entrance qualification had been a diploma in despair, the course difficult and demanding – the end a degree in determination, hope and survival. Now our group of 'post-graduates' meets weekly in a small and sparsely furnished room. None of us is able to define clearly what it is we gain or give to the group. Perhaps the group's commitment, from the very start, to the ethos that all contributions are of equal value has something to do with our success. We have proved to ourselves that there is life after despair, if you are willing to take a risk. All you need is the realisation that there are needs in your life that are not being met and that there are other people who feel the same. The rewards far outweigh the risk.

Nottingham

These stories all come from self-help groups in Nottingham – an average sort of city. It has a population of 253 227 (1991 Census) though Greater Nottingham is nearer half a million. The city population includes 10.7% of people from ethnic minority communities. The number of people in each age band is broadly similar to that of England and Wales as a whole. There are pockets of severe deprivation and in February 1994 the unemployment rate was 18%, higher than the national average.

There is a strong tradition, going back many years, of voluntary activity in the city and of support from both city and county councils. This support from both members and officers has meant there has been substantial financial and practical help to the voluntary sector and a culture of recognition and encouragement. Pressures on local authority and health service expenditure have not yet led to major cuts in grants and contracts. But voluntary organizations increasingly find it much more difficult to get realistic sums to maintain their work and people with ideas for new developments that require funding struggle to get money. The Nottingham Health Authority, unusually in the health field, gives substantial support (over £92 000 in 1994–5) to the Nottingham Self-Help Team, a voluntary agency which gives support to self-help groups and provides information about them.

The Self-Help Team

The Nottingham Self-Help Team has been part of Nottingham Council for Voluntary Service since starting as a small experiment in 1982. First its sole project worker, I am now team leader of a team of 18 paid and volunteer staff. More recently the management role has been combined with research into good practice between self-help groups and professionals. This chapter both draws on the work of the Team and brings in some of the results of the research. The research project, supported by the Joseph Rowntree Foundation, was undertaken in a wider area, that of the Trent Regional Health Authority, between 1992–93 (Wilson, 1995). In this study, group and individual interviews were carried out with a wide variety of both groups and professionals in the broad field of health and community care.

The Team's main role is to respond to requests for information and help. The pattern of demand is similar, whether people approach the Team for information or to ask for advice and help with starting up a new group. Both Figures 4.1 and 4.2, analyses of the two types of request, show the preponderance of requests in the areas of mental health, taken in a broad sense, and by people with specific physical illnesses. This has been a consistent pattern, though there is also a very wide range of other issues and needs which people feel might be helped by participation in a self-help group.

The number of groups included in the Team's annual directory has grown steadily, as Figure 4.3 shows. The groups' numbers range from those of perhaps half a dozen to over 150, the latter concentrating more

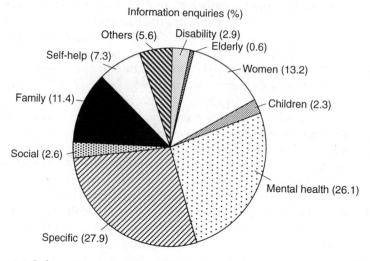

Figure 4.1 Information enquiries 1992–3, the Self-Help Team annual report 1992–3.

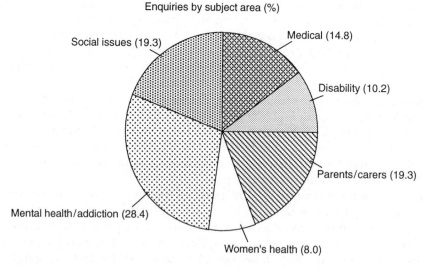

Figure 4.2 New group enquiries 1992–3, the Self-Help Team annual report 1992–3.

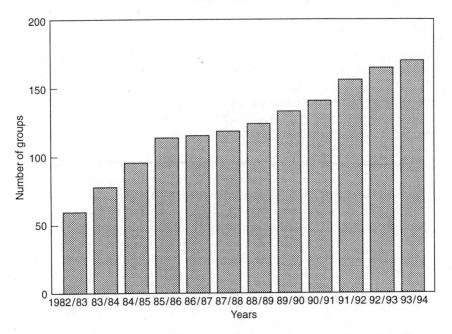

Figure 4.3 Self-help group listed in the directories in Nottingham 1982–94.

on education and information. Members come from a wide age range. A small number of groups that use the Team are largely or entirely for people from ethnic minorities – Mukti, the Divorced Asian Women's Group for example. Others such as the Lupus group include both black and white people. More women than men initiate groups and make enquiries to the Team about them, and this impression of greater involvement of women than of men is confirmed by visits to groups. No-one has yet, however, done a detailed study of membership and these are impressions rather than an accurate account.

Self-help is an idea which is put into practice in many ways. While the Team aims to have a wide spectrum of information, there is no system of affiliation, and it is not claimed that the Team's experience of self-help in the city is totally comprehensive. To give some examples, as the staff is largely white, black groups may not all be known to the Team or use its services, though the number of requests from black groups is increasing. Closed groups, meeting for a limited time, probably do not need to make themselves known. Informally organized self-help, such as the community churches, may be less visible and unlikely to feel the need to use the Team. Compared to most other towns, however, the Team's experience is considerable. The lessons learnt from 12 years' work can be considered to be sound.

Definition, values and roles

During this time the Team has come to evolve a definition of the groups with which it works, the values that underpin its work and to be clear about the role it plays. Definition, values and role are all very relevant to this account of self-help groups as a route to empowerment.

First, the definition, developed as a working tool for the Team, rather than as a prescriptive statement:

> A self-help or mutual aid group is made up of people who have personal experience of the same problem or life situation, either directly or through their family or friends. Sharing experiences enables them to give each other a unique quality of mutual support and to pool practical information and ways of coping. Groups are run by and for their members. Some self-help groups expand their activities. They may provide, for example, services for people who have the same problem or life situation; or they may campaign for change. Professionals may sometimes take part in the group in various ways, when asked to by the group.

The phrase 'self-help', though the one commonly in use, does not indicate the degree of mutual help that is an important part of these groups. In America, the term MASH groups – mutual aid self-help groups – is sometimes used to address this problem. Here, the term self-help groups is used, with the assumption that groups are based on the idea of mutual help, as a means to individual self-help.

Professionally run support groups do not fit in to the definition above. While they may well include the concept of mutual support, they are led by professionals and so are outside the definition used here. A wider study on social workers and self-help takes in this type of group and attempts to tease out some of the differences (Adams, 1990).

Second, some of the values which underpin the work of the Team:

- We believe in the value of people coming together in self-help groups, which enable members to feel empowered.
- We have an equal opportunities policy and aim to implement this by integrating its principles into our work.
- We provide a neutral, confidential and non-judgemental service.
- We believe in the value of joint working and collaboration with other agencies.

Third, the roles the Team plays – and doesn't play:

- Our practice is to react to people and organizations who are already motivated to take action. We do not start groups ourselves.

- We do not run groups or feel responsible for their decisions and actions. Our role is to offer services and support.
- Through providing services and support we aim to enable groups to be effective in realizing the goals that they want to achieve.
- We see ourselves as an intermediary, particularly between the self-help and professional worlds, and between groups.

All these – definition, values and roles – need to be worked out by anyone who is planning to work with self-help groups. This is true whether they are in the voluntary sector, professional workers in the health and social services, or researchers.

THE VALUE AND IMPORTANCE OF SELF-HELP GROUPS

The stories told by group members, quoted earlier in this chapter, bring alive the enormous life problems people face. The group members who contributed to my research also talked about the great need that they had as individuals, and the very difficult situations group members had to deal with in and outside their meetings. Several mentioned people who wanted to commit suicide coming to their group, or example. The huge impact of diagnosis of a life-threatening or chronic illness they felt was sometimes underestimated by professionals. The group was used as a trusted place to open up the distress people felt. This distress was sometimes unexpected, as a twins group found. One might think having twins would be a happy event. But:

One member phoned me and said 'Is it OK to feel this bad?'

Support from the group was the first way such distress was helped. Group support was seen as special and different from help people got from elsewhere. The long-term nature of support from people in the same situation was specially valued by a bereaved parent.

The group went on listening long after my kind family and friends had stopped.

Support from people who were further on with coping with their lives was seen as specially valuable. People saw other members as models, enabling them to feel that life could go on, that there was light at the end of the tunnel.

Second, information gained in a self-help group was felt to be particularly empowering. Group members valued the opportunity to gain knowledge about the condition or issue on which the group was based; to get information about services they could use and ask for; and to learn ways of coping. Knowledge gained from experience is different from information from families and friends, this being what one might call 'folk knowledge'. It is different too from the learned knowledge of professionals. Thomasina Borkman, an American sociologist, has written extensively about the significance, often unappreciated by people outside groups, of experiential knowledge and its effect on people's lives (Borkman, 1990). Self-help groups may be more 'adult learning groups', as a carers' group member suggested, than therapy groups.

A third benefit from membership was an increase in confidence. One of the results of gaining more information and having models to follow was that people felt more confident. One member of a chronic illness group stressed the need to go on attending.

> You can see people get more confident the longer they come.

People were aware that their increased confidence or sometimes just the existence of the group challenged existing norms and power, whether that of professionals or in the community. A group of Asian women, all single parents, wanted to be better known so other women could change their lives too.

> They are too scared. We would like to put a stop to this, make our women strong, so they can come out.

A fourth benefit from membership was the opportunity they gave to be helpful. Ann Richardson's study of self-help groups (1983) identified the concept of serial reciprocity. People in the Trent research confirmed the benefit they got from helping people currently facing problems, when they themselves were coping better. The feeling of self-worth and the pleasure of being helpful must be familiar to most volunteers. People in self-help groups are likely to have been mostly on the receiving end of help. As they progress, they can also be givers of help, often at the same time. This active role is empowering, giving the helper a sense of control, a feeling of being capable rather than impotent (Katz, 1993).

These four benefits were both consistent themes in the research and were familiar, too, to members of the Nottingham Team. But group members were also aware of their limits. They were clear that they were not providing or replacing a professional service. Theirs were small groups, largely run by people in their own time, with all the limits that any small voluntary group has and with the familiar difficulties of structure and personality problems. Self-help groups have added constraints, for people are in a group because of some difficulty in their lives. Limits of energy, lack of mobility and time affect the amount of help people can offer. Carers in particular found it difficult to give time to a group when they had full-time caring responsibilities.

Professionals and researchers, who also took part in my research, could also appreciate the value and importance of self-help groups. On the whole the benefits of support and information were clearly understood. Some researchers, however, saw the groups' most import- ant role as commenting on plans and strategies for community care. This was not seen as a major role by self-helpers. Another difference in perception was the benefits of helping others and the strong motivation people had to do so. Professionals rarely mentioned the value of being helpful, stressed by self-helpers.

It is important to be aware of such differences between the perceptions of people in the groups and those outside them. Outsiders who had made an effort to learn about groups, and it can be an effort, on the whole appreciated and understood the values and importance of self-help groups. Some professionals, politicians and researchers can, however, have very different, and sometimes inaccurate views. These can have three effects: misunderstandings; they can bring risks of co- option and diversion; and can lead to tension between what I see as the two worlds of self-help groups and professionals.

THE SELF-HELP CHALLENGE

One cause of tension between these two worlds is the challenging nature of self-help. The two major benefits of groups – increasing confidence and greater knowledge and information – can be very difficult for professionals. Growing in confidence and becoming better informed are both powerful means to empowerment for people who have felt burdened and diminished. This feeling of diminishment may come from what has happened in their lives or it may be due to the attitudes of society towards them. It is important to be aware of the effects of both, for how society perceives people with problems can be as critical as the issue itself. The motivation to form a group may not always stem from problems in people's lives. People with disabilities, gay and lesbian people, black people, for example, may well form groups in order to challenge society's perceptions and attitudes of them, rather than to focus on personal difficulties.

Assertive individuals

Membership of self-help groups enables people to challenge existing systems and practice in a variety of ways. People as individuals can become far more assertive about their needs and ways to meet them. Jean, a member of a parents group, with a severely disabled son, had been on an assertiveness course put on by the Team. She made a dramatic appearance in the office after a visit to social services.

> I've just been to see the social worker. I told her, that's not what I want. What I want for my son is a placement that's right for him. I know what he needs.

Work in the general office had to stop. Her account was so compelling and to those of us who had known her when she was first starting her group, the change in her level of confidence was very marked. Like many people who start groups, she had 'never done anything like this before'. One result, a year later, has been to challenge the perception of the social worker and to gain the help that she felt was appropriate.

A needs-led approach is now far more integrated into professional practice. For many thoughtful, progressive professionals it would be natural to work with a parent or client in this way. Professional power and knowledge is still very pervasive, however, and unless someone who finds themselves as patient or client is unusually strong, there need to be means to help them grow in strength if there is to be a creative client/professional partnership. A self-help group is one means to achieve this, as a GP recognized.

> I like it when my patients join a self-help group. I find we have much better discussions together.

The group approach

The group approach is a way of challenging authority's perceptions of needs, by working as a group rather than as an individual. Julie, the initiator of a group of partially sighted people in 1982, saw the group as a way of giving comfort and support.

> I also had an idea that we could be interested consumers and tell the authorities and the general public where they could help us best and where things could be improved . . . transport . . . spoken word cassettes in public libraries . . . traffic lights. Working together as a group to improve the quality of life for people.

Public authorities now often have consultative procedures with users on matters like this. In 1982, however, they rarely existed and groups which could take a consumer as well as a support role were particularly important. They still are, particularly in areas where the consumer view is not yet strongly valued. Where there is strong control over treatment, practice and services, self-help groups can be very important in challenging the system. Recent examples in Nottingham are groups of people coming off tranquillizers and people with eating disorders.

Consultative bodies

Some members of groups decide to take part in formal consultative bodies. Unless they are set up with proper thought and resources, it can be a daunting task for a lone individual. The mental health users scheme in Newcastle is a well-known example of good practice, but the depth of both thought and resources in the scheme is unusual.

Joining a planning group or a community health council as a member of a self-help group lessens some of the difficulties individuals face. People will have grown in confidence over time, will have a group to back them up and be able to speak authoritatively about the experience of a range of people. They will not be operating only as individuals. It is not wise, however, to assume that this is the prime task of self-help groups, nor that this is the only way groups may influence how services are provided.

The Trent research showed how groups could help increase the quality of services by good liaison with individual professionals and by contributing to their training (Wilson, 1995). For example, where their views and experience are welcomed by social workers, nurses, doctors and so on, this can be a helpful experience for everyone concerned. Where strongly entrenched attitudes make it more likely that there will be confrontation rather than mutual learning, the process will be challenging for all concerned. Indeed, some self-help groups may decide it is not worth using their limited time and energy in this way, and concentrate instead on other aspects of their activities.

There can be no assumptions that self-help groups are consumer advocacy groups. Nor can one dictate to them that this is their job. Some groups do make this role an important part of their work, choosing to look outwards and work for the benefit of everyone who shares their problem, whether they are a member or not. Others, probably a majority, choose instead to look inward and to concentrate on the needs of the people who come to the group as a means of individual growth and change.

ENCOURAGEMENT AND SUPPORT

Once one has recognized the essential nature of a self-help group, that it is run by its members, one can begin to look at whether people outside the group can be of any use. People taking part in the Trent research were eager to attend. By choosing to take part in interviews, they demonstrated their interest in developing working relationships with organizations outside their groups.

The experience of the Self-Help Team is that a majority of groups in the field of health and social needs do welcome collaborative relationships, as a means to encouragement and support. What is important is the way it is offered and the attitudes that go with it. Let us now consider who can offer support and encouragement, how it might be done and the key principles that should underpin it.

Sources of support and encouragement

In any one community, there is no one source of support and encouragement. The experience of people in self-help groups is that a wide range of people and organizations are in a position to offer this and can do so effectively. An important source is the media.

> I was standing in my kitchen with Radio Nottingham on and there was Val talking about her husband and his death from Alzheimer's Disease. It was as though she was talking to me. I phoned for details and joined the group.

Local radio not only gave this woman, desperate for help, access to the group, it promoted the idea of self-help and enabled someone who had herself benefited from membership to share her experience. It was also a way for the group to gain new members. Many self-help groups meet people's needs in a time of transition. As part of coming to terms with their situation or even coming out of the tunnel, they may need to leave the group. Most groups, to stay viable, need a continuing supply of new members. Media publicity, like a weekly column in the *Nottingham Evening Post* (Figure 4.4), is extremely important to groups which are often relatively invisible.

Community organizations, churches and other places of religious worship are other examples of bodies which can help. Where they are actively against the development of a group, refusing to acknowledge need or meet the challenge to their own status, they can make the self-help task very much more difficult. The refusal of men in a community centre to put up posters about an Asian women's single parents group is an example. In contrast, a community centre which gives free rooms to a new group is endorsing the value of the group, contributing to an increase in their self-esteem, and being practically useful.

The professional world is particularly well placed to support self-help groups based on health and social issues. Social workers, health visitors, community psychiatric nurses and many more have the potential to help. The evidence of the Trent research suggests that many of them do so, partly motivated by their individual experience and personal commitment, partly implementing the aims of their agency. A mental health team, for example, committed to the concept of users of services being involved in their own care and in the services they are offered, easily integrates support and development of groups into their normal practice.

Individuals working in agencies with a less well worked out ethos and lower commitment to the strengths and potential of clients and patients will have a harder job. 'Product champions' may wish to promote the

SELF-HELP DIARY

GROUPS with meetings in December are listed below. Please note that groups may not meet at holiday times.

Action for Epilepsy — 3rd Monday of the month, 7.30pm, International Community Centre, 61b Mansfield Road.

Aids Line (Grantham) — Telephone 01476 60192, Monday or Friday, 9-10am, or Wednesday 1-3pm.

Alanon Family Group (for relatives of alcoholics) — Mondays 7.30pm, St Nicholas Centre, 79 Maid Marian Way; Wednesdays, 10am, Adult Education Centre, Shakespeare Street; Thursdays, 7.30pm, International Community Centre, 61b Mansfield Road.

Alateen (for teenagers with alcoholic relatives) — Mondays, 7.30-9pm, St Nicholas Centre, 79 Maid Marian Way.

Alcoholics Anonymous — Meetings held daily. Telephone 941 7100, 7-10pm, for details.

Allergy Support Group — 2nd Tuesday of the month, 7.30pm, Wellbeing Centre, 11 Musters Road, West Bridgford.

Allsorts (social group for young people, 18-40 with disabilities) — 2nd Thursday of the month, 7.30-9pm, Djangoly City Technology College, Nottingham Road, Sherwood Rise.

Alzheimer's Disease Society (Nottm) (senile dementia) 2nd Wednesday of every month, 7.30pm, St Francis Main Hall, Edwards Lane.

Arnold Twins Club — 1st Tuesday of the month, 1.30-3.30pm, Sherwood Health Centre.

Arthritis Care — 4th Wednesday of the month, 7.15pm, West Bridgford Day Centre, Loughborough Road.

Arthritis Care (Clifton) — 3rd Wednesday of the month, 7.30pm, Fairham Day Centre, Summerwood Lane, Clifton.

Arthritis Care (Hucknall and District Branch) — 1st Tuesday of the month, 7.30pm, St John's Church Hall, Nottingham Road, Hucknall.

Asbestos Related Diseases Association — 1st Tuesday of the month, 7.30pm, International Community Centre, 61b Mansfield Road.

Aspley Wood Parents Group (for parents of handicapped children) — Meetings held monthly at 10am at Aspley Wood School, Robinswood Road, Aspley in term time. Tel. 929 4887 for details.

Association of Separated and Divorced Catholics (Nottm Branch) — Last Wednesday of the month, 7.30pm, The McGuinness Centre, Brooklyn Road, Bulwell, Nottingham. Not December.

Back Pain Association — 2nd Monday of the month, 7pm, West Bridgford Day Centre, Loughborough Road.

Beechdale Carers Group Drop-in Centre — Alternate Thursdays, 2.30-4pm, Beechdale Community Centre, Tel.929 3160 for details.

Beeston Mind Alert (for people over 50) — Thursdays, 2-4pm, Lads Club, Station Road, Beeston.

Beeston Mind Alive (for people over 50) — Wednesdays, 2pm, Boundary Road Community Centre, Beeston.

Beeston New Pals Club (for people 30-65) — Tuesdays, 8-11pm, White Lion, Station Road, Beeston.

British Diabetic Association (Nottm and District Branch) — December 8, 7.30pm; Self-Help Diabetes Group — 2nd Thursday of the month, 7.30pm, Diabetes Centre, Edwards Lane; Parents of children with diabetes meet at the same time as the Self- Help Diabetes Group.

British Polio Fellowship — 2nd Thursday of the month, 7.30pm, West Bridgford Day Centre, Loughborough Road. (Except January, February and August).

British Retinitis Pigmentosa Society — Meets alternate months at Sherwood Community Centre, Mansfield Road. Telephone 960 9859 or 981 9220 for details.

Burns Unit Self Help (Bush) — 3rd Monday of the month, 7.30pm, Burns Unit Day Room, City Hospital.

The Self-Help Team's information services can provide details of local and national self-help groups. Phone Nottingham 969 1212, 9.30am to 2.30pm Monday to Friday (except Wednesday when it closes at noon) or leave a message on the answerphone.

Figure 4.4 Self-help diary – *Nottingham Evening Post*, 2 December 1994.

values and benefits of self-help groups, but if they are a lone voice they may be very isolated.

Voluntary organizations with a broader brief than self-help groups, particularly those employing paid staff, can also support and develop groups. Some are national specialist organizations with a development brief, keen to see more branches grow. Other national organizations, such as Contact-a-Family and Cancerlink for example, have more of an ethos of being the centre of a network, rather than a controlling national body. Both types, however, can help.

Of special interest are local voluntary bodies, with an intermediary and development role for the voluntary sector. Councils for voluntary service (CVS), volunteer bureaux, federations of various kinds, for disability and mental health groups for example, are well placed to give support and aid development.

In the Trent region there are now a number of specialist projects with self-help workers, mostly attached to CVSs. They consistently show that the impact of local help can be increased dramatically when someone has particular responsibility for self-help group work, as part of or all of their job. They can also ensure that support and help given by other agencies are effective, contributing to a ripple effect. German research has demonstrated that where there are local centres for self-help, the numbers of groups increase.

Ways of providing it

Three major forms of help were valued by the groups in the study. The heavy use of services offered by the Nottingham Team confirms the rightness of three particular forms of help, which can be given by any of the organizations outlined above.

Giving information, the first form of help, is both a way to help individuals and to strengthen groups. Professionals, however, need to be aware that this is not a referral. Instead they can usefully and systematically put their clients and patients in touch with a self-help group. This is a more complex operation than one might think, but is both needed and valued by the groups.

The examples from the media show there are many ways to give information, however, and indirect publicity, for example noticeboards specially for groups, is a form of practice many organizations could adopt. An example of a ripple effect is the production of local directories of self-help groups, regularly updated and re-issued. When these are easily available to local professionals, they will be much more likely to put their clients in touch with a group.

Practical services and access to resources form the second way in which groups can be supported. Free or cheap meeting rooms, printing and copying, access to distribution systems, speakers for meetings, and training are appreciated by many groups. These are expressions of a general attitude of support, which may be particularly useful when groups begin.

Background support, a third form of help, may be appropriate as groups begin and as they continue. For people who have rarely done anything like this before, this type of support is often welcomed. Like putting people in touch with groups, it too is a more intricate issue than is always appreciated. A self-help worker in a CVS, even if experienced in working with new groups and with the benefit of a neutral base, will still find it difficult. A professional, untrained in community work skills, may approach this work assuming they can do it, but only later discover its complexities.

Key principles

It can be suggested that there are certain key principles which should inform the giving of support to self-help groups. The following are offered as some thoughts to date, still needing to be developed and modified, rather than being universal truths. They are closely inter-twined with attitudes and knowledge.

First, recognition of ownership is a key principle. To recall part of the definition, people in groups who have themselves experienced the situation on which the group is based, run the group. People outside the group need to recognize this and the implications for their own relationship. 'A guest at the meeting' was the description a nurse gave to his visits to a group. 'Guest' may not always be the right description, but it illustrates the way this nurse acknowledged the question of ownership and his relationship with the group.

Second, it is important for self-help groups to be valued and appreciated for what they are and how they operate, sometimes warts and all. This does not mean condoning behaviour which might harm some individuals, and this has been known. But it does imply the need to accept groups as they are, not as another form of professional help or another service provider.

Recognition of the effort it can take for someone to join is a third key principle. This has particular implications for people who provide information. Information needs to be accurate, easily accessible and offered so an individual can make an informed choice, not be prescribed as a panacea. Information also needs to be available in a form that people can keep, so they choose the timing that is right for them. It is not uncommon for people to join a group some years after they learn of its existence.

Choice is a fourth key principle. Groups have the right, I suggest, to decline offers of help or to choose the right person to give it. This can be a hard lesson for people keen to help!

Fifth is the recognition that the way help is given may need to change. This means that informal monitoring and evaluation have to be built in to any relationship. Then decisions can be reached together by the group and by those outside it, on what is best at any one time. While short-term, one-off forms of help are right at times, some forms of support require long-term commitment to be effective. This makes it particularly important that the relationship is reviewed.

Finally, there is lightness of touch. This is not easy – what might be lightness of touch to one group is control to another. Too little support could be construed by some as ignoring their value. It is very difficult to strike a balance.

To return to the main theme, does support lead to empowering self-help groups? Empowerment, as I see it, is something which people feel and take for themselves. It could be a form of contradiction in the world of self-help groups for outsiders, whatever their values, to see themselves as doing the empowering. Some self-help groups do not want support or too much interest in their activities. The evidence from many others, however, is that they do. Appropriate support makes it more likely that people and groups will do something for themselves. The right support may make it more likely too that groups will be effective, and so individuals come to feel more empowered.

CONSTRAINTS

One may argue then that supporting self-help groups contributes to people feeling empowered. It is not a simple matter and there are a number of constraints on practice, summarized briefly here.

Attitudes are of prime importance. Attitudes of communities, agencies and individuals which include acknowledgement of the value of lay and volunteer effort are fundamental to action. Alongside this has to be an awareness that there is a limit to what the professional world can do to meet people's needs. Attitudes of control and power are rarely appropriate.

A second constraint is lack of knowledge and information. Without these, individuals cannot exercise choice and groups cannot get access to resources. Nor can outsiders understand the nature of the organizations or find out where they are.

A third constraint is a lack of contact and interaction, which also has adverse effects. Where there is little contact between groups and the outside world, there is unlikely to be support and development. Different groups will benefit from different forms and degrees of interaction and contact. Even groups which prefer to be autonomous can gain. Alcoholics Anonymous, for example, has an effective system of open meetings, enabling people outside the group to find out about it without interfering in the group process. This type of interaction may be enough and lead to more people being put in touch with the group.

A fourth and final constraint on the development of the potential of self-help groups stems from current policy emphasis on service provision and contracts. Self-help groups do not easily fit into a service culture. Nor is the function of intermediaries recognized as an important service and one which is appropriate for public authorities to purchase. Self-help projects funded through the Self-Help Alliance, described in another chapter, struggled to get continued funding. Funding arrangements in the 1990s may well be holding back the contribution of self-help groups. Without intermediaries, their potential is not being fulfilled.

There are limits to what small informal self-help groups can achieve. Their contribution to people feeling empowered may not, however, be related to the limits within the groups themselves, but to the heavy constraints of attitudes, insufficient knowledge, lack of interaction and resources in the outside world.

CONCLUSION

Self-help groups can be seen as part of a much wider movement that recognizes and endorses the value of lay, citizen contributions. In eastern and central Europe, where self-help activity is blossoming, self-help groups are recognized as having a role in rebuilding a civil society. They are a means for individual citizens to play a full role in their communities, develop and use their talents and as a balance to dependence on professional care and public authorities. Participative communities are needed in the west too, a view that can be held whatever one's political colour.

To what extent are self-help groups in this country a route to empowerment? For some individuals they are undoubtedly so, though they would rarely describe their journey in such terms. The testimony of people who have benefited shows that for them, participation in self-help groups has radically altered their lives. As individuals, they have felt empowered to change or accept their situation. This change may depend, however, on them as individuals, the time they have invested in a group and the effort they have been prepared to make, as much as the group itself. The group cannot do the job for them, but it can release the latent potential people have to do things themselves.

Groups could be portrayed as all being radical, questioning, empowering organizations but this would not be universally true. Many self-help groups provide a place for friendship and social activities.

Some choose this social role as a prime activity, and one not entirely compatible with empowerment. In suggesting that self-help groups are for some a route to empowerment, one cannot conclude that all groups take this role.

It would seem that only a small minority of people affected by a problem or experiencing a difficulty in their lives are likely to actually join a self-help group. The impact of groups, however, may well be greater than numbers might indicate. The existence and visibility of groups may be enough for some people to feel courage to tackle their lives. Indirect influence by groups may be as important as strength gained by direct participation.

As consumer groups, in part, self-help groups also have a role in feeding back to policy makers and practitioners on what life has been like for them as clients and patients, and how things could be better. Users, with its connotations of drug using, is not a term commonly adopted in self-help groups. Groups are, however, part of the broad consumer, user movement in health and social care and are one means for individuals to contribute to this. Their role as consumer groups may, however, be limited through a preferred emphasis on mutual support – and this limit should be recognized. Groups must have choice in whether their role as a consumer voice becomes a significant feature of their work or not.

The yeast in the dough is an image on which to end this chapter. My perception of self-help groups is one of a raising agent, but one whose effect is not always recognized. Perhaps this is not altogether surprising. Most groups are small, concerned more with their own activities than with claiming status and reward. And those in power may not really want to see groups' contribution fostered and grow if it could mean loss of power.

When the yeast begins to work in the dough, the bulk of the bread increases. Self-help groups, if supported and valued, can be a means to greater participation in communities, an increase in knowledge and greater choice of ways in meeting need. Rather than replacing other forms of power and authority, they add to it. They can be a route to mutual benefit, to a wide range of people and aspects of community life that are growing and changing.

REFERENCES

Adams, R. (1990) *Self-Help, Social Work and Empowerment*, Macmillan, Basingstoke.
Borkman, T. (1990) Experiential, professional and lay frames of reference, in *Working with Self-help*, (ed. Thomas J. Powell), NASW Press, Silver Spring, MA.

Katz, A. (1993) *Self-help in America*, Twayne Publishers, New York.

Richardson, A. and Goodman, M. (1983) *Self-help and Social Care*, Policy Studies Institute, London.

Wilson, J. (1995) *Two Worlds: Self-Help Groups and Professionals*, Venture Press, Birmingham.

5

Self-help organizations in Germany: possibilities and constraints

Andrea Koch and Monika Reichert

The subject of 'self-help', especially the area of self-help for elderly people, is gaining increasing importance in Germany. The aim of this chapter is to present an overview of the subject. First, we give a definition of self-help. Second, the development of self-help up to the present day is outlined based on available publications on self-help for elderly people. Third, the different sectors of self-help are described and the reader is provided with information about the members of self-help organizations. Fourth, special emphasis is put on the situation in East Germany. Fifth, the position of self-help in Germany and its structural links to the social system and to the welfare state are then described. Finally constraints on self-help are discussed and some reflections regarding the future development of self-help in Germany conclude the chapter.

DEFINITION OF SELF-HELP FOR ELDERLY PEOPLE

There is a basic distinction between privately organized self-help and so-called social self-help. Privately organized self-help is developed on the basis of relations within the family and is practised outside the organized public and social system of help. In contrast, social self-help is organized in groups of different sizes and with different objectives. However, there is also a difference between voluntary activities which aim primarily at helping others – especially people in need – and work in self-help groups which is based on mutual help activities, partnership and co-operation of the members.

In Germany self-help for elderly people is organized in self-help groups, self-help projects and self-help initiatives. While self-help groups generally are created as permanent set-ups and their members mainly concentrate on helping each other, the self-help projects are normally run for a limited period of time. In addition, self-help projects are carried out by professional staff and members of the target group who together develop and try out alternative solutions to specific problems. There is also the possibility of independent working groups being initiated by self-help projects. Again the purpose of self-help initiatives is primarily to support and promote specific interests among the public and participants in such initiatives are members of the target group as well as committed others.

The common term for these three approaches to self-help for elderly people is 'the social self-help group', i.e. collective activities of older people which are not only aimed at individual needs but also at the needs of other people (Reggentin and Dettbarn-Reggentin, 1992). The characteristics of such social self-help groups according to Reggentin and Dettbarn-Reggentin are:

- common concern about the common problem,
- objectives based not only on individual needs but also on the needs of other people,
- activities that are self-determined,
- activities are not profit-oriented,
- decision-making on a democratic basis.

Furthermore, by definition the most important aim of a social self-help group is to enable members to solve a problem or at least help them to deal with it. That means members are motivated and supported to use and develop their abilities as well as everyday competence and to increase their sense of self-efficacy and self-confidence.

At this point it should be mentioned that the term 'social self-help group' is only used in academic publications. In the field of practical social work one generally speaks of 'self-help organizations', so we will use the latter term in this chapter.

THE DEVELOPMENT OF SELF-HELP ORGANIZATIONS IN GERMANY

While research on self-help in Germany is well established (Boll and Olk, 1987; Reis and Dorenburg, 1985) there is a clear deficit in research activities with regard to the area of self-help for elderly people. There are only a few studies which look at particular organizations like the 'Grey Panthers' and there are no reliable figures about how many self-help organizations for older people exist or the nature and number of their members.

The problem of gathering exact figures results especially from the fact that a distinction between self-help organizations for elders and other self-help organizations cannot be worked out exactly with respect to chronological age and also with respect to the socially organized self-help systems. In practice, there are always groups which are either intergenerational and/or which are linked to the public help system or to independent welfare organizations.

Nevertheless, there are some important aspects of self-help organizations for older people which we would like to illustrate. The first known self-help organizations in Germany were created soon after the Second World War. In 1948 the 'Bund der Ruhestandsbeamten' (Association of Retired Civil Servants) was established, followed in the 1950s by the foundation of the 'Lebensabendbewegung' (Old Age Movement), in 1962 by the 'Bundeskongreß der älteren Generation' (Federal Congress of the Elder Generation) and in 1976 by the 'Aktionsgemeinschaft der Deutschen Rentner- und Seniorenverbände' (Action Group of German Old Age Pensioners and Senior Citizens Associations). There have been others, but these are the major ones.

The self-help movement has got a new impetus since the 1980s, and in the early 1990s – according to figures based on the statistical projections of Reggentin and Dettbarn-Reggentin (1992) – approximately 3600 self-help organizations of elderly people existed in Germany, 3415 in West Germany and 185 in East Germany. In their study on self-help organizations in Northrhine-Westfalia Reggentin and Dettbarn-Reggentin analysed the socio-demographic characteristics of elders being organized in self-help organizations. With regard to age they found that the average age was 64.7 y: one third were younger than 60 y, one third between 61 and 69 y and one third older than 70. Women formed the vast majority of members – 73.5%.

The establishment of a growing number of groups, initiatives and projects in Germany during the last 15 years has been due to the following reasons:

- social political changes and reform of the welfare state in the light of diminishing financial resources,
- dissatisfaction with social services together with higher demands regarding their efficiency,
- demographic changes with an increase in the older population,
- general changes in lifestyle in modern societies,
- increasing political consciousness among the population.

With regard to elderly people, some additional developments can be mentioned. First, there have been some striking shifts in cultural images and expectations about 'ageing' and among elderly people themselves. Because people now live longer, have fewer children and longer periods of retirement, a larger part of their lives is relatively free of work and family obligations than was the case for past generations. Second, the current population of elders is better educated and therefore more self-confident about their rights and wishes. All of these contribute to higher interest and participation in self-help organizations.

When German elders are asked why they join a self-help organization the main motives are (Reggentin and Dettbarn-Reggentin, 1992): the creation or the development of social contacts and a social network, interest in the specific objectives of the self-help organization and the opportunity to meet people with the same interests, experience and problems. Additionally, the wish to extend experience and knowledge in different areas and keep active are very important motives for participation in self-help organizations. Further reasons include making provision for anticipated risks of life and structuring free time after retirement, widowhood and/or reduction of parental responsibilities (Schmelz, 1991). Evidence for the high level of motivation and satisfaction of elderly people in self-help organizations results from the fact that they invest a fair amount of time in their activities – sometimes comparable to regular employment – and membership very often lasts many years.

Self-help organizations are not part of the public and institutionalized help system (Zeman, 1988), but there are links to the health and social system, the recreational, educational and cultural sector, the labour market and politics, because in all fields of social life groups and organizations of self-help are to be found. The existing organizations can ideally be differentiated into the following six fields of activities (Reggentin and Dettbarn-Reggentin, 1992):

1. **Social sector:** In Germany self-help organizations are to be found most often in the social sector. Their particular aim is to initiate social contacts and networks in order to encourage mutual help as well as developing and improving new forms of living and housing. Examples of this kind of organization are local community groups or the foundation of communities, where young and old or healthy and disabled elderly people live together to manage problems of everyday life.

The following three sectors are of equal importance and together constitute about one half of all activities.

2. **Political sector:** The main target of self-help organizations in the political sector is the representation of their interests and participation in political decision making. There are, for example, senior

advisory boards in the communities, whose task is to look after the interests of elders. This happens in the parliament lobbies with the intention to advise and influence political decisions concerning the older generation. Senior associations of the political parties and trade unions and the most popular organization of elderly people, the 'Grey Panthers', should be included in this group.

3. **Health sector:** Groups in the health sector are focused on preventative health care in the field of health promotion such as sports activities as well as on rehabilitation measures as in the case of specific illnesses such as stroke, diabetes, rheumatism and heart disease. Apart from activities for those concerned, some of these organizations especially focus on caregivers in order to offer them relief and support and to create social networks among them.

4. **Cultural sector:** In the cultural sector activities of self-help organizations concentrate on the development of personal skills and abilities such as theatre and music groups, workshops for literature and writing which deal with contemporary history, personal history and members' experience of life.

5. **Psycho-social sector:** Although making up less than 10% of all groups, the psycho-social sector's aim is to help elders cope with suffering and illnesses, depression, and bereavement. They offer primarily emotional and social support and members are supposed to take responsibility for each other through group discussions and shared experiences.

6. **Activities related to work:** Finally, the sector of activities related to work was especially developed in the 1980s in the light of the crisis in the steel and coal mining industry where large numbers of employees were made redundant and sent into early retirement, some of them as young as 50. Members of this kind of self-help organization pursue voluntary working activities such as crafts as with the 'Kompanie des guten Willens' (Company of Good Will) or they organize information and advice centres in which elderly people are given the opportunity to pass on their experience to younger generations. Another example is the 'Senior-Experten-Service' (Senior Expert Service) by which retired experts from industry are sent into developing countries to carry out consulting, developing and social improvement activities. These organizations are financed by those who require their services. However, people who work in them only get their expenses paid.

Not surprisingly, while the 'young' old (under 65 years) are more active in areas which are related to their former job activities, those over 65 can be mainly found in social and community oriented sectors.

CARING FOR THE ELDERLY IN EAST GERMANY

The above description of self-help organizations is related mainly to West Germany. Before the unification of East and West Germany in 1989 no independent self-help organization existed in the German Democratic Republic. There social and cultural tasks with respect to the welfare of elders were carried out by two state organizations. One of them was the so-called 'Volkssolidarität' (People's Solidarity) that offered not only help and support in caregiving and housekeeping but also organized cultural events and activities. In addition there was the 'Kulturbund' (Culture Association) that concentrated mainly on local history and history of everyday life in order to keep alive customs and craft tradition. In this organization elderly people were especially valued because of their life experience and their role as 'time witnesses' (Scholz, 1992).

During the process of unification such organizations were abolished because the West German system was automatically and thoughtlessly transferred to the East. It was not evaluated whether the existing organizations could conduct their work after the unification or even whether they had advantages for the social system for the united Germany (Naegele, 1992). Though the new beginning turned out to be very difficult, a number of projects have been initiated and existing groups have merged in order to try and manage their activities through self-help and support from outside.

Apart from groups in the social and cultural sector, work based initiatives have been set up particularly in industrial regions in eastern parts of the country which have been especially affected by increasing unemployment and its corresponding problems.

Unfortunately, there are at present no up-to-date publications or studies about the subject of self-help organizations in the eastern counties. This is due to the problems and difficulties that such organizations have encountered during the restructuring process relating to the poor infrastructure including inadequate accommodation, little media coverage, a lack of financial support and difficulty in the recruitment of interested and motivated people. In addition, professional staff who are trying to set up and develop self-help organizations have hardly had enough time and opportunity to record and publish their findings and experience (Küchler and Kade, 1992).

When looking at the situation in East Germany it must be remembered that unification led to a breakdown in the life structure of many elderly people (Schwitzer, 1992) due to the sudden change of the whole social, legal, economic, and value system. Furthermore, two different lifestyles and mentalities clashed together. Former citizens of the German Democratic Republic – and especially elders – had to cope with changes in all areas of life. One East German sociologist, Schwitzer, even predicts 'dual German ageing' for the next generation. In this connection, self-help organizations have an important role in supporting elderly people to adjust to the new situation and reassuring them that they are not alone with their problems and fears.

RELATIONSHIP BETWEEN SELF-HELP ORGANIZATIONS, THE SOCIAL CARE SYSTEM AND THE WELFARE STATE

To understand the position of self-help organizations in Germany we will give an overview of relations within the social care system (Dörrie, 1985). The system consists of:

- public welfare
- independent welfare organizations
- self-help
- private help.

These four parts of the social care system have different tasks and they are supposed to complement one another. The public welfare provides offices like the public health department and offices for social affairs. They concentrate their work on administration and control: for example, they have the responsibility and supervision for health care and welfare matters. Alongside this there are six major independent welfare organizations – Arbeiterwohlfahrt, Diakonisches Werk der Evangelischen Kirche Deutschlands, Deutscher Caritasverband, Deutscher Paritätischer Wohlfahrtsverband, Deutsches Rotes Kreuz, Zentralwohlfahrtsstelle der Juden in Deutschland. These offer a wide range of social services including home health care, advice bureaux, hospitals and nursing homes and rescue services. Self-help organizations have already been described. Private help – which means help from relatives, neighbours and friends – is also an important part of the social system. Unfortunately, this kind of help is not sufficiently recognized in politics and society.

Public welfare is financed by taxes and other financial resources of the state. In contrast, independent welfare organizations are subsidized by donations, membership contributions, lotteries, and last but not least grants from official authorities. There are also variations in the funding of self-help organizations. Groups which are connected to one of the independent welfare organizations get the same kind of financial support. Most of the others find it hard to get sufficient money for their tasks because there is no legal basis which guarantees the financing of self-help organizations. Private help has not been subsidized up to now but this may change once a system of care insurance – in German called 'Pflegeversicherung' – is introduced in 1995.

As mentioned earlier self-help organizations are becoming more and more important in the social care system. A closer look at co-operation and network structures illustrates this trend quite clearly. In general, self-help organizations do not work in isolation. In order to achieve their interests and aims they try to win co-operative partnerships with agencies in other sectors – for example, self-help organizations which concentrate on health related problems co-operate with doctors, pharmacists, hospitals, health insurance institutions and of course with other organizations which pursue the same interests. Again self-help organizations which focus on cultural activities look for contacts with established institutions of adult education in order to profit from already existing resources as well as from the advice and experience of professionals. To some extent public social and health services and institutions also seek co-peration with self-help organizations, for example to help disabled elderly people.

Co-operation with independent sector welfare organizations is also very important for self-help organizations although co-operation with this traditional provider of social services is not free from problems, reservations and fears (Wagner, 1985). As long as there was a big demand for services, enough financial resources and as long as self-help organizations filled the gaps in the provision of social services (e.g. self-help for caregivers) the co-operation worked without any big problems – self-help organizations were more or less integrated in the independent welfare system. However, the constraints on public expenditure imposed by the present government make it necessary to share limited funds among more and more organizations. As self-help groups work in areas which are traditionally the concern of independent welfare organizations, there is a tendency to regard self-help organizations not only as a substitute but as a competitor – even though they recognize the positive effects of self-help and the alternatives it offers.

Furthermore, during the last few years self-help organizations have become more politically active and have often criticized the traditional welfare system, especially with regard to 'over-professionalization', hierarchical structures, bureaucracy and the disabling effects which these factors have on citizens. In contrast, independent welfare organizations and some other co-operation partners – for example, doctors – see the danger of deprofessionalization through self-help whereby lay persons might try to solve problems they are not competent for and in consequence, increase problems instead of resolving them.

However, an optimal social care network can only be developed if traditional and new structures of social work, independent welfare and self-help groups work together as constructively critical and self-confident partners. A constant dialogue seems to be essential which gives both sides the opportunity to reflect on their work. The aim should not be so much co-operation or even integration but co-existence.

At the moment, the German government is strongly supporting the self-help movement among elderly people. Politicians argue that self-help is not only cheaper but also helps those concerned to recognize their problems and activates them to find their own solutions. It looks as though the political intention is to integrate self-help and its potential into the public welfare system and save public funds at the same time.

The relationship between self-help organizations and the welfare state can be regarded as a very ambivalent one. On the one hand, it is part of the ideology of self-help groups to be independent in their work and in their objectives. On the other hand, most self-help groups need material and other support from public authorities. The dilemma is that these authorities decide which self-help organizations get subsidized and which do not and it is feared that the criteria the support is based upon are oriented towards a traditional model of public welfare, and respond more to the political opportunism of certain self-help organizations than anything else.

Critics argue that self-help groups are used to some extent for political aims (Lütke, 1985; Vilmar, 1985) because it is noticeable that self-help comes in vogue especially in times when increasing social problems are accompanied by a difficult situation in public finances. In consequence, the promotion of self-help appears as a reaction to structural deficits; it seems to take on the role of stopgap 'in the crisis of the welfare state'. Some authors refer to self-help 'as a magic trick of a cheap but effective social policy' (Lütke, 1985) or as a 'Trojan horse' (Vilmar, 1985).

However, there is no doubt that self-help can be an innovative power within the social care system and it can help to reconstruct the welfare state. But self-help organizations can neither take over tasks and services which the welfare state is responsible for nor solve the main problems of our society such as unemployment, poverty and the need for care. The welfare state should not misuse self-help to privatize problems. Rather, self-help has to be seen as a chance to motivate people to take on responsibilities for themselves, others and for their environment.

CONSTRAINTS ON SELF-HELP ORGANIZATIONS

In spite of the fact that self-help organizations are able to react more spontaneously and be more sensitive to social needs and problems, they are limited in scope and cannot be a complete substitute for professional help. A good example is in the area of health where self-help organizations can only be supportive and complementary.

It also has to be kept in mind that self-help organizations are often middle-class oriented because socially disadvantaged persons are often not able to organize and express their wishes and needs. According to various studies (Flach, 1988; Caplan, 1990) people who are involved in self-help groups already possess greater skills and competence, higher self-esteem, a sense of optimism and life purpose and therefore are more able to benefit from self-help organizations. Additionally, there are other groups of people who do not have the ability or power to initially organize or to be active in a self-help organization, for example those with severe learning difficulties, and thus it follows that self-help groups cannot be helpful for everybody. Many people still need the help of traditional welfare organizations.

Self-help organizations often rely on a few highly motivated and active people (usually the founders of the organization). If the active persons leave the self-help organization for any reason, the group very often breaks up. Hence stability, which is especially important for older people, is not guaranteed. Furthermore, because self-help organizations are very often constituted on the basis of interpersonal relations and good rapport, people who do not adapt to the existing members, their opinions and 'standards' may not have a chance to be accepted. Thus some people are still left alone with their problems in spite of the fact that self-help organizations suitable for their needs may be found in the neighbourhood.

CONCLUSION

In Germany, as in other industrial countries, we can observe two different developments which have to be taken into account when anticipating the future of self-help organizations. On the one hand, several demographic and social changes are altering the lifestyles, needs, problems and interests of older people (Naegele, 1991). On the other hand, it is expected that traditional public services for helping and supporting the elders are going to be further reduced due to economic and financial constraints. It follows that new needs of elderly people may not be met sufficiently in the future (Schmelz, 1991). Furthermore, it can be confidently stated that the potential of volunteers, especially those from religious and welfare organizations, is decreasing mainly due to increasing employment participation rates of women, less participation in religious groups and different lifestyles especially among successive groups of elderly people. Today's elders increasingly want to be independent, autonomous and self-determining without the constraints of traditional institutions and organizations.

Self-help organizations can offer a way out of this difficult situation by fulfilling tasks as follows:

- increasing participation of the older generation in politics and society and, in consequence, making changes in the society more possible from 'below';
- giving elders the possibility of contributing to society by applying skills and knowledge learned over many years not only for their own group but also for younger generations;
- postponing dependency and the need for help from others, especially from official help systems (help for self-help);
- supporting and maintaining competences and potential through active use;
- decreasing isolation and helplessness.

In conclusion, self-help organizations for elderly people are necessary for many reasons. However, there are some prerequisites to enable self-help organizations to be an innovative power in social politics and the welfare system. First, self-help organizations need to be able to work independently which means that financial support has to be guaranteed by law (Reggentin and Dettbarn-Reggentin, 1992). Second, to give more elderly people, especially the ones who, up to now, have not had access to self-help, the chance to use their potential and get involved in self-help, information about self-help must be provided. For example, which organizations already exist? What are they doing? What can I as an older person do? What needs to be done to start up a self-help organization? At the moment, the German government is supporting this idea by sponsoring so-called 'Seniorenbüros' (senior citizens offices) in which the elders find advice, contacts, and help. Third, self-help organizations are part of the welfare system but they cannot substitute for the services of the welfare state or of the independent welfare organizations. In order to find their correct position in this system, self-help organizations should not work in isolation from it but rather form a network within it whereby they exchange knowledge and experience. This would give them more influence and in turn, would help to avoid misuse by politicians and prejudice from independent welfare organizations. Finally, our society has to develop a stronger sense of solidarity and community, for self-help organizations can only be successful if their work finds recognition and acceptance among all sections of it.

REFERENCES

Boll, F. and Olk, Th. (eds) (1987) *Selbsthilfe und Wohlfahrtsverbände*, Lambertus Freiburg, Breisgau.

Caplan, G. (1990) Loss, stress and mental health. *Community Mental Health Journal*, **26**, 27–48.

Dörrie, K. (1985) Zusammenwirken von 'Selbsthilfebewegung' und sozialer Arbeit bei freien und öffentlichen Trägern, in *Selbsthilfe*, Heft 26, (eds E. Reis and H. Dorenburg), Eigenverlag des Deutschen Vereins für öffentliche und private Fürsorge, Frankfurt/M.

Flach, F. (1988) *Resilience: Discovering a New Strength in Times of Stress*, Fawcett Book Groups, New York.

Küchlur von, F. and Kade, S. (eds) (1992) *Erwachsenenbildung im Übergang*, Deutscher Hochschulverband, Frankfurt/M.

Lütke, G. (1985) Selbsthlifepolitik – Kritische Anmerkungen zur Berliner Praxis, in *Selbsthilfe*, Heft 26 (eds E. Reis and H. Dorenburg), Eigenverlag des Deutschen Vereins für öffentliche und private Fürsorge, Frankfurt/M.

Naegele, G. (1991) Anforderungen an eine zukunftsorientierte Altenpolitik unter besonderer Berücksichtigung der kommunalen Ebene. *Theorie und Praxis der sozialen Arbeit*, **11**, 418–425.

Naegele, G. (1992) 'Übergestülpt statt vernetzt' – Aus verpaßten Chancen dennoch das beste machen! Thesen zur Altenpolitik und -arbeit in Deutschland-Ost mit Rückwirkungen auf Deutschland-West, in *Vernetzung in Altenarbeit und Altenpolitik – Probleme und Perspektiven in der neuen Bundesrepublik*, (ed. H. Braun *et al.*), Kuratorium Deutsche Altershilfe, Köln.

Reggentin, H. and Dettbarn-Reggentin, J. (1992) *Selbsthilfegruppen älterer Menschen. Bestandsaufnahme im Bereich der Altenselbsthilfe*, Ministerium für Arbeit Gesundheit und Soziales, Düsseldorf.

Reis, C. and Dorenburg, H. (eds) (1985), in *Selbsthilfe*, Heft 26, Eigenverlag des Deutschen Vereins für öffentliche und private Fürsorge, Frankfurt/M.

Schmelz, C. (1991) Selbsthilfebewengung und Alter, in *Lehrbuch der psychologischen und sozialen Alternswisenschaft*, Band 3: Hilfe und Unterstützung für ältere Menschen, (ed. J. Howe *et al.*) Asanger, Heidelberg.

Scholz, R. (1992) Das Erfahrene weitergeben. Einige Gedanken zur Seniorenkulturarbeit in den neuen Bundesländern, in *Dem Alter einen Sinn geben*, (eds H. Glaser and T. Röbke), Hüthig, Heidelberg.

Schwitzer, K.P. (1992) Altern in den neuen Länder – Chancen und Aufgaben für die kommunale Altenpolitik, in *Dem Alter einen Sinn geben*, (eds H. Glaser and T. Röbke), Hüthig, Heidelberg.

Vilmer, F. (1985) Gesellschaftspolitische Bedeutung sozialer Selbsthilfe, in *Selbsthilfe*, Heft 26, (eds E. Reis and H. Dorenburg), Eigenverlag des Deutschen Vereins für öffentliche und private Fürsorge, Frankfurt/M.

Wagner, D. (1985) Konkurrenz oder Kooperation – Zur Problematik des Verhältnisses von Wohlfahrtsverbänden und 'Selbsthilfe', in *Selbsthilfe*, Heft 26, (eds E. Reis and H. Dorenburg), Eigenverlag des Deutschen Vereins für öffentliche und private Fürsorge, Frankfurt/M.

Zeman, P. (1988) *Gemeinschaftliche Altenselbsthilfe: Prozesse sozialer Integration im Alter*, Deutsches Zentrum für Altersfragen, Berlin.

6

Peer support and advocacy – international comparisons and developments

David Brandon

'It takes a man that have the blues to sing the blues.'
Leadbelly in Alan Lomax *The Land Where the Blues Began*
Methuen, 1993.

PEER SUPPORT

Peer support has been long established in areas of physical disability. People in wheelchairs, particularly those injured in accidents, assist people in similar situations recovering within the world famous spinal injuries unit at Stoke Mandeville Hospital. Alcoholics Anonymous (AA), perhaps the largest self-help organization in the world, supports tens of thousands of alcoholics. No person may be a full member except as an alcoholic, believed by AA to be a lifelong condition (Bateson, 1973).

In other areas, the experience of service users has long been recognized as an important resource. The New Careers movement, initially developed in the United States but copied over here, aimed to train offenders to become staff in penal units. It intended to recruit the poor to do paid work in the helping agencies. The scheme had six ingredients (Priestly, 1975): 'income for the poor; work for the unemployed and unemployable; status escalator for the stigmatized; manpower for human services; qualitative transformation of social work; a revolution in training design and methods.' Its full impact was successfully resisted by staff.

The Swansea Prison Listener scheme, based on American prison buddy systems, started in August 1991, uses fellow prisoners to counsel depressed and suicidal colleagues. Individual prisoners are selected for their maturity, knowledge of the system and a genuine desire to help others. The training of these 'peer counsellors' is the responsibility of the Samaritans who provide support and supervision through confidential weekly discussions within the prison.

The Midland Bank uses the mentor system. The term derives from Mentor, the revered advisor to the young Telemachus in Homer's *Odyssey* (O'Brien, 1987). A mentor became a term meaning an advisor, role model, coach and confidant. It involves someone further on, who knows the systems and problems, and who is extremely approachable and has no management responsibilities for the person being so guided.

The process of mentoring can be very powerful but sometimes the process 'overheats'. Occasionally mentors are not clear about their roles and 'mentees' make too many demands. At its best, the supporter both challenges and nourishes. Jenny, a Midland Bank trainee, said: 'My mentor wouldn't take problems from me, but turned them around and gave me options, in order to get me to think what I should do to resolve them' (Steele, 1992). Some promising British athletes have mentors. Jeoff Thompson, former world karate champion, supports Darren Campbell, would-be Olympic sprint gold medalist. Jeoff comments, 'Darren has the desire, the smile and he does the hard work. I ensure that he doesn't make the mistakes I made. The mentor scheme's objective is to show that sportspeople can take care of themselves and recycle their talents back into the community' (Liston, 1993).

One traditional and major strand of peer support lies in the self-help movement, long established in this country. There are tens of thousands of groups, working in diverse areas (Sagarin, 1969); '. . . in forming, supporting or joining a self-help group, a stigmatised person seeks either 1) to conform to the norms of society or 2) to change those norms to include acceptance of his own behaviour. In the first instance he renounces his deviant behaviour, in the second he changes not himself but the rule making order'. 'The distinctive feature about the support that a self-help network offers its members is that it is peer support, support to the disadvantaged from the disadvantaged. As oppression is a core experience, one which helps to structure an individual's sense of self, a link with others forged on the basis of a common oppression promotes a strong sense of identity which is easily translated into support' (Trevillion, 1992).

This movement is distinct from formal services in several ways: it features 'a common problem or predicament shared by all or most of the members; reciprocity of helping among members; self management of the groups'. (Robinson and Henry, 1977). One danger is that internal pressures on group members 'may result in a harsher condemnation of deviance than is found in the general population' (Henry, 1978). With the gradual weakening of stigma and increasing positive publicity, such groups have developed extensively in the mental health field, particularly in the latter half of this century.

That growth may be resisted by staff. Take this quote: 'One was painfully aware of the traditional structures and procedures at work; the supervision of movements, the subtly induced feelings of gratitude, the interference of nurses at the sight of "wrong relationships", an insistent awareness by patients that somehow we were the guinea pigs, the doctors and staff always remaining doctors and staff; a world separated by a pane of glass, a badge or nurse's uniform' (Sutherland, 1977).

An important bridge between staff and users can be the 'wounded' staff (like myself) entering the psychiatric services for treatment. They make many criticisms of their treatment. '. . . informal contact with mental illness staff/patients could be "supportive and encouraging". Incidental displays of human interest, warmth and humour on the part of staff were appreciated whenever they occurred. But the behaviour of staff, whether medical or nursing, could be extremely unhelpful. Brusqueness, rudeness, a lack of respect/consideration on the part of staff, failure to introduce themselves, or failure to specify when the next appointment would take place were all experienced as unhelpful, as was the constant turnover of staff on one ward' (Rippere and Williams, 1985).

Attempts to build bridges and make the divisions less rigid frequently battle with enemies. The introduction of volunteer programmes in the mid city psychiatric clinic in Houston, Texas, met with fairly strong staff resistance. They feared it would blur staff/patient roles and destroy long-established therapeutic alliances. The staff were too busy with direct patient activities. A one year pilot programme involved a teacher from a community college providing consultation and educational materials to support two psychiatric patient volunteers, both retired school teachers. They tutored 15 patients over nine months. Two other volunteers, both patients previously employed in the health field, provided assistance to staff and patients in the geriatric clinic. Twenty four patients were involved over 18 months, five returned to full-time work (Chacko, 1985).

Patients admitted to the San Francisco General Hospital were provided with peer counsellors – someone also suffering from mental distress who has had in-patient treatment. This is a version of the mentor system. The peer counsellor's task is to humanize the hospital environment by offering advice and information which is different from the professional hospital treatment (Church and Revell, 1990). The adolescent unit of Haverford Hospital, Pennsylvania, uses 'buddies' in the later phases of its rehabilitation programme. Buddies accompany lower phase patients and are responsible for reporting to staff any rule violations by the person they are paired with (McIver, 1991).

Early in 1971, a group of Vancouver patients treated in a psychiatric day hospital 'did not find the set up supportive, since they discovered that crises frequently arose precisely during the times when staff were unavailable (evenings and weekends), and it was against the rules for patients to see one another or to talk on the phone outside the institution. One Monday morning the patients arrived on the ward and learned that over the weekend one of their number had committed suicide. Many strong emotions were expressed, and one immediate result was the clandestine circulation of a patients' phone list.

As time went on, some of the patients discovered that they were relying on these 'illegal' phone calls far more than on the therapy they were receiving during day hospital hours, and they began to talk among themselves about the kinds of "help" that were truly useful. By the time all of them had been discharged from the hospital they felt that their informal network was the one form of real support they had' (Patmore, 1988).

They formed a group called the Mental Patients Association. They ran a seven day a week drop in centre and five co-operative residences.

Chamberlin notes that 'Many professionals deeply resent being excluded from meetings and activities of the group. In fact, this is one of the organisational problems with which any group attempting to set up an alternative service will probably have to deal early in its existence . . . Those professionals and other non-patients who fight attempts by ex-patients to exclude them from some meetings are precisely the same people who will probably attempt to control and direct the group' (Chamberlin, 1988).

Adams describes similar problems in the general relationships between professionals and self-help groups. '. . . problematic relationships between self-helpers and social workers, questioning of their autonomy and the authority of professionals by consumers.' '. . . corruption by professionals of the challenge; exploitation of non-professional helpers; professionalisation of self-helpers; co-option by professionals' (Adams, 1990).

One considerable and particular problem is what Chamberlin calls 'mentalism', expressing itself in many forms (Chamberlin, 1988). This means the pervasive tendency to see service users as inferior people, sometimes actively encouraged on professional training courses. Users complain of not being treated seriously: 'Legitimate complaints are seen as part of the illness. Doctors' diagnoses are not always satisfactory and sufferers' views on their needs and treatment are not given sufficient consideration. Doctors don't treat people as human beings. There is no sense of partnership between staff and patients. Staff control is too great, and often proves insensitive to individual needs' (South Glamorgan Mental Health Users Alliance, 1991).

Service users' experiences are inevitably pathologized. For example, 'If a user is angry, it is seen as something unresolved in their mental distress, not a reaction to the way they've been treated' (Kelville, 1992). More recently the Ashworth Hospital enquiry report quotes a staff member: 'Within this environment patients' behaviours and characters are constantly under scrutiny. They are placed in a "no win" situation. If they express their needs, they are "attention seeking". If they adapt to the system, they are "manipulative". If they conform, it is surface compliance. If they rebel, they are suppressed. If they form relationships, they are construed as unhealthy and conspiratorial. If they keep to themselves, they are isolated, withdrawn and "deep". Patients are condemned for being institutionalised and criticised if they try to exert some control over their lives' (Williams, 1992).

Staff are often over-protective. 'They often feel that they should shield patients for as long as possible from the delays or uncertainties which inevitably occur in the transitional process. This view is not shared by patients who feel less worried by being involved in the ups and downs of negotiation for property and places than being subject to last minute announcement of changes' (Braisby, 1983).

A woman in her mid-fifties talked of staff who cared for her in a long stay hospital: 'They meant well, don't get me wrong. I'm not criticising them. They thought it was all for the best, for our own good, but they treated us like children. They made your mind up for you and you stopped thinking for yourself. They said we could not be expected to cope with the ups and downs of life. It did me no good, I lost confidence altogether' (Camden Consortium, 1988). Unintentionally, staff developed a passive culture.

Professional jargon can reveal mentalist attitudes and act as a considerable and intended barrier to understanding. A survey of 100 service users examined the common understanding of terms in regular use by the social services profession. Asked what they understood by 'gender', 'criteria', and 'equitable manner', most users did not know what they meant. They understood that a 'format' was something you wiped your feet on (Jowell, 1991). It is vital to use terms that users can understand.

Changes require a revolution in attitudes. 'Our awareness of the reality of disability is limited because we live in a society geared towards people whose bodies and minds are fully functioning. This may seem strange when one considers that disability or illness can happen to anyone at any moment of their lives – it is an inevitable part of the human experience. Nevertheless, society is organised in such a way as to treat disability as an exceptional circumstance that requires special and, in the main, separate provision which is often inadequate and serves only to maintain the divisions and lack of understanding between able-bodied and disabled people' (Bynoe, Oliver and Barnes, 1991).

Some changes present fresh problems. 'Most disabled people now have more access to more services and, on the whole, are less likely to end up in a segregated institution. However, they generally pay a price for those services – for example, invasions of privacy by a veritable army of professionals and having to accept services that the state thinks they should have or can afford, rather than those they know they need. There is often a further price to pay: being socialised into dependency – because services are provided for rather than with disabled people . . .' (Gillespie-Sells and Campbell, 1991).

Chamberlin goes further than advocacy and peer support and argues a powerful case for user-led services. She identifies three distinct service models: first, 'Partnership model where professionals and non-professionals work together to provide services. The recipients are told that they are partners in the service. However, the distinction between those who give help and those who receive it remains clearly defined'. Second, 'Supportive model where membership is open to all people who want to use the service for mutual support. Non-patients and ex-patients are seen as equals . . . professionals are excluded from this model'. Third, 'Separatist model – ex-patients provide support for one another and run the service. All non-patients and professionals are excluded because they interfere with consciousness raising and because they usually have mentalist attitudes' (Chamberlin, 1988).

She outlines some principles for patient-led services:

- provide help with needs as defined by the clients,
- participation must be completely voluntary,
- clients must be free to participate in some parts of the service without being required to participate in others,
- help comes from members to one another and is seen as a human attribute and nothing to do with formal qualifications,
- the direction of the service is in the hands of the service recipients,
- service clients must decide whether participation is limited to ex-patients or open to all,
- responsibility of the service is to the client alone.

For example, 'Project Release in New York operates a seven day a week community centre that is entirely patient directed. No one is designated as staff. It feels that members could not be equal if some were paid to be there . . . In order to discourage anyone from becoming a passive recipient, all members are required to serve on one or more of the committees (fund raising, community centre, newsletter, and so on)' (Chamberlin, 1988).

Progress towards this kind of increased user involvement has been extremely slow in this country. For example, each local mental health group in Bassetlaw in Derbyshire has a development worker, none has a mental health professional. They organize groups on a drop in basis for one day a week. The main activity is social talk in a sympathetic but cheerful atmosphere. 'These groups are not intended to cater for people whose regular behaviour was disruptive . . .' Initially, agency professionals constituted the management committee but they were to be replaced in phases by elected group representatives. The Harworth group has now reached full self-management. Decisions are taken round the table and recorded in a log book. Two women take care of the cash box. The recent verdict was that 'Things get done, even if it does take twice as long as before' (Pymn, 1989). Notice that some potential service users are still excluded as a matter of policy.

In most of these mentor and peer support schemes, there is massive control by professionals. Some resemble 'star prisoner' systems where 'trusties' are given special status and privileges. Their training, relationships and structures are all dominated by the needs of professionals.

Perhaps the most detailed and revealing description of peer support is that of Brian Keenan (Keenan, 1992). He describes the blossoming relationship between himself and John McCarthy when they were both imprisoned and tortured as hostages in Lebanon. He draws out the distinctive nature of the support of someone in the same position, undergoing the same sort of suffering.

A survivor friend writes of supporting a distressed woman. 'A woman I am close to from a co-counselling support group for mental health system survivors, recently started not being able to sleep. After a week with no sleep at all, she became badly frightened and started having racing thoughts and experiences which seemed like reality but which she later thought were not real. Having been to a psychiatric hospital before, where she had been forcibly injected, she did not want to go back and was very reluctant to consult her new GP, whom she had never met.

She asked me and other co-counsellors, some of whom were also friends, for help and we organised a rota of people so that someone could be with her nearly all the time. After she had spent a night at my house, still not sleeping, I went with her to her GP, who prescribed Melleril. He was concerned at leaving the situation like that, but agreed to leave it up to her as to how much of the drug she took, after we had explained the support system. The first 2 or 3 days of taking the drug, she ended up taking 225 mls only at night, which enabled her to sleep. But this made her drowsy through the day so she cut down gradually and within two weeks was down to 50 mls. A week later she had stopped altogether.

She spent over a week at my house. A lot of the time was spent not in counselling as such, especially early on, as we wanted to get her attention away from irrational thoughts and fears and on to what was good about the present situation. We used massage, swimming, relaxation, cooking, country walks, listening to music, interspersed with some counselling when she seemed about to release some of the real underlying terror. We were also physically very close, hugging her a lot and telling her how much we loved and valued her. After she had gone back to her own family, we made sure she had regular counselling sessions with us, several times a week.

She said that the experience was incomparably better than the two previous occasions when she had had similar problems and went into hospital. She said that the key factors were that we were not frightened of her and the situation. She had a "safe place" to go where she could forget about day to day problems and where people were loving and supportive, and that her new GP listened to her and treated her with respect, allowing her to decide about taking the drug. Otherwise she feels that she would have landed up in hospital.

If we had been involved with her at an earlier stage, she would not have needed drugs. I have had similar experiences supporting someone close to me who had been under mental health section more than once. She came off chlorpromazine very quickly and no longer uses it. She prefers to monitor herself closely, using counselling, aromatherapy and massage.' Co-counselling is a therapeutic system, where each person in a pair plays a role, in turn, thus helping the emotions of the other.

Peter Campbell of Survivors Speak Out, with a vast experience of supporting and of being supported, asks a number of pertinent questions. 'Is there a way to provide the necessary support for peer support without some sort of professionalized take over? What are the tensions between formal and informal structures? What will the role be for activists who are very critical of systemized care? The best support comes from friendship. It is shared one to one support during the wobbly periods. Some people's networks are already dominated by survivors. Survivors have similar experiences and backgrounds. Is that feeling of common experiences real? In a way there is a legend of collective experience when people's experiences of distress and service use may be, in reality, extremely different.' As the survivors' movements develop, schisms are inevitable. Groups will increasingly emphasize differences rather than commonalities.

However for most service users in most parts of the world, there is a very long way to go towards any sort of user involvement. The World Health Organization sounds a note of caution and realism. 'For hospitalized patients the ward is their daily environment. Yet the influence of patients on the rules of the environment remains small.

Institutional rules and bureaucratic procedures often lead to situations in which the individual cannot develop and ultimately becomes alienated . . . the patient is expected to adapt to the needs of the institution rather than the other way round' (WHO, 1989). Changing that imbalance will take many decades.

PEER ADVOCACY

Peer advocacy involves individual support by recovering or recovered users in helping other service users to express and fulfil their individual wishes. It differs radically from conventional citizen advocacy, described earlier, in that the advocates are not so-called 'valued persons' but people who are also mental health service survivors. They share the social stigmatization of what is sometimes called the 'spoiled identity' of those they support. Peer advocacy is an important and powerful confluence of both the peer support and advocacy movements, probably beginning, in the formal sense, with John Perceval in the early 19th century (Brandon, 1990).

As we have seen in this study, users are frequently encouraged to feel bad about themselves. Their essential experience of living is grossly invalidated by the very definition of 'mental illness'. The psychiatric labelling process tends to cover the whole being of the individual in the eyes of others who feel superior. Both the devaluing services and the 'mentalist' staff assist users to internalize negative feelings. Survivors may blame themselves entirely and their personal weaknesses for their distressed condition rather than more powerful others and massive changes in socio-economic structures.

Chamberlin notes that 'the crippling stereotypes about mental illness have often been internalized by ex-patients, many of whom believe (at least some of the time) that they are weak, incapable, untrustworthy, "sick", "crazy", or whatever. It is difficult or impossible to go through the experience of mental institutionalization without beginning, to some extent, to hate oneself. Part of the process of institutional "treatment" is convincing the patient that his or her former ideas, beliefs, and behaviours were wrong' (Chamberlain, 1988).

Peer support and advocacy is one way to counteract some of those powerful processes and to help users to see both themselves and their experiences in a much more positive light. It carries the idea that they are valuable people with useful experiences. They can be both advocates and also colleagues of the powerful mental health professionals. They can be taken seriously, learn increased skills and receive respect from powerful others. But the essential test is whether peer advocacy is 'effective' and if it has both distinctive and positive features.

Peter Campbell describes one incident in his long experience of peer advocacy. 'I have used the mental health system for twenty five years, and I am pretty articulate and know fairly well the ins and outs of the system. Last autumn when I was on section 3 for a month and was in an acute ward in London, I had a friend of mine, a fellow user, acting as my advocate. It was the first time . . . and it made a really big difference to me. She spoke on my behalf and supported me and it transformed the nature of that meeting. It was quite a learning experience for the other people and the mental health workers. All I can say is that it made a real difference to my feelings of empowerment.

She was someone who was in complete sympathy/empathy with me. She knew the "power trip" from the inside. It was "inside" her too. She was emotionally involved which I saw as a plus. We were reciprocally involved. I expected that I would act as her advocate at some point. This strengthened us both *vis à vis* the system. That reciprocity establishes a particular bond with a potential for deeper benefits. For example, it made a difference for me that this peer advocacy had grown out of friendship. The solidarity issue means that there is a "piquancy" when the advocacy relationship is clearly connected to a common and clear approach to wider issues. She was realistic. She had an instinctive knowledge of what was on and what was not on. She was aware of the essential limits of advocacy and of my powerlessness from her direct experience.'

Shuresh Patel, a survivor working on the development of patients' councils in Lancashire, found that staff ridiculed his ideas about advocacy; also there was a resistance from other patients who felt overwhelmed by the power of the staff. If patients don't assert their rights, they will just get walked over by the psychiatric system. Discussions involving staff met with hostility: some staff were actually disgusted. For example, some referred to the embryonic patients' council as a 'witch hunt'.

'In taking up allegations of racism in a psychiatric setting, I was always told that it was just my delusions. I was allegedly hearing things in my head. But on one occasion I had a witness. I was called a "Pakki" by a hospital staff member, complained and he got disciplined. I have just given up my job in Unravel Mills, an industrial therapy unit. It's just an extended mental institution in the community. Packing things into boxes was humiliating and there was also no heating in the part of the building where I worked. I made friends with the only other coloured user who complained that he couldn't get a vegetarian meal, needed on religious grounds. I served as his advocate. The staff responded "He should change his religion". Like me he was a Hindu and we were both supposed to change to Christianity to solve the menu problem! Their whole attitude was very hostile.'

I have also faced some of the dilemmas of advocacy over many years. I have been an advocate for fellow mental health service users, both inside and outside MIND. Often I had the more formal paid role of a social worker or MIND regional director, acting on behalf of patients. Such advocacy roles were frequently made extremely difficult. For example, it was made difficult to get access to records and other written material, which would be readily available in my straight social work role. I was resented personally and seen as betraying my colleagues. I was perceived as a deviant member of the established club. I had gone over the wall. As a professional, you were supposed to make some kind of choice, to be reliable and, above all, loyalty was crucial, to share an unquestioned faith in colleagues, at least publicly. Choosing to be on the side of the users was to make both a deviant and disloyal decision which needed some sort of punishment.

I had made no secret of my experience of psychiatric treatment, writing about it in various books and professional journals. Colleagues would comment on that experience as an explanation for my subsequently perceived deviant behaviour. My unusual interest in the experiences of users would be explained in terms of individual deviancy. One particular psychiatrist talked openly of me 'going native' in a hospital case conference. Another talked at a case conference of me being 'untrustworthy'.

When I was more obviously involved in peer advocacy, I was perceived as 'crossing boundaries', of 'getting emotionally over-involved', of 'letting my passions rule my head', of 'over-identifying with clients and patients'. I should keep private my experience of being a fellow patient. A charge nurse told me that it was harmful to tell users that I had been in their situation. 'It blurs professional/patient boundaries. You should save that sort of communication for your own psychotherapy sessions. You shouldn't bring it in to the work.' It was suggested in various letters from professionals that my peer advocacy was a result of my instability and, a much more subtle assault, 'actually working against the best interests of the patients concerned'. I had apparently 'lost all objectivity'. Certain patients were being 'penalized' because of my damaged support. Sometimes they were really being penalized, usually by others.

When Perceval (Brandon, 1990) mounted a systematic assault on conditions in Northampton county asylum, incidentally where the poet John Clare had been incarcerated for many years, he was attacked by a hospital official. The official stated in a local newspaper that Perceval's sympathies with the insane 'are of a very morbid character and his judgement to the last feeble and weak' (Podvoll, 1990). This attack on Perceval involved re-clientizing him.

I recall representing some patients on a long stay hospital ward and talking to both them and other professionals about some of their experiences as being similar to my own. A nurse said to me during a coffee break 'Remember David, they're only mental patients. They complain about conditions and you represent them. But they don't really understand things in the way you and I both do. Their decision making processes are permanently damaged. Don't ever confuse their situation with your own. We go home at the end of every day and they stay right here. They don't have our helicopter view of the world. They don't have either our education or professional discipline'.

Such a course of action was always difficult. There were no established pathways for the peer advocate as Perceval discovered. 'I resolved – I was necessitated – to pit my strength and abilities against a system (of lunacy), to fail in no duty to myself and to my country; but at the risk of my life, or my health, and even my understanding, to become thoroughly acquainted with its windings, in order to expose and unravel the wickedness and the folly that maintained it, and to unmask the plausible villainy that carries it on' (Podvoll, 1990). He paid a huge personal cost for this heroic struggle.

Like Perceval, Karen Campbell, a staff member at Fulbourn psychiatric hospital, Cambridge, had experience as a user and worked to develop her influence. She says that on a ward level, complaints can get ignored or false assurances given that the matter is being dealt with, when in fact it is being ignored or buried. Similarly, buckpassing such as 'That is not our responsibility . . . we have no say on that . . .' also occurs. Lack of information, refusal to make information available or denying any knowledge of means of access to information can be a problem.

The most blatant form of obstructionism our (peer) advocates have met with is staff apathy and indifference; staff failing to inform users that the advocates will be visiting the ward and that they are available on a regular basis. Staff can feel threatened and undermined by 'patients' operating outside their usual roles, and in what they perceive as quasi staff roles. When people have been defined as unskilled and inferior, it is usually difficult to accept them in more equal and skilled roles.

As in the Perceval example, some professionals fight back by re-clientizing peer advocates. They may try to continue a dominant relationship which has characteristically emphasized the clients' personal difficulties and not valued their strengths, qualities and insights. Professionals will need considerable help and training to see peer supporters as equals instead of seeing them as a threat to their livelihoods. Feelings of traditional territoriality and ownership can be extremely powerful. Professionals too have fragile egos although usually rather more money than mental health survivors.

Campbell notes that the user advocate can be made to feel intimidated by the hierarchy within the hospital and health authority. He or she may be asked to meet with very senior managers or consultants. The advocate may be expected to give a formal presentation in staff teaching sessions on advocacy. This process of intimidation is integral to the existing power structures in the mental health services, with the user at the bottom of the pile. The user advocate is made to feel unqualified to question or deal with 'the professionals'. The user advocate has very little credibility with paid workers, and can be made to feel very much alone. He or she is frequently seen as in some way representative of all users' views, as if he or she had some invisible direct line to other patients!

Karen Campbell said 'I recently had an extremely uncomfortable conversation with a powerful consultant psychiatrist, who made clear his objections to user advocates. It would mean "unscrutinised people" coming on to "his" ward and stirring up dissent. Wielding power means excluding others from sharing that power, thus the consultant was defining his territory. He would have no power over the advocates therefore he objected to their presence. User advocacy challenges the traditional paternalistic ethos of psychiatry, it threatens the exclusivity and integrity of the professional carers. The response is to devalue the threat. User advocates face indifference, hostility and scorn. Not many hospital based staff are prepared to take user advocates seriously'. The peer advocacy movement can rely on considerable resistance from psychiatric staff who feel threatened and demoralized. They cannot be expected to welcome the work with such a new and radical movement without help and support from the psychiatric system.

Peer advocacy shouldn't simply be a personal and *ad hoc* arrangement. One exciting new development is that some citizen advocacy projects now recruit users as advocates. The Birmingham Citizen Advocacy Project was set up late in 1987 by the local association for mental health. It grew out of a consultation exercise with mental health users, who saw the need for such advocacy. It received funding for three years and was based in a south Birmingham psychiatric hospital, a particularly unsuitable location. Lorraine Lewis, currently a user of mental health services, was appointed co-ordinator in February 1990 and the office moved to the Community Enterprise centre.

With her assistant co-ordinator Andrew Dunning, Lorraine sees advocacy as a fundamentally anti-discriminatory activity in complete contrast to the experiences described earlier. They have deliberately set aside the traditional 'valued citizen' condition. They see an advocate as 'anybody who can make things happen'. They give considerable support to the matches between the advocate and the partner. Currently 50% are peer advocates, which means that both the partners have a direct experience of mental health services. Lorraine has a very extensive network in Birmingham, particularly amongst users, so that new advocates with mental health backgrounds are coming forward all the time.

Bernard also has experience of psychiatric in-patient facilities. He went on an advocacy training day and met Lorraine who felt he needed an advocate, possibly because his son has cerebral palsy. Bernard wanted someone for himself. He already knew Bali Gill, also a mental health user who had trained in advocacy. All three felt that their partnership would be good. The formalizing of the relationship through Lorraine increased the power.

Bernard feels peer advocates are the best. 'Bali understands my problems because she's been through similar crap. She doesn't see herself as an advocate and me as the partner. We share a deep care and concern for each other which is both equal and reciprocal.' He and Bali have developed a self advocacy group based on the Soho psychiatric day centre and edit *The Pioneer Voice*, a mental health users' magazine which is very critical of traditional psychiatry.

Lorraine sees the practice of equality as vital in advocacy. She encourages reciprocity and the sharing of personal stories and other experiences. She agrees with Bernard that it often improves matches where both people have a mental health problem. 'Many things just don't have to be explained. There is an increased intuitive understanding when someone has been through a similar process themselves.'

Peer advocacy can be very diverse. It may involve 'wounded staff' taking up issues on behalf of people they identify with, in their spare time. It may also involve long-term friendships between people on a reasonably equal footing where both may have an advocacy role for each other at different times. Peers may represent each other, for example, at formal case conferences when it is difficult for the survivor to speak out because he or she feels under considerable pressure from the professionals. Peer advocacy can come less equally from more experienced peers who act more like mentors, with some training in representation and whose life is more together, at least at that particular time. That may be reversed at some future time.

Advocacy may involve a long-term relationship as in conventional citizen advocacy or a coming together for a brief period during some particular crisis: so-called crisis advocacy. For example, I have represented, on an informal basis, a large number of people who were mentally ill and homeless or facing the prospect of compulsory admission to hospital.

Paula was unwilling to take the psychiatrist's advice, refusing to take the prescribed medication in particular. 'It makes me feel awful, dopey and stupid. How am I supposed to take care of the children and do my part-time cleaning job if I'm asleep all the time?' The psychiatrist threatened her with compulsory admission and then with abandonment

('I'll wash my hands of you completely . . .') unless she carried out his instructions. She trusted me because we had shared some common experiences of psychiatric treatment. We attended a case conference together and I helped her express her views. Some staff were very unhappy at her being represented, including the psychiatrist. However, we managed to talk them out of compulsory admission and they continued to provide some form of treatment which was much more acceptable to Paula. They saw more easily that she had strong views with some justice in them and not necessarily a symptom of her mental illness. Although of course, it is always very possible to be 'crazy' as well as right!

All these variants involve certain important and common features:

- The relationship is entirely unpaid and completely independent of service provision.
- Both partners have been at some time or are currently mental health service users. They share that experience readily with one another.
- Both have an essential understanding of the meaning of what representation of another involves.
- The purpose of the advocacy is to develop and express the wishes of the partner, not those of the advocate, with both passion and discipline.
- It involves staying close to feelings of equality and similarity firmly based in respect and affection.
- It avoids any copying of professionalism and remains proudly amateur, literally meaning 'stemming from love'.
- The advocate is committed to developing both the knowledge and skills necessary to bear better witness to the complaints of his/her partner.

All this leaves important and largely unanswered questions about the future of peer advocacy. Can it be both developed and extended without coming under the dominant control of the various professionals? That would be a difficult journey. Can the peer advocates be supported and trained without becoming pseudo professionals? Can peer advocates provide an effective advocacy service when some experience suggests otherwise? That raises essential questions about what advocacy is and is not. Can advocates be respected by the professionals; be seen as colleagues and equals? The mental health services are full of fear, especially on the staff side, and people easily get defensive and angry.

We are not arguing here for peer advocacy as some sort of exclusive service but suggesting that it has some unique possibilities as well as some special difficulties. Mental health service survivors may well need other forms of advocacy, seen by them as more relevant. They may also use several different forms of advocacy all at the same time. In this next section we need to look more closely at the more practical aspects of how this kind of advocacy can be effectively organized.

IMPLEMENTATION

'The true neighbour will risk his position, his prestige, and even his life for the welfare of others. In dangerous valleys and hazardous pathways, he will lift some bruised and beaten brother to a higher and more noble life.' (Martin Luther King Jr)

Peer advocacy is one important aspect of peer support for 'bruised and beaten brothers' as well as sisters. It could help to promote a number of changes in the psychiatric service. It could help staff to recognize that service users have relevant and valuable experiences, gifts and skills. It helps the development of assertion and speaking out, gradually changing the suffocating environment of passivity. Service users could become, at the very least, active partners in their recovery. Peer advocacy challenges the whole negative process of 'mentalism', particularly in staff and carers. When they are seen increasingly as people of value, who have something important to contribute, it is easier for users to come in from the margins. It is easier for them to be included rather than socially and economically excluded. They can once again be perceived as unique and valued individuals.

Despite vigorous projects like those in Birmingham, work involving users as supporters and advocates remains largely unexplored. Service users have a direct experience of psychological disability, the relevant services and the roles of different professionals. Many have left hospitals and hostels and now live independently and successfully. They have personal knowledge of the themes of rehabilitation, resettlement and recovery from the inside. Some users may want to act as practical guides, positive role models, counsellors. As we have seen, they are given few opportunities to make positive contributions except in the fringe areas of alcoholism and drug dependency.

Peer support would extend the already considerable influence of the blossoming self-help movement. Groups of people getting together, because they have in common some perplexing or devaluing experience or condition, can be immensely worthwhile. Peer support could provide another avenue for that river of wisdom and goodwill. It could help both relatives and survivors. In each case the person would have to have had a similar experience to the person supported.

A lot of peer support already happens on an informal and *ad hoc* basis. A clinical psychologist introduces a man who was in mental hospital until last year to help another just coming out who has no friends. They have meals together and attend the occasional football match. They share personal notes about the competence of the various professionals. They tell each other what the mental health services were and are really like.

A woman with a long history of depression, whose husband left her and the two children, is introduced by a social worker to another who has had a very similar experience who is now feeling better. The second woman represents the first at case conferences. In speaking out for the other, she gains increased confidence and skills for herself. After some experience of advocacy, she trains for counselling and finds a way of making a living after years of unemployment. The first sees a possible positive way ahead in the eyes of the advocate. There is life after depression after all.

Peer advocacy would offer individual help and friendship to users in contrast to the mostly group work of self-help. It would require considerable changes in staff attitudes; changes in relevant structures; much support and some training in specific areas like welfare rights, practical counselling and listening skills as well as in advocacy. The purpose of training would be to supplement their already extensive direct knowledge and personal qualities rather than to turn them into substitutes for a professional, which would be a sad irony.

Training

Lorraine and Andrew from the Birmingham Citizen Advocacy Project are involved in training mental health professionals, which has implications for staff and relatives and even users. They concentrate on presenting a serious challenge to the stereotypes held by professionals. Training professionals should involve looking at areas of mentalism; the development of negative imagery from films like *Psycho* and the newspapers. It should involve negative attitudes induced by training; feelings that professionals are in some way 'superior beings', reinforced by ten thousand things inside the services, everything from the ward round to the offices.

For example, Podvoll, a psychiatrist, notes that there is an injurious barrier frequently created in professionals and volunteers. He describes this as 'I am different from him; it is he who is unhealthy, not me; he feels his own pain and I feel mine; it is he who is indulging in extreme autism and I am the witness'. But this barrier is unstable, it naturally breaks down – one becomes identified with the other's pain. And then out of some kind of fear, one tries to justify and fortify one's differences again by further elaboration of thoughts. This results in 'increasing speed and impatience, which eventually manifest in the therapeutic aggression of asylum mentality' (Podvoll, 1990).

Such training should only be undertaken by those with a direct experience of mental health services. That direct experience of suffering and treatment is vital to understanding of the nature of oppression at depth. One report on disability makes this point very clearly and outlines some ideas for content. 'Only those who experience disability as a form of social oppression really understand thoroughly enough to teach about its reality. It was decided by the Trainers Forum that training around disability should only be carried out by disabled people, equipped with professional training techniques and a thorough understanding of all disabled people's lifestyles within the context of a social model theory of disability' (Gillespie-Sells and Campbell, 1991).

Gillespie-Sells and Campbell outline their objectives for a training course:

1. to reach a social model of disability as opposed to an individual, medical model,
2. challenge some of the common myths and false distinctions,
3. demonstrate practical application of equal opportunities,
4. recognize that black disabled people, disabled women, disabled lesbians and gays experience multiple oppression,
5. to draft action plan for constructive changes,
6. equip participants with a working knowledge of disability which will enable them to recognize discriminatory language and stereotypical visual images (Gillespie-Sells and Campbell, 1991).

The Birmingham Citizen Advocacy Project confronts mentalism head on. Each new advocate gets a training pack in three basic sections. New advocates work with the co-ordinator. The first section defines what a mental health problem is in a valued way. What is society's response? What are our basic needs? The second section defines different types of advocacy: its history and basic principles; who needs it and who does it; what are the various roles of a citizen advocate? It looks at various conflicts and pressures. What to expect from the Citizen Advocacy Office? Why do people need advocates? The various roles of service providers. Who are advocates? What do they do? The sorts of needs advocates can meet. The third section is much more challenging. New advocates are given four scenarios to work on by themselves. They have to write their gut reaction to each story. They work through their written comments with the co-ordinator. This encourages them to look more deeply at themselves and their attitudes, many of which may be negative. Service users must examine their own internalization of social negatives about mental illness. They are certainly not immune from the effects of mentalism.

Staff training must necessarily include the increased awareness of both sexism and racism. Women and men have different experiences of psychiatry. It is often difficult for women to find their own voices in mixed sex groups. Racism is rife in the mental health services as we saw from the experience of Shuresh Patel (NHS Training Directorate, 1991). Part of this battle must include the struggle against those two evils.

Advocates' training needs will vary greatly. They may need help in listening skills and in being assertive. They may need to understand more of the labyrinth of services and what the various professionals are doing. They may need more particular help, for example, in understanding the side effects of the various drugs prescribed. They will certainly need to acquire more knowledge about the labyrinth of service systems and more skilful ways to travel round them. Mostly their training needs will be specific to the experiences of the person they support.

John Southgate defines five major roles for advocacy (Southgate, 1990):

- nurturing
- witnessing
- protesting
- translating
- supporting.

He believes that the advocate has an important nurturing function. He or she must learn to give emotional and also practical nourishment to the distressed person in ways in which they are willing and able to accept. They have been through intense periods of deprivation and loneliness and now need to be appreciated and listened to and, above all, taken extremely seriously. Frequently they will be people who are lonely and cut off from relatives with few friends and with little money. They have few reasons to trust others. The effective 'match' may involve doing things together like going to the cinema or pub, learning how the other person really is, learning to share and to trust, outside the often difficult and pathological world of psychiatric treatment. They are nourished within the advocacy relationship. They have a secure setting in which to acquire increased skills and develop confidence, this mysterious human quality. This doesn't involve getting into 'deep counselling mode', but the sustenance from ordinary friendship.

The advocate must also bear effective witness to the suffering and maltreatment of the person he or she supports. They too know what it has been like to be mistreated and now they stand in solidarity with the other and his or her pain. The survivor has someone else to watch out for him, to record the nature of the indignities. He or she has someone to watch over them. The task of the witness is to note and record what happens to the partner, who has hitherto not been believed by powerful others. Lord Shaftesbury noted the central dilemma in the early 19th century. 'What an awful condition that of a lunatic! His words are generally disbelieved, and his most innocent peculiarities perverted; it is natural that it should be so; we know him to be insane; at least we are told that he is so; and we place ourselves on guard – that is, we give to every word, look, gesture a value and meaning which oftentimes it cannot bear, and which it would never bear in ordinary life' (Skulkans, 1979).

Out of this watching, the advocate makes a protest against what has been done to the person; about how he or she has been devalued and diminished. They amplify both the nature and degree of the suffering and give a loud and clear voice to the vulnerability of the other so that people can hear who have the power to change things and understand the nature of the changes which are necessary. They are saying that the destructive things which have been happening to that person must cease. The person must be seen as being a valued individual. The 'devalued' person is no longer alone but has an impassioned and articulate defender. There is no place for the neutral in advocacy.

They translate and interpret the words and feelings of the person who is suffering to others. Not only do they know what it is like to suffer but they must also know how to make that suffering understandable to those with power. They have learned some of the professional terms and language which the powerful can understand. This language and terminology is the dominant mode. They understand some of the immense complexity of the repressive psychiatric systems. Another important interpreting function may be to help the partner understand what has happened to them in much more ordinary language and terms than offered by mental health professionals. They may need help in explaining to themselves what a 'breakdown' really means in non-psychiatric language.

Advocates must also support the inner advocacy and creativity of the individual. They nourish the belief inside him or her that things can change for the better; that something can be done to improve their situation; that there is a way out of despair and powerlessness. They support the power of the individual to speak out, his or her creative power. They encourage increased individual responsibility and power, not culpability. Peer advocates need a thorough training in all these five major roles.

Fresh structures

It is no good designing more three pin plugs if there are no appropriate power points in which to fit them. Advocates battle for a better deal for service users. Unless they are just to develop duodenal ulcers, they must meet with a sensitive service system which fully appreciates their function, or at the very least, one which is not actively hostile. Services must develop ways of seeing feedback, often very critical, as useful and even important. Accepting criticism with good grace is an important and extremely rare skill.

Professionals must also develop a variety of different roles for both current and former users, so their unique experience of the psychiatric services is seen as valued, especially by professionals. For example, in Newcastle upon Tyne, users act as consultants to keep them central to service purchasing work. The Mental Health Services Consumer group provides a small honorarium for each member. It has a monitoring role, completing some written reports on rehabilitation wards. One benefit has been the abolition of individual packages of sauce, butter and jam, all very difficult to open for many elderly residents (Barker, 1991). Lambeth Link in London has been influential in a large number of ways in the local services. For example, it is rightly concerned about the domination of the assessment process by professionals, so has designed 'community self assessment forms' to help users formulate how they see their own needs.

We must begin to involve users in the processes of selection, training and assessment of student professionals. In one imaginative venture, 21 patients helped to assess medical candidates for a psychiatric examination (Persaud and Meux, 1990). However, a sizeable minority of these patients were distressed by taking part in the examination. It seemed that patients were looking for different qualities in the medical students as compared with the professional examiners. For example, patients were seeking candidates who gave good advice, a skill not formally assessed by the examiners.

However, one study is very critical of the methodologies of much user involvement and research. It sees four major issues in collecting user feedback: obtaining a representative sample of users; asking the right questions; asking questions in an appropriate manner; understanding and interpreting the data correctly. It emphasizes methods which stress qualitative evaluation (McIver, 1991). Diversity is essential. For example, a mental health unit in East Surrey is implementing the following steps: a user group comprising past and present users; staff development and awareness training across the range of health care, social services and voluntary groups involved; customer sampling approaches including suggestion boxes, patient's satisfaction questionnaires; formation of a quality assurance group including all stakeholders; feedback information collated and made available to the planning and policy teams (McIver, 1991).

Peer advocates need formal ways of taking up issues (Beresford and Croft, 1993). They need easy and relaxed access to senior managers who can make real changes; appropriate recognition and respect from relevant professionals; a melting of traditionally defensive attitudes; as well as formal complaints procedures which work. In most of these areas, we have still much to learn from our Dutch colleagues (Brandon, 1990).

Advocacy systems

Some peer advocacy will need more formal systems and an organization. It is much too valuable a process just to be left to a few dedicated professionals or services who 'just happen to know someone who . . .' The organization must be local and comprise exclusively people who have had experience of mental health services, except for some sympathetic supporters and advisors where relevant expertise is required, as with lawyers and accountants. As Peter Campbell hinted earlier, such a formal organization brings many problems, already experienced in the citizen advocacy movement. It may stifle natural friendships; it may drift away from the formal advocacy towards informal befriending as Brighton discovered. It may tend to suffocate in petty bureaucracy, death through a million rules. That has already become a problem in the Netherlands.

Not everyone who is a mental health survivor is necessarily a suitable advocate. Some people may be too introverted, lack passion and not have the assertion skills, just like the rest of the population. A major test will be their efficacy as advocates. Mostly, the needs of the survivor will dictate the nature of the advocacy. Does this particular person have the passion, skills and discipline to get a better deal for current service users? Sometimes the answer will be no. Co-ordinators will have to exclude some people as well as encourage others.

In a recent note Peter Campbell writes: 'Any advocacy system needs to be bedded within not separated from "campaigning" type approaches. It needs to be objective but clearly committed'. There must be a close link between concerns about individuals and what is happening to them and concerns about entire systems and how we change them.

Any structure would need full co-operation from existing mental illness services whilst remaining completely independent. This will mean service structures, outlined earlier, into which feedback from advocacy can fit without too much resistance. Such structures would provide for the continuing independence of the advocacy systems and simultaneously welcome its observations. That is not an easy balance. We naturally seek to control things which cause us pain.

The schemes would offer one-to-one volunteers, both people having in common a direct experience of mental illness and the services. Paid co-ordinators, also with an experience of using services, would identify people in need of advocacy. They would recruit individual advocates with relevant experience and skills. They would also make the introductions and develop the matches. Part of the matching would lie in the similarity of experiences of the services and their 'treatment'. The co-ordinators would provide a bank of information for the use of the advocates and provide information about relevant workshops. Advocates could meet other advocates to share both triumphs and disasters.

Peer advocates would need considerable support, to see the world through the eyes of the other. Coming into this kind of advocacy might involve some of them in fierce struggles with former enemies and re-awaken old and personal battles, particularly about medication and electro-convulsive therapy (ECT). They must avoid fighting some of their particularly personal struggles at the expense of the person currently being supported. Powerful professionals may fight back with all sorts of accusations, especially that the advocate is harmful for the survivor. Advocates are ordinary human beings. They may over-identify, fail to appreciate fully the differences between the person they are supporting and their own situation. They may sexually and financially exploit their partners. Just because you've taken major tranquillisers doesn't mean you're Sir Lancelot! Just because you've tried to kill yourself doesn't mean you necessarily understand what is going through the head of another individual who has also tried it.

Advocates will need the kind of passionate and yet thoughtful support which the Birmingham service currently offers. They may also need advice from sympathetic professionals, both inside and outside the mental health services, to redress some of the immense power imbalance observed throughout this study. The advocacy organization will need an advisory board comprising people with specific skills and expertise, required by both the co-ordinator and the advocates. These skills and knowledge could be called on whenever needed. John Perceval got such early and expert advice from Dr Jean-Etienne Esquirol, the leading figure in the reform of French asylums, in Paris in the 1830s (Podvoll, 1990). It seems to have made a deep impression on him.

The core of this support would come from a local committee of other survivors. Those without direct psychiatric experience would be excluded or serve on the various advisory committees. The core group would work on their common experiences and suffering and give support to those now in similar situations. This emphasis on the common experience of oppression and distress would provide a strong ballast to the advocacy movement.

Inclusion from exclusion

Peer advocacy could be an important element in the struggle to include rather than exclude people from mainstream society. It involves a form of judo which begins to value those qualities which were hitherto devalued and dismissed. We have tens of thousands of people who have had an experience of considerable importance and relevance – of being a psychiatric patient. We must learn to use those experiences in creative ways. It might be one crucial element in a *'rite de passage'* such as Alcoholics Anonymous provides for some alcoholics, to find a useful expression for a hitherto devalued experience.

The peer support movement must be careful not to exclude some of the most marginalized, the poor and homeless as well as those who are black and female. For example, Sayal comments 'It is my belief that there is an indissoluble link between the politics of racial oppression and its psychological effects on black women . . . The use of psychiatry as a method of control and punishment of black people is on the increase and there is more encroachment of psychiatric expertise into prisons and courtrooms' (Sayal, 1990). Racism is a particular and difficult problem within the special hospital psychiatric system where some significant numbers of staff have declared links with the National Front. For example, 'The culture at the Ashworth hospital nurtures and fosters covert racism' (HMSO, 1992).

Not only ideas of mental illness but notions of positive mental health within the psychiatric world are essentially sexist and racist as well as mentalist. Mental health ideas are centred around uncovering and developing personal power, achieving personal goals. All with more than a whiff of western industrial machismo. Those seen as drastically failing these targets are frequently processed with heavy psychiatric labels.

For example, interviews with 35 Afro-Caribbean service users in Lewisham found that only four hadn't got the serious psychiatric diagnosis of schizophrenia. They felt overwhelmed by feelings of isolation. Many had been humiliated and intimidated by hospital staff and experienced direct racist abuse (Frederick, 1991). In another study, 139 practising psychiatrists completed a questionnaire showing evidence of 'race thinking' – the stereotyping of black patients which 'could lead to inappropriate management' (Lewis *et al.*, 1990). It will prove a very considerable challenge to see that these groups and others find a full voice in the new self-advocacy movement and a major role in peer advocacy. It will require fresh structures rather than the traditional white middle class committee and conference systems, which have dominated this area for so long.

Peer advocacy could be one small but significant segment in re-adjusting the enormous power imbalance between staff and service users. Paul Sayer writes powerfully of that imbalance in a beautifully moving and perceptive novel (Sayer, 1988): 'Where did they find the initiative, this animated desire to take me apart, build me up, re-invent me? I had no satisfactory answer, save the recurrent notion that somehow they were really attempting reconstruction of their own selves, imposing on me an image of the way they thought they were, or should be'.

Peer advocacy could be so important in many people's lives. There are those who could find a strong new voice on behalf of others and those who could feel that, at last, they are not alone; that there is someone beside them who can speak with skill on their behalf and at the same time knows roughly what it has been like to stand where they presently stand. Some of those will look at the peer advocate and think, if he or she can do this, then one day so could I.

REFERENCES

Adams, R. (1990) *Self-Help, Social Work and Empowerment*, Macmillan, London.
Barker, I. (1991) Agents for change. *Open Mind*, October/November.
Bateson, G. (1973) The cybernetics of 'self' – a theory of alcoholism, in *Steps to an Ecology of Mind*, Paladin, London.
Beresford, P. and Croft, S. (1993) *Citizen Involvement – A Practical Guide for Change*, Macmillan, London.
Braisby, D. (1983) *Moving Out From the Large Hospitals* (eds A. Davis and D. Towell), King's Fund, London.
Brandon, D. (1990) *Innovation without Change? Consumer Power in Psychiatric Services*, Macmillan, London.
Bynoe, I., Oliver, M. and Barnes, C. (1991) *Equal Rights for Disabled People – The Case for a New Law*, Institute for Public Policy Research.
Camden Consortium (1986) *Treated Well? A Code of Practice for Mental Hospitals.*
Chacko, R.C. (1985) The chronic patient in a community context, in *The Patient Volunteer*, American Psychiatric Press.
Chamberlin, J. (1988) *On our Own*, MIND, p. 102.
Church, K. and Revell, D. (1990) User involvement in mental health services in Canada, in *Report of Common Concerns: International Conference of User Involvement in Mental Health Services*, MIND.
Frederick, J. (1991) *Positive Thinking for Mental Health*, Black Mental Health Group.
Gillespie-Sells, K. and Campbell, J. (1991) *Disability Equality Training – Trainers Guide*, CCETSW and the London Borough Disability Resource Team.
Henry, S. (1978) The dangers of self-help groups. *New Society*, 22 June.
HMSO (1992) *Ashworth Hospital Enquiry*, pp. 148–151.
Jowell, J. (1991) *Community Care – A Prospectus for the Task*, Joseph Rowntree Foundation, York.
Keenan, B. (1992) *An Evil Cradling*, Hutchinson, London.
Keville, H. (1992) The best qualified trainers of all. *Care Weekly*, 12 November.
Lewis, G. *et al.* (1990) Are British psychiatrists racist? *British Journal of Psychiatry*, **157**, pp 410–415.
Liston, R. (1993) Campbell on the track of glory. *The Observer*, 17 January 1993.
McIver, S. (1991) *Obtaining the Views of Users of Mental Health Services*, King's Fund, London.
NHS Training Directorate (1991) *Training and User Involvement in Mental Health Services.*

O'Brien, J. (1987) *Learning from Citizen Advocacy Programs*. Georgia Advocacy Office, p. 5.

Patmore, C. (1988) Is patient power coming to Britain? *Community Psychiatry – its Practice and Management*, 3, November.

Persaud, R.D. and Meux, C.J. (1990) Clinical examinations for professional qualification in psychiatry: the patient's view. *Psychiatric Bulletin*, **14**, pp. 65–71.

Podvoll, E.M. (1990) *The Seduction of Madness*, Harper Collins, London.

Priestly, P. (1975) New careers: power sharing in social work, in *Towards a New Social Work*, (ed. H. Jones), Routledge & Kegan Paul, London.

Pymn, B. (1989) Run it your own way. *Community Care*, 6 April.

Rippere, V. and Williams, R. (eds) (1985) *Wounded Healers – Mental Health Workers Experiences of Depression*, John Wiley, Chichester.

Robinson, D. and Henry, S. *Self-Help and Health, Mutual Aid for Modern Problems*, Martin Robertson, Oxford.

Sagarin, E. (1969) *Odd Man In: Societies of Deviants in America*, Quadrangle Books, Chicago.

Sayal, A. (1990) Black women and mental health. *The Psychologist*, January.

Sayer, P. (1988) *The Comforts of Madness*, Sceptre Books, Sevenoaks.

Skulkans, V. (1979) *English Madness: Ideas on Insanity 1580–1890*, Routledge & Kegan Paul, London.

A Manifesto for Change: The User's Viewpoint (1991) South Glamorgan Mental Health Users Alliance.

Southgate, J. (1990) Towards a dictionary of advocacy based self analysis. *Journal of the Institute for Self Analysis*, **4** (1), December.

Steele, T. (1992) Friends and mentors. *Midland News*, March, pp. 12–13.

Sutherland, S. (1977) *Breakdown*, Paladin, London.

Trevillion, S. (1992) *Caring in the Community – A Networking Approach to Community Participation*, Longman, Harlow.

Williams, K. (1992) in *The Ashworth Hospital Enquiry Report*. HMSO, p. 146.

World Health Organization (1989) *Consumer Involvement in Mental Health and Rehabilitation Services*, Division of Mental Health, WHO, Geneva.

7

The third age: a consideration of groups and their activities

Tony Chiva

INTRODUCTION

This section will provide an overview of third age self-help groups. It proposes that these groups work to meet the fundamental needs of participants and that they impact in a variety of ways on society as a whole.

A third age self-help group is a group set up by or established to meet the needs of people in the third age, i.e. people in their 50s and beyond. They may be of a self-help or mutual support kind. These groups may be relatively short-lived in operational terms. Self-help and mutual support groups can be seen as voluntary, small group structures for mutual aid and the accomplishment of a purpose (Katz and Bender, 1976). The benefits to the members of the group are not consistent, and can be of variable quality (Wenger, 1993).

Third agers have been variously described. In the context of this chapter the third age can be considered as the period in a person's life when their main form of occupation is no longer economic activity or child-rearing. There is no upper age limit to the third age since mental and physical ability can remain with people until their death, at any age. A fourth age is not obligatory, and its commencement is not chronologically determined (Laslett, 1989). This contrasts with the Carnegie Inquiry which has placed an upper limit of 74 years on the third age (Carnegie, 1993).

This chapter will not seek to identify all the third age groups that currently operate, but will rather focus on some examples of main kinds and their roles. It will emphasize the integrative function of these groups and the holistic way they allow/enable people to maintain or develop a way of life or role within their community. These groups therefore have or can have an empowering function. However, some self-help groups which may be organized autocratically using directive processes may be helpful in some aspects of an individual's life, but not necessarily empowering (Caserta and Lund, 1993).

Generally speaking there are not many different self-help and mutual support groups for older people. In most geographical areas there are a few key groups which have often been successfully operating in other areas. The self-help groups (SHGs) most frequently encountered are: socially based groups such as residential groups or dinner clubs, universities of the third age (U3A), pensioners' forums or conventions, retired members/fellowship groups such as Transport and General Workers Union retired members group or Friends in Retirement (FIRcones).

Third agers often have key roles in other self-help groups, though these groups are not solely dedicated to third agers. In a voluntary capacity, many third agers commit themselves to supporting self-help groups in which they have an interest and which are not solely dedicated to third age issues.

THIRD AGE GROUPS

The typology that will be used to subdivide third age self-help groups is based on their overall functions (Adams, 1990). There are three basic kinds: problem-solving; self-development; and consciousness-raising, though it must be borne in mind that there will be overlaps between the functions of groups within these categories.

- Problem-solving self-help groups undertake activities to help individuals or others face specific problems.
- Self-development self-help groups have a wide variety of activities with an educational, social and personal development focus.
- Consciousness-raising self-help groups benefit the individual and may
  involve a social change aspect.

Functions of the three main kinds of self-help groups

There are some functions that the three main kinds of third age groups have in common and some which are mainly found in consciousness-raising and not problem-solving self-help groups. It is important to remember that third age self-help groups are not static; the membership of groups varies from time to time, some groups can change the services or benefits of membership as they evolve, officers on the executive or management group may change or the group may alter in response to changes in the wider community.

The responsiveness of self-help groups to these factors is very variable and may depend on the organizational structure of the self-help group. For example, the way the self-help group sees itself and its membership: is it a democratically led group? Does it see itself as responding to the changing needs of its members? Does it see itself as providing some core functions which are relatively fixed in nature and scope?

All three kinds of self-help groups: have the following in common: they provide mutual support to people in a similar position; they develop ways (perhaps of different existing provision) to meet the needs of their members; they disseminate information; they maintain contacts with other organizations and fundraise.

Functions that are more likely to be the prerogative of the problem-solving self-help groups are: dissatisfaction with services currently made available, e.g. public health or social services; this relates to their need to maintain a 'watch-dog' function; and the desire to raise funds to improve knowledge and concern about the issues involved.

The consciousness-raising groups have a dissatisfaction related to their area of concern. This is based around the need for a major change in the social systems that have constructed a particular view which the consciousness-raising self-help groups challenge. Therefore they operate to influence socio-political perceptions and seek positive action in the areas of their concern.

Both problem-solving and self-development groups will provide some services and practical help to their members, as may the consciousness-raising group. The self-development group will be providing information which seeks to enable members of the group to make changes themselves.

Main types of third age groups in each category

Some examples of self-help groups within the problem-solving category are the Alzheimer's group, Age Well groups, peer health volunteer groups, senior health mentors, and dinner clubs. The Age Well, peer health, senior health mentors and dinner clubs may, for some of the functions, become more like a self-development group.

In the self-development category some examples are Older Women's Networks, culturally bound social groups, University of the Third Age (U3A), retired person associations and groups, Association of Retired Persons, pensioners' rights groups, and grandparenting groups. Older Women's Network, U3As and pensioners' rights groups may for some of their functions become more like the consciousness-raising group.

The consciousness-raising category includes such groups as

pensioners' elderly forums, Pensioners' Voice, Pensioners' Convention, Pensioner Action Group (Sheffield) and older lesbian women groups.

Exploring the problem-solving category

This category contains the numerous groups which are established to help people, such as patients, their friends or relatives, cope with a particular problem. Often the particular problem is a health problem, though few health problems are solely limited to third agers. Third agers are the group that either experience the problem first hand because they face the health issue in themselves or because they are the carers. Additionally, and this applies to the other categories, third agers often establish or are the key players in many self-help or mutual support groups because of their valuable life experience, and frequent desire to give something back to others or to the community.

Problem-solving groups arise and are sometimes established by professionals because the individuals need greater support than can be or is provided by statutory or agency services. The self-help groups' main purposes are support of people with particular conditions or their relatives. Often the groups become expert in their understanding and knowledge of the condition. At this point they can become political, seeking to influence current medical practice, governmental allocation of resources and research undertaken. This is then a raising of the profile of the condition – a raising of the general public's awareness with the associated raising of priority in people's consciousness (at this point there is a connection with the functions of the consciousness-raising group). The individual member will probably gain an identity with others and a greater sense of self.

In summary, these groups then seek to support their members, mobilize specialist and public opinion, increase the body of knowledge concerning the condition and gain financial support for improving the situation for people facing the problem, the 'sufferers'.

At this stage in the development/evolution of a problem-solving self-help group they may have some of the characteristics of the self-development or consciousness-raising categories – depending on the emphasis and ways the self-help group seeks to 'influence' their members, and social and political systems.

From a holistic point of view, these groups may or may not consider the person as more than their condition. However, generally because of the likely discrimination against the group, an advocacy element relating to the whole person will probably become linked to the problem-solving self-help group.

Exploring the self-development category

It would appear that the majority of third age groups are within this category which includes the main elements of social contact and education.

This includes Older Women's Network, culturally bound social groups, U3A, Association of Retired Persons (ARP), pensioners' rights groups, and grandparenting groups.

The main groups that will be considered in this category are:

- Jubilados – social function (mainly),
- U3A – educational function (largely),
- Retired persons associations or groups – support, welfare and campaigning functions.

Club de Jubilados Espanoles de Londres

Jubilados group in London was established in co-operation with the Spanish Embassy to be a focus for social and cultural events for Spanish elders living in London. Jubilados is the Spanish word for pensioner. The group meets to be 'jubilant' about their age, several times in the week and has both afternoon and evening activities. This group, like other culturally bound groups, enables its members to participate and share their own culture and language. In providing this support Spanish elders who may feel isolated within a broader community gain a greater sense of themselves.

The Jubilados group has an executive committee consisting of third agers. The club provides a friendly meeting place for Spanish people. They can attend when they wish, and participate in a range of general activities, ranging from card games to discussion on relevant issues.

The Jubilados arrange special events such as meals/celebrations, trips in England and Spain. Some financial and practical support to the Jubilados Espanoles is provided by the Spanish Embassy. Additionally, contacts with other organizations, like Pensioners' Link, has enabled native (Spanish) speakers to learn to speak and write English more effectively.

In summary, Jubilados has increased its membership and has a mainly social function; this function underpins the value placed on the sharing arising from cultural identity. There are comparable groups to this for many other cultures, usually located in the larger cities.

University of the Third Age (U3A)

This has been established in England, Scotland, Wales and Northern Ireland for 11 years, and within Europe for 21 years. U3A, in the UK, has been expanding rapidly and has increased by 25% both in terms of membership and new groups established in the last few years.

U3A is organized locally and there are currently 245 local autonomous groups with 40 000 members in total, composed mainly of people over 50 years old. Each local group establishes its own programmes, electing representatives to a national executive committee.

Local U3As charge a low annual fee to attend or participate in as many 'groups' as they wish. The fee is kept low to increase access to older people and because the 'group' convenors and programme organizers give their time freely and are older people themselves.

U3A groups around the UK seek to offer a balance within their programmes to include social, educational and physical elements. Socially, meetings are established for purposes of friendship, organization and administration of the U3A. The educational activities may range from the practical such as crafts, to the aesthetic such as creative writing and art history, to the academic such as philosophy, technology and environmental studies. Physical activities may include walking, swimming, yoga and badminton.

U3A groups do not award qualifications in the UK, though its members sometimes choose to attend award-bearing courses. The purpose of U3A groups in the view of Peter Laslett (1989) is shared learning; where the 'teacher' is the 'learner' and the 'learner' is the 'teacher'. This democratic, student-centred approach is reflected in the movement as a whole.

More recently in the U3A at the national level, a number of developments are taking place. A third age newspaper is produced. An annual conference with a summer school is run. National subject networks are being established to link U3A members from local groups; these include pen friends, art and music, languages, walking, bird watching, and science and technology. Networks develop seminars, field trips, papers and local meetings. An interpreter and translation network available to the community was especially established for the European Year of Older People and Solidarity between Generations which took place in 1993. Local U3As are piloting Open University courses. The practice of shared learning is being applied currently to science and technology without an 'expert' convenor. This particularly is a challenge to perceived views on education where it is assumed that an 'expert' is needed to explore complex issues, such as science. Shared learning is about people sharing experience and understanding and relating this to the context of their lives. Certainly to understand complex issues there will be a need for clear information and some clarity of understanding. U3As assume that people can achieve this with some focused attention. It is locally and nationally seeking to evaluate its own effectiveness and is undertaking research into different aspects of its function, including the process of shared learning.

U3A is a special example of a self-help group, which has retained its autonomy and volunteer status despite conflicting pressures and demands. In doing so they have retained a democratic style with shared learning as the desired goal, a holistic approach to older people and their developmental needs.

Retired persons' groups/associations

Retired persons' associations (RPA) often arise because of a perceived common background and the need, under the pressure of life change, to maintain existing and develop new contacts with people in a similar position (PRA, 1992; PRA and ReAction Trust, 1994). On this basis retired persons' groups often arise at places of employment. These are sometimes supported and encouraged by employers, especially if they have post-retirement policies for their ex-employees.

Usually RPAs are established by the retirees themselves often as a consequence of a pre-retirement course, though frequently welfare, personnel or pensions officers within companies play a key role in their initial establishment of RPAs. Some RPAs arise from other kinds of 'collective' such as those of trade unions or professional bodies.

The main purposes of RPAs are to provide a means for members to remain in social contact and to develop shared interests. The RPAs can vary in responsiveness to their members. Some local RPAs may have very small memberships whilst others can include many thousands.

RPAs that remain connected to former employers can provide useful feedback to the employer on conditions, human resource policies and may be able to provide functional consultancy. RPAs receive feedback from their membership so that factors that ex-employees identify as unhelpful can now be raised through the RPA officers with the human resource staff of the employer. This has happened, for example, in connection with information on pensions being given to employees prior to their attendance at pre-retirement courses, the need for earlier preparation for retirement and how ex-employees from the RPA can be used on short-term or part-time contracts for specific purposes.

Consciousness-raising category

This category includes groups which benefit individuals and have a social action function. An implicit and explicit role is therefore changing the circumstances in which members of the group find themselves. These circumstances may be social, political or economic. Socially constructed values can limit a group, their opportunities and potential.

Through social action by a particular group, currently held negative 'world views' can be deconstructed and changed to more positive ones. In this context many groupings of older people with a 'campaigning' element operate, including pensioners' forums, pensioners' conventions, pension action groups (pensioners' rights) and many of the trade union retired members' groups.

The broad focus of these groups is seeking to raise awareness and to change the way older people are treated socially, politically or economically. In many ways later 20th century society does not value the 'spirit' of older people. The elder within the elderly is largely being forgotten or dismissed. Our task-oriented, problem-focused culture devalues the multiple 'unseen' and forgotten qualities inherent among older people. The social construction of retirement and early retirement reduces the 'permitted' economic contribution of older people to the negligible (Itzin and Phillipson, 1993). The convenient stereotypes of older people as non-citizens, non-active, withdrawn, with an irrelevant contribution means they can remain unseen and unheard, voiceless participants in a multigenerational society. It is against this backdrop that these consciousness-raising third age groups campaign for the basic rights of older people. The campaign is necessarily fought with all age groups and political and economic systems. Sheffield Pensioners Action Group have stated 'We have the power to change things and to be seen as a democratic force across a broad spectrum'. Unfortunately, because of discriminatory stereotyping, older people sometimes see themselves as limited and ineffective aged beings. Pensioners' forums and action groups, for example, have to work equally hard, or harder, to encourage active participation of older people as to generate the effective use and allocation of resources on behalf of older people, and other groups.

This aspect of consciousness raising for the group or membership is part of the major task for these self-help groups. Sheffield Pensioners Action Group widely circulate their own paper called *Senior Citizen*. Other groups do the same.

The Older Women's Lesbian Group indicate that society's consciousness concerning the rights of lesbian women is impoverished and that normative beliefs inhibit and label older lesbian women. This discounting puts a pressure on lesbians to conform and can create devalued and unhappy older women, increasing the sense of isolation and dependency already part of the social construction of old age, and indeed lesbianism.

The consciousness-raising self-help group in many ways can be seen as the final product of self-help groups if the essential element of social action is included. Not that holistic self-help groups move inevitably from problem solving through self-development to consciousness raising. The challenge of social action may be greater or less than the challenge to other types of self-help groups. Inevitably social action implies a change in social values and norms, a reconstruction of societal perceptions. This is a major challenge for any group and yet there have been detectable shifts in societal perceptions due to the action of groups. Pensioners' forums have, within their local areas, created changes in the attitudes of local government decision makers. This has applied particularly with respect to consultation where the existence of a pensioners' forum has influenced local authority perceptions, so that they now automatically think 'We need to find out what our older residents think of this' (Carter and Nash, 1992). Peer health has positively influenced attitudes of older people to activity and increased their self-confidence (Nash and Chiva, 1993). They also feel more satisfied with their own lives and believe they are giving something back to the community. These may not be major societal shifts in attitudes but on a local microeconomic level can be significant in themselves.

SUMMARY

The need for third age self-help or mutual support groups will only arise as an awareness of need is perceived by the individual or group. The majority of local third age groups are based around a social function rather than the political or social change aspect. Third agers have a lifetime of experience which they choose to invest in activities and interests which please them and satisfy their needs. The imperative for forming a self-help group to meet a fundamental need will only arise when individuals either have a pre-existing awareness of the benefits of such groupings or where the motivation to form such a group is very high.

Third age self-help groups, like other self-help groups, vary in the length of time they exist and flourish. Dynamic shifts take place in short periods of time.

The social and economic patterns of the late 20th century have involved drastic changes and will create different needs for existing and later cohorts of third agers (Laslett and Fishkin, 1992). In consequence where third agers express or have a perceived need, relevant self-help and mutual support groups will arise.

There are still areas where there is a lack of groups such as those involving men; social contacts for the very isolated, depressed and lonely; and networks for new widows or widowers.

Problems with the natural holistic evolution of self-help and mutual support groups are many. These include: the natural reticence of many (older) people; the commonly held belief that things are 'fixed' and unchangeable; the uncertainty of relating to others as opposed to being solely reliant on self; and the 'energy' needed to commit oneself to such a group.

These factors inhibit the development of third age mutual support and self-help groups. Indeed the culture of third age groups has tended towards isolation or purely social groupings, apart from those in military service, strong labour unions, brother/sisterhoods and professional groupings. This has mostly created negative perceptions of individual and collective power and unfortunately does not reflect the enormous latent and potential power within the group known as the third agers or the economic, social and political power and influence of older people as a whole.

Third age self-help and mutual support groups have mainly arisen by the focused and consistent efforts of individuals/groups committed to the establishment of particular educational or social activities for others. This element of consciousness among third agers creates positive trends, and the successful establishment of local groups committed to particular activities as action. The University of the Third Age is a good example of the way a movement can spread when a need is expressed or perceived.

The future of third age self-help and mutual support groups is certain. Clearly, the changing socio-economic climate will create the need for new 'routes' to achieve and maintain the distinctive values inherent in particular third age groups.

The nature of a third age group in itself is misleading, implying a suggestion of homogeneity; this is not the case. It may be that within a particular subculture of a group certain beliefs or values predominate. This would not hold true for the rest of that group where very different beliefs and values may be current.

This makes the effects of third age groups on society even more challenging because the society being influenced includes other third agers. The challenge to third agers generally and to third age self-help groups in particular is to recreate an image of their valuable role within a multigenerational society. The building of confidence and purpose among third agers is a positive effect of many self-development and consciousness-raising groups. Some third age groups encourage inter-generational activities such as 'adopt a grandparent' for school children.

A concern of third age self-help groups is the impact they can have on changing the way the media negatively presents older people. The more impact third agers have the greater will be shifts in societal attitudes to the positive value of persons of all ages.

The role of third age self-help groups is becoming clearer but the message is not always easy to convey. The need for commitment and insight is demanding, and challenging for third agers. However, the need to empower and support all ages within our multigenerational society cannot only be the responsibility of these third age self-help groups.

REFERENCES

Adams, R. (1990) *Self-Help, Social Work and Empowerment*. Macmillan Educational Ltd, Basingstoke.

Carnegie Inquiry into the Third Age (1993) *Life, Work and Livelihood in the Third Age*, Carnegie United Kingdom Trust, Dunfermline.

Carter, T. and Nash, C. (1992) *Pensioners' Forums: An Active Voice*, Pre-Retirement Association, Guildford, Surrey.

Caserta, M.S. and Lund, D.A. (1993) Intrapersonal resources and the effectiveness of self-help groups for bereaved older adults. *Gerontologist*, **33** (5), pp. 619–629.

Itzin, C. and Phillipson, C. (1993) *Age Barriers at Work – Maximising the Potential of Mature and Older People*, Metropolitan Authorities Recruitment Board, London.

Katz, A.H. and Bender, E.I. (1976) *The Strength in Us – Self-help Groups in the Modern World*, New Viewpoints, New York.

Laslett, P. (1989) *A Fresh Map of Life – the Emergence of the Third Age*, Weidenfeld and Nicolson, London.

Laslett, P. and Fishkin, J.S. (1992) *Justice Between Age Groups and Generations*, Yale University Press, London.

Nash, C. and Chiva, A. (1993) Older volunteers as change agents. Paper given at conference on *Caring for the Elderly in the Community*, Community Research Institute, Plymouth University, April 13–16, Plymouth, UK.

Pre-Retirement Association (1992) *Work in Later Life*. Conference report, occasional paper No 6, Pre-Retirement Association, Guildford, Surrey.

Pre-Retirement Association and ReAction Trust (1994) *The Challenge of Carnegie – Strategies for Work in Later Life*, Standing Conference, Pre-Retirement Association and ReAction Trust, Guildford, Surrey.

Wenger, G.C. (1993) The formation of social networks: self-help, mutual aid and old people in contemporary Britain. *Journal of Ageing Studies*, **7** (1), pp. 25–40.

8

Not too 'grey' power

Jack Thain

THE HISTORY

Perhaps it would be justified to explain why the title of this chapter tries to take away the image of 'grey power' that seems synonymous with other pensioner movements across the world.

There are several movements of older people, although mainly in America and Australia, some very politically active and some very wealthy, calling themselves Grey Panthers, Grey Power or similar names. The British movement has never tried to emulate them, especially if there is political or commercial dominance in the original organizations. Yet it is in complete solidarity with all who are engaged in a genuine fight for the justice and the pride of their country's elder citizens. A magazine called *Grey Power* is even a serious and influential outlet for trade union and other retired people's associations in Britain, which is distributed mainly in the North.

The National Pensioners' Convention (NPC) is the only umbrella group for most of the main pensioners' movements in the UK. The NPC brings together the following organizations: active trade union retired members' associations, called RMAs; large county-based pensioner movements such as those of East Anglia; national independent pensioner organizations such as Pensioners' Voice and Pensioners' Rights and a combined independent trade union and non-union members' organization under the name of the British Pensioners and Trade Union Action Association. In addition, there are a multitude of Pensioner Forums, which bring together other groups of active pensioners, covering the whole UK.

We now have, in the NPC, something that many governments have longed to obtain: a unification of many organizations with entirely differing structures and backgrounds, being able to speak with one voice and move in one direction to support a very vulnerable section of our society.

However, the ramifications of the National Pensioners' Convention go beyond these islands with connections in other parts of Europe and the world, about which more will be said later.

The aims of the NPC are to bring equality of basic living standards to all European elderly people, in particular those of the UK. Where these conditions fall below a given level for human dignity, the NPC aims to fight, within the law, to put matters right. To do this the organization is stated as being across party political boundaries but as a campaigning group falls foul of the British charity laws, which state, in approximate terms, 'that any organization that sets itself up to oppose political acts of government, no matter that they may be seen as supporting those disadvantaged by such acts, cannot be deemed to be a charity'. Such activities have to be funded by themselves and preclude them from charitable grants. In that context the NPC is completely worked by volunteers erasing the idea that the elders of this country are a grey cloud in the background of the life of the community to be ignored by all, and, in particular, governments.

The question that is often debated is: How did it all start?

There are many organizations bringing together elderly people, some of which have been in existence for a number of years, while others are quite young. Although they work hard for their members it was soon realized, by one man in particular, that scattered movements were not going to be listened to, more so as the British political thought seemed to be becoming more polarized and the Conservative Party was starting to show a leaning to the extreme right of the political spectrum. Therefore, before he retired from his position as General Secretary of the Transport and General Workers Union, Jack Jones laid plans for an amalgamation of pensioner movements under one very powerful, but democratically run umbrella organization.

Upon retirement he was appointed president of his union's retired members section. Scorning offered honours for his work as a trade union leader, he set about the task of bringing together first of all the very important retired members sections of other unions and later on, the even more scattered self-governing organizations within the larger field of retirees.

'Our Jack', a name of endearment given to Jack Jones by his union colleagues, or as he was once headlined: 'That Old Fox of Smith Square', knew his business when it came to persuasion. He enlisted the support of his many very powerful friends, both in office and retirement.

The founding document of the National Pensioners' Convention was made public on 26 March 1979 at a press conference authorized by the then general secretary of the Trades Union Congress (TUC), Lionel Murray.

The TUC's press officer released the information to the main press, radio and television networks that the first ever National Pensioners' Convention would be held at the Central Hall, Westminster, on Thursday 14 June 1979 and the following affirmation would form the opening of the debate, 'That every pensioner has the right to choice, dignity, independence and security as an integral and valued member of society'.

About 2000 people were expected at this assembly and the attendance exceeded even this estimation.

At that first press conference, besides Lionel Murray and Jack Jones, were Donald Hobman of Age Concern, Hugh Falkner of Help the Aged, Fred Baker of the British Pensioners and Trade Union Action Committee and George Dunn of the National Federation of Old Age Pensioners. This attested to the paramount desire of the key elders' organizations to have one co-ordinated voice speaking for the older citizens of this country.

PENSIONERS AND POLITICS

It must be remembered that at this time in the history of the NPC, the TUC was playing the main part as not only provider but motivator. In fact up until 3 March 1988 the chairmanship of the NPC was held by the then General Secretary of the TUC, with Jack Jones holding the position of vice chairman.

The time was fast approaching when the NPC must stand on its own, if it was to survive and become a powerful mediator. At the same time, it was also recognized that to attract organizations that were not of trade union origin or attached to any political party, it had to declare the intention of being divorced from party political leanings. This would allow it to carry out a campaign to right the wrongs being done to those already retired, yet allow it to disregard the colour of any government.

The critics of the above idea suggested that to have such a programme would put it into the political spotlight, because any change asked for or given must be made within political restraints. Yet one does not say that teachers of religion in multi-racial schools are biased towards any one religion, just because they have to work within that wide field.

The NPC knew their critics would try to label them, so they set out to prove such people wrong, a very difficult task when one government has been in office so long.

The political pendulum was once again swinging to the right. In April 1979, the leader of the Conservative government, Mrs Thatcher, was to alter drastically the income of state pensioners, by removing the link with the average wage index and instead attaching any rise to the retail price index. The result was to deny the elder citizens their rightful share in the country's still growing wealth which they had done more than most to ensure.

At 1993/1994 entitlement, the state pension was £89.80 per week for a couple and £56.10 for a single person. This follows the adjustment from the average wage index to the retail price index. We can equate the loss to a married couple, the wife having a pension of the husband's national insurance contributions, of approximately £20 per week. This point was recognized not only by the NPC but also the TUC speaking for its member trade unions. Later on the non-trade union retired members associations wanted to take up the fight.

Unwittingly Mrs Thatcher did more to unite these other pensioner movements than anybody else, by allegedly saying 'Pensioner movements? Let them organize and speak with one voice, then and only then will I listen'. This seemingly arrogant remark spread like wildfire. The NPC was now firmly in place with support from not only trade union retired members sections but from the faster evolving county and national organizations. In a two-day congress hosted by the Birmingham City Council, Jack Jones was confirmed as President with Joan Hall of the British Trade Union Action Association and Wilf Page of the Norfolk and Norwich Pensioners Association as supporting Vice Presidents. To complete the team were an already elected general secretary, Jack Thain, treasurer, Cyril Marshal, and minute secretary, Christine Osborne.

At this congress the Declaration of Intent was formed, placing on record the objectives and basis of all future actions of the NPC. This left people outside the organization in no doubt about the parameters within which the fight was to be held to promote a better quality of life for state pensioners.

The NPC's Declaration clearly describes the principles it holds dear, not only for its members but for all those elders who are not in a position to speak for themselves.

THE PRINCIPLES

The Declaration of Intent was formed on 24 April 1992 and with additions as agreed by full council on 2 September 1992.

THIS CONVENTION DECLARES THAT every pensioner has the right to choice, dignity, independence and security as an integral and valued member of society.

These rights require an adequate State Retirement Pension. Although we seek concessions, we adhere to this central aim of an adequate pension to enable pensioners to pay their way.

There must be an immediate commitment to a pension level of

not less than one half of average gross earnings for a married couple, equal to £152 per week (1993 values) and not less than one third of average gross earnings for a single person, equal to £101 per week (1993 values). This to be up-rated at six monthly intervals by the increase in gross average earnings or the increase in the cost of living index, whichever is the greater. (These required incomes should not be confused with the loss figure as shown previously as they hold an additional requirement to remove means testing.) There should be an additional flat-rate pension, non-means tested, for those over 75 years of age, and a further payment at the age of 80 years, to be increased annually in line with the RPI or average wage index, whichever is the greater. Other benefit levels should be adjusted accordingly. Further, as soon as possible, ALL ELDERLY PEOPLE SHOULD RECEIVE THE FULL BASIC PENSION, REGARDLESS OF SEX OR MARITAL STATUS. In addition to an adequate income pensioners should as right:

i) Live in accommodation which is appropriate to personal needs and circumstances, with a reasonable degree of choice, including sheltered housing.

ii) Be able to call upon the full range of non-means tested community and personal services to give full support as the need arises, e.g. home care (including domestic help), 'meals on wheels', chiropody, television and telephone.

iii) Be able to use national schemes for free travel facilities on all public transport and in all parts of the country, with appropriate facilities for disabled people. (In view of the wide disparity in the availability and types of existing travel concessions throughout the country, a national scheme be introduced involving the levelling-up of the existing arrangements to the same equality of the best schemes in operation.)

iv) Have access to comprehensive free health care on demand.

v) Be able to maintain a warm and well lit home with additional heating payments for all pensioner households from October to March of each year.

vi) Be paid a tax-free Christmas bonus restored to its 1972 purchasing power and adjusted annually in line with inflation.

vii) Be eligible for an adequate retirement pension on ceasing work at any time of his or her choice after the age of 60 years.

viii) Be entitled to an adequate death grant irrespective of age.

ix) Be relieved of standing charges on gas, telephone, electricity and water.

x) Have the right to be consulted by central or local government and public utilities over plans that might affect their lives.

THE ACTIVITIES

The NPC's movement now consolidated and started to increase in membership numbers as it became more widely recognized as 'the pensioner authority'. Meetings were held with Ministers, the All-Party Parliamentary Pensioner Committee of the House of Commons, the Carnegie Third Age Enquiry, the British Medical Association, and many other authoritative bodies relating to the elderly and their place in society.

Age Concern England gave a valuable measure of support when the NPC was in its embryonic stage by helping to arrange meetings, offering committee rooms and office facilities. They continue to do so to this day by gathering information, specialized data and statistics. Their regional offices have given the same backing in the field, by sharing their knowledge, publications and statistical material with the NPC's member organizations.

By now, the associated individual members were in excess of one million and the ramifications of the movement stretched across the country into Wales, Scotland and Northern Ireland. As events and actions took place in the form of controlled marches, rallies and public meetings, held in the name of the NPC or its associate member organizations, the media took more interest. From that source of information, applications came in from other campaigning pensioner groups asking to join. The NPC now outstripped, in associated numbers of people, any of the main political parties and yet it had not tested the mettle of the government in confrontation. This was yet to come.

With an arrogance, or an ignorance, which only political historians will be able to untangle, the government of this period appeared to ignore or only pay lip-service to this massive body of voters by pushing through such measures as VAT on domestic fuel and power, knowing that the elderly would be a group who would suffer the most, since they require ample supplies of each to survive any harsh winter. True, an offering was made from the government for small sums of money to ease the burden imposed; these were not sufficient to meet all of the new costs and there was no guarantee they would last for ever. During this period the state pension, although increased by inflation figures on a yearly basis, was losing its value against the average pay in the country. Many newspapers and experts in elderly affairs were predicting that by the year 2010, the purchasing value of the state pension will have moved so far down in relation to wage earning purchasing power that it will be hardly worth having. The NPC gave voice to these fears whenever it could and kept up its demand to return the yearly increases to the average wage index.

While continuing its campaigning role, the NPC turned its sights to instruction forums for its members and, hesitatingly, it tested these waters with friends in the academic field. But it had to leave it to the individual member organizations to start up educational forums and schools due to the lack of grants to fund central facilities and pay staff.

The aim was that every retired person, no matter what their background or educational level, should have the opportunity to learn how to run an organization, speak in public or to the media. Also to be able to approach, with the confidence of true knowledge, those in public life who hold the power over their actions and lives. Above all, to use their training to break through the red tape of bureaucracy. With training and confidence many more retired people would be able to use their hidden talents for the good of the many.

The NPC has never said that all they want is just the 'good life' for their members. What they advocate is that all those who retire, for whatever purpose, and at whatever age, after a lifetime of work, should have sufficient, secure financial means, leaving them to live their retirement in dignity and with pride of place in our society. At the same time they should be able to benefit from a secure health and community care system.

Great Britain needs all the help it can get to hold its place in the future world and alongside its diminishing workforce should stand a back-up force of retirees, similar in concept to that of the Territorial Army; well-trained, well-looked after and paid. They would be proud of their place and should not be taken for granted or as semi-slave labour to be used or thrown aside at the will of politicians who only see them as a drain on the economy and the resources of those still working.

Unfortunately, the NPC was diverted a little from its path in 1993. That year, as many will remember, was designated the 'European Year of the Elder Person and Solidarity between Generations'. It was a great idea emanating from the EC Commission and supported by the Department of Health. The officers and associate members of the NPC gave a great deal of time to its ideals and many functions took place. There were exchanges with European countries and most of the charities within this country played a part, alongside the younger generation through schools and clubs. For the organizers, within the confines of Age Concern England who worked so very hard, and the participants it was a success and the onward theme is worth progressing. However, for the NPC this pretty picture must end as 1993 could be also called 'The year of an attack on the welfare state', since it stretched the resources of campaigning bodies to the limit.

Two successive Chancellors of the government, seeing a large public sector debt, took the time-honoured path of easing the burden by curbing public spending, in one way or another, on the poorest in the land, since it is they, according to the government, who through no fault of their own use more of the country's welfare resources than it is claimed the country can afford. As an explanation: when the great Beveridge plan was conceived and implemented to take care of the people of this country, no matter what their station in life, from the 'cradle to the grave', much of the wealth to cover this great high water mark in social history, which included the state pension, came from the pay packets of the workers and the employers. Nobody in the political spectrum seemed to look ahead to say what would happen if there were not enough pay packets or employers to foot the bill. Also nobody looked far enough ahead to see that medical science would advance so much that people could live longer. Nobody foresaw the statistical bulge in numbers of elderly people seeking retirement or the diminishing of the large family unit. Faced with all these facts and a large public spending budget, it was decided that the poor could not be looked after in the manner required by an earlier generation, in either health or wealth.

Lower interest rates were hitting those just above the targeted benefit level, while the rich were enjoying lower tax rates and giving themselves larger and larger incomes and perks. As an example of the changes between 1979 and 1993 a Member of Parliament's salary rose from £9450 per annum to £30 854, trying to keep in line with civil service pay scales. At the same time their office cost allowance rose from £4600 per year to £39 960. Over the same period the state pensioners had a reported 42% increase up to £2917 per annum for a single person and for a married couple £4669. The percentage figure was not strictly accurate as it appeared to contain rises in additional benefit monies as well as the basic pension. It will be noted that *pro rata* any increase in the basic costs of such things as telephones, gas, water, electricity, public transport fares, clothes, footware or food would be a greater burden to the pensioners than, say, an MP or a captain of industry.

The overwhelming sidetracking of the NPC's plans for that year came about not only because they had to fight those problems mentioned above, but the heaviest blow of all was the imposition over the two years 1994 and 1995 of value added tax on domestic fuel, power and their standing charges. This unfeeling act had to be fought tooth and nail and on 29 June 1993, after much planning and research plus a vast amount of mailing and advertising, the NPC had the support of 14 000 elderly people to lobby Parliament. They came from the far corners of the UK, and on that day some 4000 squeezed into the Central Hall at Westminster to hear Jack Jones, their leader, MPs and officers of various sections of the movement tell them to make as much fuss and speak with as many of their own Members of Parliament as possible.

The response was magnificent, the cheering could be heard right across Westminster, while outside the House of Commons people queued in the sunshine waiting to get in to have their say.

Then tragedy struck. Around Westminster, Central Hall and in Parliament itself thronged the media. Television cameras were pointed at people who, in their normal lives, might never have been seen on television, radio broadcasts were being prepared, while reporters asked thousands of questions. Yet the drama for the NPC was unfolding in another place. Michael Mates MP, junior minister for Northern Ireland, had resigned his post over a thoughtless gesture in support of somebody he thought had been wronged. On 29 June he got up in the House of Commons and made his resignation speech. We lost 95% of our media coverage, so once again the pensioners' protest was outflanked by an unforeseen event.

Despite this setback the foregoing shows the strength of this umbrella grouping of the nation's campaigning pensioner movements, because on 20 October of the same year, they, with the support of the *Sunday Mirror*, Age Concern and Help the Aged, mounted another onslaught by a lobby of Parliament. This time the leader of the Labour Party came in to speak on their behalf, as well as leading members of the other two parties and high officers of various charities.

The NPC can, and will, mount similar protests no matter the colour of the government of the day, if it sees, as at present, an unjustified attack from any quarter on the people it represents. The future could be bright, if the politicians would try a little harder to listen to the NPC.

The influence of the NPC is growing in many fields such as in local government, health, and community care committees. Its opinion is being sought by the more discerning and progressive of consultative groups. We have added our voice of experience to the Carnegie Institute's findings, the British Medical Association's community care consultation document and we are a member of the National Council of Voluntary Organizations.

The many programmes now in the planning stage are keeping the various working parties busy. These include large conferences and petitioning Her Majesty the Queen. The latter is to remind her ministers that we are asking them for changes in the state pension, VAT on fuel and the National Health Service.

The NPC also steps into Europe, by being a large influence in the pensioners' parliaments, set up in the first place by the socialist MEP group and carried forward in 1993 by the all-party MEPs of the European Parliament.

Reaching out across the European Community of the 12 member nations, 500 delegates were selected, one for each of the elected members of the established European Parliament. The meeting was in Luxembourg under the same conditions as would be seen within the main EC Parliament. There they discussed the conditions and welfare of the elders of each country, trying to reach an agreement for care and welfare for all, bearing in mind that each country does not have the same economy or social structure as the others.

Great strides have been made, and at the 1993 pensioners' parliament the following incomes policy was adopted by both the political right and left.

1. The statutory pension should remain as the fundamental basis of retirement provision throughout the European Community and its member states.
2. The retention and improvement of basic pensions is urged along with determined efforts to ensure workers, at the end of their working lives, receive an income that will allow them a decent standard of living. This basic pension to be related to a substantial percentage of the national average wage.
3. The introduction in each member state of a guaranteed minimum pension for every person who has reached retirement age but is not entitled to receive the basic pension. This minimum pension to be fixed at a substantial level of the basic pension and to be seen as a measure to fight poverty which for the greater part affects older people, in particular older women.
4. Special consideration should be given to provide substantial extra payments and services to older people suffering from any form of invalidity, in addition to their guaranteed rights to a basic or minimum pension. Also the rules governing invalidity should be harmonized, given the current wide differences between member states on the rights to invalidity pensions.
5. Regular, and not less than yearly, adjustments should be made to the basic pension and the minimum pension in line with national average wages or the cost of living, whichever is the greater.
6. With regard to the operation of occupational pension funds and recent cases of fraud and misuse, the NPC demands action at Community and national level. This is to ensure tighter regulatory supervision and proper protection of contributors and beneficiaries against the dangers of insolvency, fraud and misuse as well as for adequate representation of contributors and pensioners on the management boards of such funds.
7. The NPC welcomes the resolution recently adopted by the European Parliament inviting the council and the member states to apply fully the council recommendation on the common criteria on minimum resources in the social protection systems and the council recommendation on the convergence of national social security systems.

8. The NPC urges, furthermore, that national governments refrain from measures which disproportionately impose burdens on pensioners.

The above was approved by the full (plenary) session, 24 November 1993.

Many of the NPC affiliated organizations sent representatives as well as all officers of NPC being there. The NPC's President Jack Jones acted as one of the 'rapporteurs' guiding the findings of the incomes group to its successful conclusions.

The NPC is a grouping of many campaigning pensioners organizations, who know from bitter experience that the strength of unity is the only way forward.

It is true of any organization, no matter what its base, that there will from time to time spring forth 'kings for a day', people who tend to flare up like 'Roman candle' fireworks, leaving little trace behind. In the NPC there is a functional body that will still be looking after and reacting to the interests of the elders of this country far, far into the 21st century and like any solid foundation it will stand the storms of time.

THE FUTURE

The actual fight for a retirement pension started in 1898 to get rid of the stigma of 'poor law relief' that put honest, hardworking men and women, many well beyond the age of 70, into segregated workhouses and institutions until they met their end as the unwanted and forgotten in paupers' graves. In 1908 that great struggle ended in partial success. Many of the excuses heard today, to hold back the state pension and reduce its call upon the wealth of the nation, are the same as in those far off days. So, the present is part of the past and the future will tell the story of today's struggle for the poorest of our time.

Where now is the NPC going and what does it plan?

We have submitted a petition to Her Majesty the Queen asking the following:

The undersigned petitioners pray that your Majesty will urge your Ministers to:

i) Improve the position of all pensioners by a substantial increase in basic retirement pension, also to ensure that all future increases be related to the annual average wage index, or retail price index whichever is greater.

ii) Stop any further VAT on domestic fuel and power, and refrain from any other form of financial burden, which will discriminate unfairly against the elderly, the poor and the infirm.

iii) Provide substantial extra national resources in the health and care of the elderly.

The NPC collected one and a half million signatures and in September 1994, after a set piece rally in Westminster Central Hall, handed it in to Buckingham Palace, believing that, if Her Majesty's Government has not the political will to alter and improve the pensioner's well-being, then perhaps a plea to the Head of State might produce a better hearing.

Whatever happened between Her Majesty and Her Ministers will be only a matter of historical record, but in the House of Commons during the November debate on the Budget, the Opposition managed to defeat the government's proposals to enlarge the 8% VAT on fuel and power to 17½% and we believe that our contribution in the form of the petition helped in that turnaround.

Following on into 1995, and not withstanding the continuous meetings with politicians, we have a programme to stage a 'Pensioners Parliament' between 16–18 May. As we cannot get our present government to back the wishes of the last Elder Citizens Parliament in Luxembourg, the National Pensioners Convention decided to host it themselves to allow our elder people a voice so long denied.

Until that aim is achieved the NPC has taken up other issues such as women's retirement and pension rights, ageism, care in the community, standing charges on bills for domestic essentials, many times in co-operation with other organizations such as the Fawcet Society, Cespa and Age Concern England.

We will continue to lead and counsel all who are genuine in their desire to return the whole of the retired pensioner population of this great country to pride of place in its society.

The elderly population dilemma is not an original to this country and we can learn a great deal in cross-border dialogue. We need far more forums where the voices of those who have the wisdom of age can be heard and acted upon in an equality with those generations which follow. After all, the true wealth and power of any country is in its people, young and old.

9

Pensioners' forums –
a voice for older people

Tony Carter and Caroline Nash

HOW FORUMS DEVELOPED

National organizations representing pensioners' interests historically arose mainly around the demand for adequate retirement pensions. Such demands go back to the early years of the century. As early as 1902 a national conference was called by the Co-operative Union Congress and the Trades Union Congress to call for an old age pension and to save 'aged Britons . . . from disfranchisement and pauperism, from the ignominy of "charity" or from actual starvation'. Thus started an historic link between the trade unions and pensioners. In 1939, a petition to raise the old age pension from 10/- to £1 gained two million signatures.

It was not until the 1930s that organizations with a pensioner membership began to appear – some of these early organizations, like the National Federation of Retirement Pensioners Associations (known as Pensioners' Voice; founded in 1940) and the Scottish Old Age Pensioners' Association, are still in existence.

The early concentration on economic demands soon widened to include other national issues. These have included, in recent years, transport issues, such as concessions for older people; standing charges in the bills of public utilities and campaigns on ways to provide adequate heating in winter for older people on income support. More recently still, government policy to place care back in the community has produced anxiety and debate within pensioners' organizations (Thornton and Tozer 1994), not the least because older women tend to be one of the main groups affected. This area of concern has not so far produced clear campaigning objectives.

Issues raised nationally, such as pensions and welfare improvements, are typically matters for national decision by government and the concern of pensioners' organizations has been, therefore, to influence or change government policy, largely by campaigning. Where representations to government ministers have been made, these have typically been in the form of deputations, and have been seen as an extension to campaigning rather than as detailed discussion on points at issue with a view to seeking an agreed conclusion. Pensioners' organizations, from their early days, have stressed their political independence and have not abated their demands when a Labour government has been in power, even though the rhetoric of the Labour Party is often perceived as being more sympathetic towards the problems of older people than that of the Conservatives.

Undoubtedly, national campaigning which involves criticism of government policies has been congenial to many activists in pensioners' organizations. Frequently, such activists were formerly involved in trade union work and they brought to pensioners' organizations valuable organizational experience and a robust approach to authority. They also brought, however, a Labour (or at any rate, non-Conservative) political outlook. Thus, although the organizations themselves were politically independent, many of the active members involved showed enthusiasm for attacking government, particularly, it might be said, a Conservative government. Not all organizations demonstrated this characteristic; the oldest established national organization, Pensioners' Voice, remained non-partisan in its approach. One of the newest, the Association of Retired Persons, is determinedly independent politically, although with strong commercial links, and has a leadership which includes a variety of political views, including active members of the Conservative party. The recently formed National Pensioners' Convention, founded to be an umbrella for all organizations with older people in membership, asserts vigorously its non-party political stance.

National campaigning, although arguably necessary to highlight major issues of poverty and discrimination affecting older people, has its limitations. It restricts local activity by members of pensioners' groups and supporters of older people to mere support of the national objective, even though this may find active expression in local demonstrations, lobbying of local MPs and public activity such as meetings and petitions. More significantly, national campaigning frequently does not address local issues, perhaps seemingly more mundane, but about which there might be strong feeling in the locality and which have direct impact upon the day-to-day lives of older people. National capaigning often has long-term objectives, such as the campaign to re-establish the link between pensions increases and wages rises – a link broken by a Conservative government in 1980 in favour of simple inflation proofing.

So, a certain amount of battle fatigue can set in, allied to a feeling of powerlessness on those many local issues having a strong impact upon older people.

Moreover, there is some evidence (see Carter and Nash, 1993) that concentration upon a militant national approach can produce a wary response among sections of retired people who do not espouse strong political views. As in any section of society, these sections constitute a majority, which is thereby cut off from expression of their interests and needs.

A further factor is that not all retired people are 'pensioners', in the sense of those in receipt of the state retirement pension. With changing economic circumstances, people are leaving paid employment much earlier. Economic activity rates are estimated to have fallen between 1971 and 1991 from 71% to 67% at ages 55–59 and from 54% to 39% at 60–64 (Phillipson, 1993).

National campaigning to raise the state retirement pension may be therefore less attractive to many pensioners than lower key attempts to improve local facilities for older people. Concentration upon 'economic' demands, such as better pensions, may not mobilize retired people who are not 'pensioners' or who feel themselves relatively well off, perhaps because of other income such as an occupational pension. Such groups may respond more immediately to issues such as safety, crime, loneliness, improved facilities and such concerns which can be addressed at a local level.

Another factor making for changing approaches has been a growth in local organization among pensioners in the 1980s. In part this was a response to what were perceived to be growing problems of older people; inevitably these included pensions, particularly as a result of the breaking by the government of the link between rises in earnings and pensions increases but also included poverty issues with local impact, such as housing and keeping warm in winter. It also coincided with a new surge of interest in campaigning about these problems especially by trade unions, leading in very many instances to the setting up of union retired members' sections. In response to these perceived problems voluntary bodies concerned with older people also began to adopt a more campaigning style. With a greater and more effective level of organization locally came the possibility of raising meaningful local demands. The move towards getting to grips with issues affecting older people locally did not replace national campaigning, but was an addition to it, as a response to the expressed needs of older people in the locality.

This approach has not been opposed by national leaders of pensioners' organizations; rather it has been adopted by them. Thus, an aim of the National Pensioners' Convention is to establish standing machinery for discussion with the government of issues of concern to older people and it has encouraged local organizations with which it is in contact to take action in support of local demands. (Its co-operation with the Pensioners' Forums Project carried out in 1992–93 by the authors was enthusiastic and the NPC sponsored a national conference in February 1994 specifically to consider how older people can influence public policy.) The Association of Retired Persons, an organization with a largely middle-class membership which tends to stand aside from the main-stream pensioners' groups, has urged its local centres 'to become pressure groups used to achieve members' common aims and goals'. (*ARP Reporter*, Winter 1993). The January 1994 issue of *Pensioners' Voice*, publication and usual name of the National Federation of Retirement Pensioners Associations, quotes its Wellingborough Branch: 'Not only are we campaigning for a better pension, but we campaigned against the removal of beds from the local hospital (and won); and we have campaigned for better bus services and safer buses, as well as cheaper fares'.

A major manifestation of this developing trend has been the setting up of pensioners' forums (or 'elderly' or 'older people', etc).

WHY FORUMS?

True to its Roman origins a forum is a place where people can gather together to discuss public policies and to have their own views heard. Beyond this there should be some mechanism by which the results of discussion, and particularly any consensus reached, will be brought to the attention of those in authority.

Today's society is vast and complex with populations so great that, unlike in ancient Rome, they generally preclude each individual from having direct access to decision-making bodies. Pensioners' forums exist to provide a voice for older people in representing views to authority. Such a collective organization allows the less confident and less vocal to make their opinion felt by electing a representative who will have a chance to express the views of the smaller group and vote within the forum.

Although constituted in different ways, the main purpose of pensioners' forums is to provide a non-threatening space where older people, directly or through their organizations, discuss their views and then make a consensus of their opinions known to the authorities – those bodies of people whose decisions concerning the environment in which we live affect us all. These may include local authorities, health authorities and trusts, transport undertakings, sports and leisure providers, education providers and, with the current emphasis upon reducing the scope of local authorities' work, commercial and voluntary organizations with contracts from the public sector.

In many instances, notably in Greater London, forums are umbrella organizations made up of one or two representatives of the other local groups of older people in the vicinity or those groups concerned in some way with older people, such as from the voluntary sector. Their views are made known to the public body concerned by letter, frequently followed up by meetings which are business-like in character, seeking results rather than confrontation. In some instances, these meetings are of a regular kind, with a predetermined periodicity.

Where the forum is of the umbrella type, relevant groups, including those organizations with a major interest in older people, are invited to participate in the forum. These are likely to include voluntary organizations, such as Age Concern groups or the local branch of the Carers National Association, membership organizations of retired people, such as pensioners' action groups, associations of retired members, whether of unions or employers (such as the Civil Service or Post Office), luncheon clubs, sheltered housing tenants associations, ethnic elders, discussion groups, and so on. Often they will include other organizations whose interest in older people is less specific, such as churches.

In order to ensure that everyone has a chance to make him/herself heard, some of these umbrella type of forums also permit individual membership for those older people who shun 'clubs' of any kind or, for one reason or another, are not attracted to the traditional type of pensioner organization.

To facilitate meaningful representation, such umbrella forums are usually based upon the area of a local authority and relate to that authority or other public bodies, e.g. NHS, within that geographical area. This is overwhelmingly the case in Greater London. Difficulties can arise, however, when health authority and social service areas do not coincide, as is frequently the case. Goodwill can overcome such difficulties although differences can be advantageous in that agreement reached with one authority can then be quoted to the other.

Other forums are based entirely upon individual membership, within a geographical area, which may correspond to the local authority area or may be community based. In Scotland the local forums are locality or neighbourhood based, although coming together in a regional forum, such as the Strathclyde Elderly Forum or the Fife EF. In such instances, representations might be locally directed, for instance to local councillors, or the social services patch office, or they might be forwarded to the umbrella organizations for representations at a higher level, usually the region. This form of forum has great strengths, being related to an area which is immediately identifiable to older people, many of whom will know each other because of use of other local facilities, but it is apparent that difficulties of representation could arise. (Potential problems of this nature arising from local government reorganization in Scotland have been recognized by Strathclyde Elderly Forum.)

TYPES OF FORUM

Four basic patterns in setting up a forum may be identified. These are:

- pensioner initiative
- local authority initiative
- overlap
- collaborative.

Pensioner initiative

Examples include Greater London Forum for the Elderly (GLFE), Strathclyde Elderly Forum (SEF), Midlands Pensioners' Convention and National Pensioners' Convention (NPC). In this case representatives of local (or national as well in the case of NPC) pensioner groups have joined together under an umbrella organization so that the views of their members can be passed on via a recognized and acceptable channel to public bodies.

Local authority initiative

An example is Nottingham City Council's 'Elderly Voices'. Here the City Council decided it would like direct access to the opinions of its older residents. It therefore invites all older people to an open meeting. Transport is provided free of charge if required. After a welcoming coffee and biscuits and the formal part of the day with speeches from, for example, the Leader of the Council or a local pensioners' leader, groups of older people meet together to air their views with council staff representatives, each from a department whose functions have an impact upon the lives of older people. The staff members take notes which are analysed together with the other group opinions and this then forms the basis of discussion for the following year by a joint group of council representatives and voluntary and pensioners' organizations. The following year's meeting, which has a report of the year's work as its agenda, allows older people to take their council to task if their wishes have been ignored.

Overlap

In this case a member of a forum is also a member of the local council and thereby constitutes him/herself a channel by which older people's views reach the decision-makers. An example is Sheffield Pensioners' Action Group where a member has also been elected as a councillor.

Collaboration

An example is Barking and Dagenham Forum for the Elderly. Here the council and representatives of older people's groups joined together to form the Elderly Forum. The council assists the forum by providing office and meeting rooms plus administrative support. Being on the same premises facilitates lines of communication, although the forum does operate independently.

In some areas regional forums have been set up. In these cases, the local forums send representatives to the regional body. This tiered system works well in areas like Greater London, with London borough-based forums, and in Strathclyde, with local or 'neighbourhood' forums. In London, the Greater London Forum for the Elderly was set up when the GLC still existed; now, in the absence of all-London government, it acts as a forum for the exchange of views and co-ordination of strategy, as a resource and development agency in setting up new forums, as well as making representations on London-wide issues, such as transport. In Strathclyde (and other Scottish regions) the umbrella organization makes representations to the regional council, responsible for policy on a range of important issues concerning older people, such as care in the community. (This role may change with the proposed setting up of smaller unitary authorities in Scotland.) The SEF also has an important role in addressing and campaigning upon national issues, whether in Scotland or Great Britain as a whole.

There are many pensioner groups which make representation to their local councils and other public bodies which do not consider or call themselves forums and which might have a broader view of their role as a part of a national movement. These might be, for instance, a local pensioner action group or a branch of the Transport and General Workers' Union Retired Members' Association. Other groups which do call themselves forums act more as discussion groups without any recognized channel of representation to bodies in authority.

The type of local forums discussed here usually associate themselves with national campaigning on major issues of general interest to older people. An example was the campaign in 1993 against the proposal to impose VAT upon fuel bills. Local forums were drawn into this national campaign through links with the national pensioners' organizations but also by the strength of local feeling among older people. (Bromley Forum in south east London felt constrained in its annual report to draw attention to a role it clearly felt a bit uncomfortable about; commenting that despite its non-political stance it had no option but to respond to the local strength of feeling on this issue.)

All the varieties of pensioner organization discussed have an important information dissemination role, using their own locally produced newspapers or newsletters to provide news of local facilities available to older people, local and national campaigns and, in some instances, official information. Some of these local publications have achieved wide and influential coverage, for example *Lewisham Pensioners' Press*, produced by Pensioners' Link which is affiliated to Lewisham Pensioners' Forum, and which contains important information for retired people in the borough, including (paid for) official council announcements. It has achieved a 10 000 circulation.

Some forums offer individual welfare advice to older people, such as Kirkcaldy in Fife or Wolverhampton, where the local Pensioners' Convention has a volunteer force carrying out minor maintenance and repairs. In Strathclyde, PAGE (Pensioners' Action Glasgow East) runs an advice shop.

SETTING UP A FORUM

Our research has shown that the most successful way to establish a new forum in 'virgin' territory seems to be to start by inviting everyone to an open meeting. Obviously it helps if a small group of people get together to plan this, but it would be feasible for one person to do it. Usually a large hall can be found at little or no cost. The council, community centres and church halls are possibilities. Money to cover costs can be earned by serving tea and biscuits to participants. Publicity can generally be had in the local free newspapers/radio and posters can be placed in libraries, doctors' surgeries and Post Offices. There will also be certain organizations of particular relevance which can be invited individually – such as Age Concern, local councillors and social service and transport representatives. Some of these may well be asked to speak.

At the meeting (which may well attract large numbers of people) a list of everyone's name and address is taken so that future contact with interested parties is made easy. A request is usually made for those interested in actually doing some 'work' and becoming part of a steering group to set the forum up officially to stay behind at the end (or at least to make their interest known) so that progress can be made.

This steering group will then meet to organize the forum, with such tasks as drawing up a constitution, suggesting what form membership should take and planning future meetings. Costs are usually minimal and are met by members' subscriptions, small grants and council (or other) contributions in kind (such as free photocopying or postage).

WAYS TO SUCCESS

Local organizations which concentrate on national, particularly economic, issues such as increasing pensions and removing standing charges can become discouraged when they see no results for their campaigning. It thus becomes important to address smaller scale, locally important issues so as to maintain the morale and the support of the local membership as well as providing a way of building alliances with retired people who are not involved in the mainstream pensioners' movement. A diet of rallies and petitions on major national issues is not found sustaining by all. Success in pursuing such national issues is not always apparent either (sometimes it is, of course; the VAT on fuel campaign resulted in the government at any rate recognizing the principle of compensation for all pensioners). Addressing local issues, which can secure wide local and cross-party support, can result in a degree of success, although government-imposed financial constraints may inhibit major improvements in community care, for instance.

It must be pointed out, however, that the very existence of a local representative group of older people in itself constitutes some degree of success. Authoritative bodies do not wish to create conflict. If there is a vocal group in the area its possible reactions are likely to be considered at some level before decisions are made and even unpopular policy decisions can be tailored to deflect a possibly adverse response.

In order to have an impact on local consciousness and to achieve something with tangible results, some local forums have found it wise to concentrate, at least in part, on something small-scale and non-controversial such as street lighting or location of bus stops. Improvements here are likely to benefit a large proportion of the population and support from all sections of society will therefore be more readily enlisted. Success on such issues heightens corporate feelings and support and encourages further action.

Examples of such local activity on relatively small issues but which nonetheless have bearing on the quality of life for older people include the state of pavements (Southwark), layout of the bus station (Glenrothes), community alarms (Kirkcaldy), seating in a shopping area (Dumfries and Galloway), safety in the home (Bromley), re-siting of a post box (Meadway, East Birmingham).

Success at this level is profile raising, builds community feeling and increases self-confidence to tackle more substantial issues. Thus, Lewisham co-operated with the local council to produce a health pack for older people. Midlands Pensioners' Convention was represented on a council committee which produced a Birmingham City strategy for the elderly. Oxford Pensioners' Action Group has an annual meeting with the council at which issues, both small and large, are given an airing.

If something is usable and acceptable by an older person, then it is likely to also be usable and accepted by other, potentially less able, people in society. Thus, a crossing which gives an older person time to cross the road will also allow more time for those with heavy bags of shopping or small children; an easy-open jam pot will be welcomed by all of us who do not possess Herculean muscles; and clearly lit streets will make women as well as older people feel safer at night.

Such activity provides a high profile in the locality and acceptability by the population as a whole. This can lead to intergenerational under-standing and activity with important consequences for social cohesion.

RELATIONSHIPS WITH AUTHORITY

Some issues are likely to be much more controversial and harder to resolve; frequently these are matters in the borders between national and local responsibility, such as care in the community. They involve the council in having to reconsider its own priorities. It follows that councils are far from uniform in their attitude towards forums. Some have formal machinery for discussions. These may take the form of regular meetings, scheduled, with a council officer having the respons-ibility to agree an agenda with the forum and to ensure that those of her/ his colleagues necessary to deal with the items listed are present (this happened in Strathclyde and Fife). At the extreme end of the spectrum is Lewisham, where the council has set up a standing committee, including representatives of the forum, to discuss matters of concern to older people; as a result, the council invariably goes out of its way to acknowledge publicly its support for older people. Of course, it has to be acknowledged that financial constraints may not allow specific action in every case.

At the opposite end, there are councils whose tolerance extends little further than polite acknowledgement of the forum's existence. No doubt, the majority of councils fall somewhere in between, operating uneasily in the area between bureaucratic distaste for pressure groups and the realities of electoral politics.

UNDER-REPRESENTED GROUPS OF OLDER PEOPLE

There are more women of retirement age than men. Although they are not always at home in the often male-dominated environment of the traditional pensioners' organization, significant examples exist in which women have reached a prominent position within forums. Strathcylde Elderly Forum, West Midlands Pensioners' Convention, Mansfield Pensioners' Action Group and Norfolk and Norwich Pensioners' Associations all boast female officers with vision and authority.

It might be expected that such shining examples of leadership would encourage other women to step forward into similar roles, but this does not seem to be the case – or it is happening very slowly. Most of the women alluded to tend themselves to have a strong background in the trade union movement and are therefore more comfortable than most with current, rather formal, ways of working. Like Mrs Thatcher as Prime Minister, their leading role tends to heighten masculine rather than feminine qualities. The strength and assertiveness of the women leaders may actually make less forthright women less likely to step forward.

It seems that a gentler approach is more likely to attract the majority of older women. Setting up less obviously politically motivated discussion groups may be a way to arouse their interest and obtain their views. They too might respond to locally based initiatives alert to issues of importance to them, for instance, the role of older women as carers. Women only groups might be a necessary first step; one such in London, the Association of Greater London Older Women (AGLOW), has attracted support.

The other group, or rather groups, of older people under-represented in the pensioner movement tend to be from the minority ethnic groups. To some extent what goes above for women applies equally to ethnic elders although reinforced by feelings of exclusion derived from experienced or perceived racial discrimination. Older people from a different culture usually lack a strong trade union tradition and have tended to be less active in a representative capacity during their working lives. Again, there are examples to the contrary, such as Wandsworth Pensioners' Forum, but again these, because of a perceived contrast inability, can make the more silent majority feel less equipped to speak out.

Ideas for attracting older ethnic support are similar to those suggested for women. Discussion groups regarding issues of interest are a good start, but it may well be necessary for certain groups to be conducted in an appropriate language and by an ethnic elder, as some ethnic elders are not proficient in English. A more confident elder can then bring the group's views to the larger geographical representative forum. (It is worth noting that some cultures – particularly Muslim – will not permit the free mix of men and women so that posters, speakers, etc. must be appropriate or no one will turn up.)

For both older women and ethnic elders, conscious decisions by existing pensioners' groups to make specific efforts to end under-representation are needed.

FUTURE DEVELOPMENTS

Following Age Concern England's 1992 campaign *A Voice for Older People* and the work of the Pensioners' Forum Project, a number of new forums have started up, in addition to almost complete coverage in the cases of London boroughs and very wide coverage in the Scottish regions.

Although no complete survey has been undertaken, there appears to be growing interest across the spectrum of pensioners' organizations in finding ways of getting to grips with day-to-day issues of concern to older people. One may speculate that this is a trend which may well continue. Government policy may be having an effect; the rhetoric of consumer consultation and citizen's charters may help to rouse people's consciousness that their views can be made to count. The possibility of effecting local change will help to politicize the older population, making for a more effective voice nationally. The campaign around the imposition of VAT on fuel in 1993 was largely undertaken by organizations either representing or with an interest in older people and clearly had some effect upon the government's approach to compensation for the increases.

The outlook of the younger retired person may be important to the future of this movement. An active local organization of the retired, offering representation on a broad spectrum of issues of concern to older people, local and national, could help to counter feelings of powerlessness when the mutual support mechanisms of the shop floor or management team, union or chamber of commerce, are lost. In turn, the younger retired can bring up-to-date relevant skills to traditional pensioners' organizations, in areas such as computerization, accounting, even perhaps market research.

Much depends upon the organizations of older people themselves. A unified body or even an effective, broadly based umbrella organization has not yet arrived and the progress of the the National Pensioners' Convention in fulfilling that role is inevitably very slow because of the diverse interests to be taken into account. Hence, leadership or advice from national level may not be forthcoming. In the face of the growing number of problems likely to be faced by older people, they have yet to find a universally suitable response. The growth of the forum movement may be one pointer to the future.

APPENDIX: SOME USEFUL ADDRESSES

Greater London Forum for the Elderly,
54 Chalton Street,
London NW1 1JR
Director: Carole Newman

Midland Pensioners' Convention,
37 Woodfield Road,
Birmingham 13
Secretary: Helen Grew

National Pensioners' Convention,
4 Stevens Street,
Lowestoft,
Suffolk   NR32 2JE
General Secretary: Jack Thain

Nottingham Elderly Voices,
Council House,
Nottingham NG1 4BT
Chair: Councillor Sylvia Parsons

Strathclyde Elderly Forum,
Block 6 Unit E2,
Templeton Business Centre,
Glasgow G40 1DA

REFERENCES

Carter, A. and Nash, C. (1993) *Pensioners' Forums: An Active Voice*, Pre-Retirement Association (University of Surrey), Guildford, Surrey.
Phillipson, C. (1993) Older workers and retirement: a review of current trends. *Benefits*, (8) September/October.
Thornton, P. and Tozer, R. (1994) *Involving Older People in Planning and Evaluating Community Care*, SPRU, University of York.
L. Wynn (ed) (1992) *Power to the People*, King's Fund Centre for Health Services Development, London.

10

Gaining confidence – speaking out

Zelda Curtis

The ageism rife in our society heaps insults on older women, which, too often, drains their confidence. It robs them of their voice and renders them invisible. It was as a counter to the oppression of ageism that the Older Women's Project was formed in 1985. The Older Women's Project of Pensioners' Link was the forerunner of AGLOW (Association of Greater London Older Women).

By bringing together older women of different cultures and backgrounds to discuss and campaign around issues affecting their lives, the project aimed to help them gain the confidence to speak out and become guerillas in the battle for a brighter future.

To fulfil this aim the project set out to arm the women with information and offered them the opportunity to share their experiences and learn from each other. By doing so it sought to help them gain the confidence to demand representation on bodies making decisions about their lives.

The project provided a forum through which their collective voice could be heard demanding recognition that gender, age, race, disability and sexuality were issues that must not be ignored. It encouraged older women to seek involvement in the planning and monitoring of services, to make certain they were appropriate and relevant to their specific needs.

'The needs of older women have been neglected by professionals who have not found them rewarding to work with, and policy-makers who do not rate their needs as a priority', claims the Women's National Commission, an advisory committee to the government, in a report *Older Women – Myths and Strategies. An Agenda for Action*, brought out at the start of the European Year of Older People 1993. Here we are now, two years on, and despite the Commission's recommendations to enable older women to enjoy the 'sort of future they richly deserve', little advance had been made in that respect.

The report went on to state that 'while much can be done by government, responsibility also rests with women themselves', and went on to say that 'current generations of older women may lack the assertiveness and confidence needed to express their needs and that they should therefore be encouraged to do this'. To understand why older women lack confidence we must examine their position in society.

THE POSITION OF OLDER WOMEN

There are around seven million women aged over 60 in Britain, and the great contribution they make to the economy through their unpaid work in the home, as childminders within the extended family, as volunteers staffing the charities, as carers and 'good neighbours', goes unrecognized. This society devalues women once they are past their child-bearing, child-rearing age. Low priority is given to their needs and too little research is done into the specific issues that affect their lives. Society values individuals for their wealth and conspicuous consumption, and most older women are poor and have no flash status symbols. They suffer low self-esteem and have low expectations because they are made second-class citizens by the ageism in our society.

Women today who have reached the age of 70 are of a generation that suffered from the negative social attitudes towards the education of women. Many of them left school at 14 and they feel the lack of education has rendered them powerless. That was why it was important in setting up the Older Women's Project that, from the start, it was older women themselves who formed the management committee and who planned and monitored the work of the project. Black and white older women of differing backgrounds, lesbians, and women with disabilities were all encouraged to shape the work of the project to meet their different needs. They planned a programme of participative conferences to discuss all those issues that affected the lives of older women, robbing them of confidence, such as the rundown of the health service, the cuts in benefits, the increasing deprivation and discrimination. Having been made to feel like second-class citizens, they lacked self-esteem and had little will to take action. With the project's support, however, they began to take more control over their own lives.

WHY A PROJECT FOR OLDER WOMEN?

Older women are among the most disadvantaged members of our society, with 80% of all lone women over 60 suffering poverty, living in poor housing, many in poor health, and feeling isolated and lonely.

At the age of 60 there are twice as many women as men, and four times as many after 75, so we say that public policy for elderly people must take into account their specific needs. Yet, despite their large numbers, little attention is paid to them. The Carnegie Inquiry into the Third Age recorded in its report that 'For those with health, enough money, and the personal skills and resources to build a lifestyle of their own choosing, this freedom (retirement from paid employment) can bring a fulfilling life, including the opportunity to give more attention to themselves', but for the more disadvantaged older women, particularly those who are carers, the opportunity to lead a fulfilling life or pay more attention to themselves is very limited.

Many women who were members of pensioners' action groups had to be convinced of the need for an Older Women's Project. Our argument was that the pensioners' movement had shown little interest in campaigning on women's issues. The women's demands were subsumed within the national demands of the male pensioners, who saw no need for a separate women's project. Therefore the Older Women's Project was set up to empower the most disadvantaged, helping them to make their voices heard in the corridors of power.

Many of the participants in the conferences organized by the Older Women's Project were drawn from among the most disadvantaged women – those living in poverty in the inner city, often in poor housing and alone. To enable them to find their voices we provided assertiveness training; classes on communication skills; advocacy, information and any resources needed; setting up health courses, and study days, and resourcing support groups. We felt we were beginning to succeed when 50 older women went to the House of Commons to meet with Jo Richardson MP (then the Shadow Minister for Women) to tell her what they felt should be included in Labour's policies. That day the older women began to sense their power to bring about change. The ease with which they spoke to Jo Richardson showed how confident they felt.

WHY THE EMPHASIS ON HEALTH?

To remain independent and active, it is essential that older women look after their health. Self-health care is crucial to maintain their well-being, and, therefore, the older women wished to be involved in health-related activities. When we launched the Older Women's Project with the first-ever London-wide festival, over 500 older women came for the weekend to take advantage of the opportunity to share their experiences, learn new skills and, above all, to enjoy themselves. The activities ranged from self-defence and yoga classes to video and computer training; discussions were held on health, racism, and other issues of special importance to older women.

It was from a workshop at that festival that the suggestion came to hold a London-wide health festival. The aim was first, to consult with older women on what they perceive as their main health concerns and to provide a forum for older women from all cultures to explore and discuss issues relating to their health care and to learn from each other. Second, to generate enthusiasm and information that could then be used to start up local health initiatives for older women, based on their needs and with their involvement.

Over 400 older women from right across London attended that first weekend health festival. Campaigning and self-help were the major themes for the weekend and the programme took in practical advice, information sharing, exercise and swimming sessions and exhibitions.

Areas of health looked at were diet, blood pressure, arthritis, diabetes, sickle cell anaemia and the safe use of drugs and medicines. The sessions on stress, relaxation and massage were very popular and sent everyone home in a rested mood. Then having been shown how to massage each other, the women could use this new skill to help other older women. The discussion groups gave older women the chance to talk about their own health needs with the emphasis on how to change things for the better, including sessions on how to get the best out of your doctor, and how to campaign for a health service more relevant to the needs of older women.

A planning group of older Caribbean women organized similar events for black and ethnic older women, to discuss the racism they suffer and how best to confront it and they also pinpointed the lack of research into the specific illnesses that affect their lives.

The points made on the general health issues discussed in all the conferences were incorporated in a leaflet that was widely distributed to MPs, councillors, service providers and health authorities. One of the points they made was that 'older women experience trivialization and dismissal of their treatable health problems with the common response of "it's your age" and are fobbed off with tranquillizers'. They also pointed out the need for routine smear tests for older women and called for the upper age limit at present imposed to be abolished, because of the high percentage of elderly women that die of cervical cancer. They complained of the lack of preventive health care and alternative treatments. They called for more well-women clinics with greater emphasis on older women's health, more women-only facilities, and for funding for self-help health groups.

To fulfil the second of the aims of the health festival (that the project should encourage local health initiatives), health days were planned in several localities.

LOCAL OLDER WOMEN'S GROUPS

Finding an interest among some older women in Waltham Forest and Hackney, it was decided to help them set up groups in their localities. In Waltham Forest we found support for the project from the women's committee. With a grant of £6000 per year, the help of one of their women's unit staff, and with the Waltham Forest Women's Centre as a venue for planning meetings, the first of many successful day conferences on different themes was organized around health. The local Mencap members gave us support and district nurses worked hard on the day giving general advice, testing blood pressure and advising on diabetes. Other health workers spoke on arthritis and the yoga and keep fit sessions were very popular.

The Waltham Forest Older Women's Group became firmly established and invited service providers to their regular Wednesday meetings to hear their views on education, community transport, pollution and sheltered housing and they followed up with further official meetings at the town hall. Their intervention helped retain a public convenience for women that was about to be closed and their well-argued case for different bus routes was listened to sympathetically by London Transport and some changes were made.

Other interesting days organized were on environmental issues; on housing with a session on 'living alone and loving it'; and probably the most enjoyable one focused on arts activities, where the women exhibited their talents. Their paintings were displayed, their poems read, their embroidery, crochet and patchwork draped, and they also had the opportunity to acquire new skills such as jewellery making, photography, drumming, flamenco dancing, henna handpainting, etc. The Waltham Forest older women were very interested in their local history and to add to their cultural experience they visited many museums and galleries.

In Hackney, we were only able to get a small start-up grant from the women's committee to enable the older women to form a group and hold a health day in a local community centre. There were sessions on art therapy, on yoga, keep fit, nutrition and massage, as well as information stalls and exhibitions. The group of women in Hackney went on to do a reminiscence project out of which they produced a booklet and a drama presentation. They performed it in day centres and community halls, to pensioners' organizations. It portrayed the experiences of Caribbean women coming to Britain in the 1950s to work as nurses here.

In Newham we worked together with Age Concern locally to organize an older women's day with sessions on health, education and transport. The majority of the participants were older Asian women. At the end of the day they danced for us and encouraged all of us to join in with them. For some of those Asian women it was their first experience of going out unchaperoned.

FUNDRAISING FOR HEALTH GROUPS

Having shown our experience of organizing groups locally, perhaps it would be helpful to others who are thinking of forming a local group to know of funding sources (see Appendix A) and to learn of some of the difficulties our group members had to face. One lesson we learned was that too large an amount of funding can create as many problems as too little.

One group found it very worrying to have to administer large sums of money, and after some years they hadn't enough active members to enable them to use the funds as designated. The grant was supposed to be used to organize two conferences, regular meetings with speakers, and two outings in a year. Finding they could no longer cope with that level of work, they had to ask their funders to cut the grant to cover only their regular meetings and outings. They are now coasting along quite happily.

Another group remained basically self-financing. Members paid just 25p each meeting and 10p for a raffle ticket, and with the use of a free room and a kettle in their local women's centre, they met regularly to chat over a cup of tea, and fundraised only if they had some special project in mind.

Fundraising can take up so much time and energy that some members gave up disconsolately. The main encouragement to give you is don't be frightened of the funders; many of them can be very helpful – try them. AGLOW can also give you advice and some administrative or publicity support if needed. Advice could also be had from your equalities officer in the civic centre or from your local women's centre. The mayor usually has a small pot of gold to give to deserving causes and the local police station also has a small fund to be tapped. High street stores can be generous too. But for meaningful work you need to have three-year funding and, therefore, have to tackle the larger funding organizations whose preference is to fund self-help health groups.

EDUCATION AND HEALTH

Due to the interest shown in health issues, the Older Women's Education Group (of which the project was a founder member) organized a study day on 'older women and health'. Dr Moya Sidell described the research she had undertaken for the Open University on gender differences in health in later life; in a workshop on 'hormones and health', the menopause and HRT were discussed; another workshop dealt with 'bereavement and loss'; and another looked at 'coping with change'. Dr Joyce Leeson summed up by declaring that 'the combination of woman power and grey power had great potential to exert influence on society'.

As many of the participants were members of other women's organizations such as the Co-operative Women's Guild, the Fawcett Society and the Older Feminist Network, Dr Leeson's words were reported widely.

Since then we have moved into a new area of work with older women users of the mental health services.

OLDER WOMEN AND MENTAL HEALTH

Older users of the mental health services with whom we consulted showed us how great the need was for support groups for older women suffering depression and mental distress. Many older women, living in poverty, in poor housing and suffering isolation and loneliness, also suffer from depression. The 'cure' offered them by GPs is tranquillizers and statistics show that there is a steady increase in sleeping pill prescription with increasing age. One in five over 65 regularly takes sleeping pills. Older women's mental symptoms are not treated as seriously as older men's and they are rarely offered the 'talking treatments'. They complain of lack of choice allowed them in treatment, and of lack of appropriate community care services.

With this knowledge, the Older Women's Project decided to organize 'get togethers' of users in various localities, with the aim of setting up support groups. The planning of these 'get togethers' has been in co-operation with MIND and other local community groups. At the first, held in Ealing, the discussion centred around depression and tranquillizers and a group of participants showed interest in forming a support group for older women with depression, which we helped them set up. All of them had complaints about the treatment they had received in hospital and feared having to go back.

We were then asked to organize a 'get together' in Brent, where a flourishing support group has since been formed. As there is little research done into the specific needs of older women users of mental health services, we are planning to follow this up and publish our findings. Meanwhile we offer information, advice and advocacy. However, we have consulted with older women users to find out what they consider to be good or bad practice in the mental health services and we are contributing our findings to a booklet being produced by a core group of the World Federation for Mental Health looking at good practice in mental health for women in the UK. One thing the women emphasized was the need to change attitudes towards those suffering mental health problems. The stigma attached continues to affect their lives long after they are discharged from hospital and it requires a public awareness exercise to give people an understanding of mental distress. Health promotion units are essential for such work, yet no new funding has been allocated for health promotion.

WHO CARES?

In all the work we have described, the project has been endeavouring to give older women the support and information they need to gain more control over their lives. It was felt that information was the key to being able to make proper choices. Thus, after our inaugural meeting setting up AGLOW it was not surprising that we should organize a conference on 'community care – six months on' so that our members could be well informed and, armed with the knowledge imparted by the speakers, continue to campaign to improve that care.

On the very day of that conference, the newspapers reported on a British Medical Association survey which stated that care in the community was failing, with few homes available for the mentally ill. They called for an urgent review of the government changes made in April 1993 which were intended to improve care for the mentally handicapped and old people, yet 85% of the doctors questioned said there had been no improvement in services to patients and 40% felt they had deteriorated. The chairman of the BMA community care committee said they were concerned that a large burden is being placed on carers who are looking after relatives with little or no respite. There are 6.8 million carers in the UK and an analysis by Arber and Ginn (1991) shows that people over 65 provide 35% of the informal care needed by other elderly people. It is hard to tell exactly how many older women carers there are because they accept the role without asking for any help, as they have done all their lives, and they don't get registered. Traditionally, women have borne every burden stoically and never asked for help. They always put themselves last and they are adamant that they wouldn't wish to be a burden on their family.

The community care services are intended primarily to enable people to continue to live in their own homes independently or with the support of carers, and the aim is to provide appropriate support for people's needs. The cornerstone of the Community Care Act, therefore, is the assessment of needs. The older women at the conference expressed concern about the process. They pointed out the complexity of the assessment and the confusing jargon used. They were also deeply worried about the questions on finance. They don't like being asked about their personal finances and certainly they dislike the element of means testing for services. In some cases, older people are having to wait many weeks for assessment. The worthy aim of the Act – to have a needs-led approach rather than resources-led – is not being achieved because there are insufficient resources to meet the needs.

To enable older people to remain in their own homes, it is necessary to provide them with affordable help with repairs, decoration, odd jobs, window cleaning and gardening, said our members. And they were all concerned about the increasing number of homeless older women living on the streets, many of them suffering from alcoholism.

The women were also worried that the cuts in adult education generally would affect adults with learning difficulties who attend courses as part of their package of activities. Concern was also shown about the withdrawal of funds from black and ethnic community groups in a number of boroughs, because they were so necessary to facilitate self-help advocacy, campaigning and community development.

One of the most poignant moments of the conference was when one older woman stood up and said 'I don't want to be made to be a carer', but was obviously worried about the failing health of her older sister. The women all agreed that the opportunity should be given to them to pay attention to their own needs and aspirations for the first time in their lives. They wanted to develop their own creativity and increase their knowledge and skills, to be able to offer more to society.

AGLOW has published a report of the conference on community care and distributed it to councillors and health authority officials as well as local authority officers. We had some replies saying that they agreed with our criticisms and all of them were pleased to have the women's views and said they were considering them. Our views were also being sought at conferences organized by other organizations both in and outside of London.

In a recently published book entitled *Women Come of Age* (Bernard and Meade, 1993) it is stated that:

> Under community care policies, joint planning between social services and health services is a primary objective. But we question whether this goes far enough. Key contributors to enabling older women to remain independent, for example housing, leisure and education departments, transport and town planners, may not be part of the process. Environmental solutions, such as designing and equipping accommodation with low-cost aids, ensuring that local shops and post offices stay open, making the most of local community centres for keep fit sessions, a lunch club and a mobile chiropody service, or putting more accessible buses on the roads,

are as much part of the fabric of living in the community as home-care services. Mechanisms for facilitating this sort of 'neighbour-hood based' planning, in partnership with older women, need to be developed.

The members of AGLOW endorse this wider view and they seek to improve the quality of life for all older women, offering them dignity in old age and a continuing role in society.

LIFE TO YEARS

We feel we have rightly placed an emphasis on health in pursuing our aim to help older women gain confidence. But, though women are survivors, even they cannot 'live by bread alone'. So while women are living longer and many in good health, it is imperative that we don't just add years to their life but also add life to their years!

For that their minds as well as their bodies must be nurtured, their self-esteem boosted and encouragement given them to play an active role in society. Through the study days organized by the Older Women's Education Group, in which AGLOW plays a planning and organizing role, many interesting subjects have been raised for the women to discuss. 'Older women organizing: then and now' gave a history of women organizing themselves from the Chartist movement to the Suffragettes, through to the match girls strike and Asian women on strike in Southall, to abortion demonstrations and Greenham, and to today's tenants' groups and activist groups in local neighbourhoods. In 'As others see us' the women looked at the roles and images of older women in the media and how these reinforce ageist, sexist and racist stereotypes and limit their own expectations.

In 'Public places, future spaces' we examined older women's use of, and safety in, public spaces. We heard how a group in Southwark were involving people, in partnership with local authorities and government agencies, in improving safety in the underground passes leading to the Elephant and Castle shopping centre and the surrounding areas. We were also inspired by a woman living in Clones (population 2000) on the border between the north and south of Ireland. She described movingly the cross-border co-operation. She, and the other women there, have achieved a regeneration of the economy in the area. With that in mind, the women then discussed what they wanted from the urban planners. In 'Older women into Europe' we looked at what the issues are for older women in the single European market; learned of the history and powers of the European Community and how it works; found out the organizations that might further our objectives for a richer and more fulfilled older age. And now we are looking forward to our next study which is going to be on peace.

GOING INTO EUROPE

In Lewisham an Older Women's Project was set up through the good offices of Lewisham Council and their equalities unit. The women decided to exchange information about their daily lives and experiences with older women in Perugia, Italy. Out of that, exchange visits developed, and videos and photographic exhibitions were made and shown at other older women's events in Belfast, Bonn, Charlottenburg, Copenhagen and Utrecht. Gradually the informal network spread to also embrace older women from Belgium, Greece, Portugal and Spain, resolutions were sent to the European Commission and the network formalized into the Older Women's Network, Europe.

AGLOW's own programme also offers, as a contribution to empowering older women, some courses on 'the media', on 'how your council works', and on 'public speaking'. For the summer term a music course and a communications course are being planned.

The project aims to give the women the information and confidence they need to make informed choices and to deal with the professionals who have the power to affect their lives. Since the Community Care Act, local authorities are supposed to consult and involve users in the planning and provision of services, but what is being done cannot be described as genuine consultation. It might even be described as manipulation.

Older women need to be alert to this and armed with the assertion that they are the best people to judge what their needs are; they have to convince service providers that they have much to offer in any discussion on policy or planning. Once confident enough to speak out, I have seen, in committee situations, how a quiet-voiced older woman can cut through all the jargon and double-talk with a simple but effective suggestion. The ideas they put forward are based on long and hard experience of life in their local community and understanding of the people within it. As users of the services they can often see where the best laid plans can go astray. They might also more easily see how to cut corners and costs or make the services more appropriate to their needs.

WHAT CAN OLDER WOMEN OFFER?

Older women are already contributing their skills to many community projects and charities. Traditionally they have staffed Oxfam shops and organized jumble sales and bazaars to raise money. Or they make tea at the local drop-in. They have been the 'good neighbours' in their parish and baby-sitters in their family. But now are also serving on community health councils, as governors of schools, as chairs of management committees of local projects, and on forums for the elderly.

An older woman has been co-opted onto the Women's Committee of Islington, having been nominated from AGLOW. It gives us the opportunity to raise many of the issues that concern older women, and at the moment, the committee is very concerned about the safety of women in the borough.

But much as one would like to think that our wisdom and experience enable us to fill all these roles admirably, the women themselves would be the first to say that they need some training to enable them to play their part to their own satisfaction. They feel that it is essential that they be given the same training opportunities as the paid staff get in the organization. They also see the need in this fast-moving world to keep up with the new technology. Whilst we have sometimes had a 'computer taster' session at our conferences, we realize that it is insufficient and so AGLOW will be organizing some computing classes. We ran a six-week course on 'producing a newsletter', taking in design, layout, editing, editorial decision-taking, writing skills, etc. A newsletter is vitally important to encourage other older women through example. We want to pass on the word to others that older women are finding their voices and are beginning to be heard. They are not all powerless victims. Some are standing up for their rights in the face of the government's assault. Active in their local pensioners' organizations, they are fighting to defend the welfare state.

But, perhaps what I am happiest to see, after all these years since we first started the Older Women's Project, is the personal growth of the women we have worked with, the flowering of their talents, and the pleasure and support they have found through friendships with other women. They have grown strong.

APPENDIX A: FUNDERS' ADDRESSES

Age Concern England, Astral House, 1268 London Road, London SW16 4EJ

BT Community Programme, PO Box 72, Southampton SO9 7ET

Charity Projects Ltd., First Floor, 74 New Oxford Street, London WC1A 1EF

City Parochial Foundation, 6 Middle Street, London EC1A 7PH

Co-operative Community Awards Scheme, Member Relations Dept., Co-op Retail Services, 78–102 The Broadway, Stratford, London E15 1NL

Department of the Environment, 2 Marsham Street, London SW1P 3EP

Department of Health, Richmond House, 79 Whitehall, London SW1

Gulbenkian Foundation, 98 Portland Place, London W1N 4ET

Hampstead Wells and Campden Trust, 62 Rosslyn Hill, London NW3 1ND

Help the Aged, Head Office, St James Walk, London EC1
London Borough Grants Committee, Fifth Floor, Regal House, London
    Road, London TW1 3QS
LWT Telethon, London TV Centre, Upper Ground, London SE1 9PP
Rowntrees Memorial Family Fund, Beverley House, Shipton Road, York
Tudor Trust, 7 Ladbroke Grove, London W11

APPENDIX B: ADDRESSES OF WOMEN'S GROUPS

AGLOW Association of Greater London Older Women, c/o 6–9 Manor
    Gardens, London N7 6LA
Asian Women's Resource Centre, 134 Minet Avenue, London NW10
    8AP
Bangladesh Women's Association, Community Centre, Stanley Road,
    London N15
Fawcett Society, 46 Haileyford Road, London SE11 5AY
Gemma, Box BM 5700, London WC1 3XX
London Irish Women's Centre, 59 Church Street, London N16
London Lesbian Line, Box BM 1514, London WC1 3XX
London Women's Centre, 4 Wild Court, London WC2B 4AU
National Alliance of Women's Organizations, 279/281 Whitechapel
    Road, London E1 1BY
National Council of Women, 36 Danbury Street, Islington, London N1
    8JU
Older Feminist Network, c/o Astra, 54 Gordon Road, London N3 1P
Older Lesbian Network, c/o London Women's Centre, 4 Wild Court,
    London WC2B 4AU
Older Women's Project Lewisham, c/o E. Sclater, Civic Centre, Catford,
    London SE6
Rights of Women, 52 Featherstone Street, London EC1Y 8RT
Union of Turkish Women, 110 Clarence Road, London E5 8JA
Women's Therapy Centre, c/o 6–9 Manor Gardens, London N7 6LA

REFERENCES

Arber, S. and Ginn, J. (1991) Gender, class and income: inequalities in later life.
    British Journal of Sociology, **42** (3), pp. 369–396.
Bernard, M. and Meade, K. (1993) *Women Come of Age: Perspectives on the Lives of
    Older Women*, Pandora Press, London.

FURTHER READING

Curtis, Z. (1989) Older women and feminism: don't say sorry. *Feminist Review*,
    31 (Spring), pp. 143–147.

Ford, J. and Sinclair, M. (1987) *Sixty Years On: Women Talk About Old Age*, Women,s Press, London.

Forster, M. (1989) *Have The Men Had Enough?* Penguin, Harmondsworth.

Franks, H. (1987) *What Every Woman Should Know About Retirement*, Age Concern England, London.

Gibson, M.J. (1985) *Older Women Around the World*, International Federation on Ageing, Washington DC.

Hemmings, S. (1985) *A Wealth of Experience: The Lives of Older Women*, Pandora Press, London.

Johnson, J. and Slater, R. (1994) *Ageing and Later Life*, Sage, London.

Macdonald, B. and Rich, C. (1984) *Look Me in the Eye: Old Women, Ageing and Ageism*, Spinsters Book Co., San Francisco.

Meigs, M. (1991) *In the Company of Strangers*, Talonbooks, Canada.

Neild, S. and Pearson, R. (1992) *Women Like Us*, Women,s Press, London.

Olsen, T. (1980) *Tell Me a Riddle*, Virago Press, London.

Shapiro, J. (1989) *Ourselves Growing Older*, Fontana, London.

Sidell, M. (1991) *Gender Differences in the Health of Older People*, Research Report, Open University, Milton Keynes.

11

Practical projects for empowering people in health and social welfare

Vera Ivers

INTRODUCTION

Self-health Care in Old Age began as an identified project in 1986 after a successful bid to the European Commission for funds under the second programme to combat poverty. The initiative had evolved, however, as a result of work undertaken over a number of years at the Beth Johnson Foundation.

The Beth Johnson Foundation is a small charitable trust with a commitment to working in innovative ways towards improving the quality of life for older people. A total of 50% of the necessary funds for the self-health care initiative came from the second poverty programme sponsored by the European Community and 50% from the Foundation. The project identified circumstances in which people who might benefit from the programme could be deemed to be disadvantaged and experiencing poverty of access to health and welfare services.

Meaning of Poverty – 1

> More than material deprivation, it is a lack of access to the kinds of information, knowledge, social contact, recreational, educational and health care opportunities which might enhance well-being in later years.

Meaning of Poverty – 2

> As a consequence, many older people may feel a sense of powerlessness, lack of confidence and self-esteem, feel isolated,

helpless and apathetic – feelings which are hostile to good physical and mental health.

Over a number of years the Foundation has worked in partnership with older people in determining which issues affected their quality of life. During this working partnership which began in the early 1980s positive health and well-being were identified as priorities. Foundation staff were able to meet with people before retirement when it was clear that anxieties were often about income maintenance and the ability to meet commitments. These anxieties were addressed and appropriate information obtained. Other topics such as health, activity, personal development and relationships were introduced and were continued in discussion post-retirement.

It was at this stage that the issue of health and well-being became the predominant topic for discussion. There was a demand for specific information about various conditions and advice about diet, activity and stress control. Clearly the question of remaining independent was of great concern and comments echoed those of participants in a survey on independence (Sixsmith, 1986): 'Take away your independence and you are finished. You just deteriorate and that's it'. Independence for our group members was closely linked with remaining active in body and mind, being able to look after themselves. Some participants were worried about the public discussion concerning the cost of health and welfare services and the proposition that increasing numbers of elderly people were proving an unacceptable burden on the working population. Most people had believed that contributions during their lifetime to the National Insurance scheme and through their efforts at work and at home during those years entitled them to the services they might need in old age. There was sometimes anger that their needs might not be met and sometimes unhappy acceptance that if resources were scarce, the old would be last in a list of priorities.

SEEKING AND COLLECTING INFORMATION

During one series of discussions in 1984, the group considered the information they would need in order to make personal plans for maintenance of health and well-being. As an exercise between weekly meetings they were asked to seek out the information that had been identified as necessary for them to be able to make informed decisions about personal health plans. Six women undertook to research available information and advice, each agreeing to approach different agencies. The topics of most interest were:

- Informed advice about sensible diets.
- Information about exercise with advice about what was and was not sensible.

- Dealing with stress and crisis; where to go for help.
- Specific information about conditions which are associated with ageing. In particular, what help and treatments are available. High on everyone's list in this category were arthritis and rheumatic conditions.

After a period of two weeks the research resulted in only four leaflets being found, obtained at a health centre and at a chemist. Perhaps even more interesting was the fact that where participants had identified professional health workers who they felt might have offered information or advice, none was forthcoming. Following the exercise an eminent local rheumatology consultant was asked to attend a session to talk about treatments now available and answer questions. Members were very grateful and impressed by the consultant's expertise in traditional medicine but disappointed that their attempts to raise questions on alternative ways to deal with arthritis and rheumatism were not answered. Similarly an alternative therapist invited to a later meeting was only able to discuss herbal mixtures.

It was as a result of this work and numerous other health discussions with older people (Bernard and Ivers, 1986) that the Self-help Care Proposal was formulated. Although it concentrates on health, in the process it addresses other issues such as poverty, access to information and opportunity, feelings of powerlessness and isolation and lack of social contact.

SELF-HEALTH CARE

The aim was to provide an accessible, attractive and popular means of furthering health education and promotion among older people. The underlying principles were identified as follows:

- To raise older people's awareness of the need for health care and maintenance.
- To encourage involvement of more older people in health care programmes.
- To assist older people to identify their health needs and to develop the skills and strategies required to obtain the resources to meet their needs.

Definitions of what was to be included in the project were also clearly set out as follows:

- All the actions and decisions that an individual takes to prevent, diagnose and treat personal ill health.
- All individual behaviour calculated to improve and maintain health.
- All decisions taken by individuals to gain access to, or use, both informal support systems and formal medical services.

The work began with four components:

- a senior health shop
- peer health counselling
- a care line
- health-related activities.

The development of peer health counselling enabled the work to expand so that it later included:

- reminiscence groups
- advocacy
- support groups for Alzheimer sufferers
- senior citizens involved in public services, health and advocacy (SCIPSHA).

THE SENIOR HEALTH SHOP

This was to be at the very core of the project – a place where people over 50 years of age could drop in on any weekday, offering information, advice and practical help in a relaxed and friendly atmosphere. It was important that people should feel free and comfortable to use the facility and that it would be attractive to all backgrounds, particularly those who were experiencing poverty or in some other way disadvantaged. The shop had to be accessible in two respects. Firstly, in geography so that people could reach the shop easily, finding it accessible by public transport and by car. Secondly, it should be situated where they would normally be visiting.

The city of Stoke-on-Trent is an affiliation of six towns, all of which have their own history and identity. It was not going to be possible to site a shop in each of the six town centres, but the city commercial centre is Hanley, where the senior health shop is sited. It seemed likely that many people from the other towns would use the city centre's extended facilities at least occasionally. Finding suitable premises in a high rent area was not easy but eventually the demise of another charity allowed us to move into a small shop which is less than five minutes walk from the bus station, car parks and shopping centre.

Access also had to be considered in terms of persuading people to cross the threshold. The shop had to be comfortable, warm, attractive and have a friendly and non-clinical atmosphere. The decision to make the front of the shop into a small and attractive healthy eating cafeteria was perhaps the most important element in considering access. While some people would come for specific information, it was hoped that others would come in for refreshments and be influenced by the health information material of which there is an extensive stock displayed all around the shop. The window display is changed monthly, carrying topical health messages. The senior health shop manager is a qualified nurse and offers blood pressure and weight checks as well as personal and confidential consultations.

The cafeteria offers drinks and snacks using ingredients recommended by the district dietician. The menu is small and simple with occasional special items. The recipes for items served are printed and on display. Customers are encouraged to take them away and try them at home. Perhaps the most interesting development with regard to the cafeteria concerns the older volunteers who prepare and serve the food. They are interested in their own health and make use of the information available. They receive training and support from the project staff and become very good at helping customers to take the step between coming in to take refreshments and making use of the shop as a health facility.

At the planning stage it was hoped that premises would be found which would accommodate all that is described above plus a small seminar room where health discussion groups could take place. However, the availability and cost of city centre shops made that impossible, so that it was particularly pleasing to observe discussions taking place between customers at different tables, often the result of an enquiry and the volunteer or staff member pointing to a leaflet or book. Other people would be interested and join in the discussion.

Monitoring of the senior health shop users is achieved by means of a questionnaire which is completed for a full week, in the early days on a three monthly basis, and later at six monthly intervals. Data collected offer sociodemographic material as well as health issues. For example, in 1988 more than half of respondents were single or widowed and 88% were not working. Incomes were generally less than £99 per week. Tables 11.1 and 11.2 show respondents' comparisons with more formal health services, and topics discussed with peer health counsellors and clients.

Numbers using the shop increased over the first three years with 1988 showing the greatest use at 11 036. Inevitably, many customers return several times – sometimes as a regular weekly visit. However, there has been a consistent recording of 20% new users year on year. There is no doubt that the cafeteria is a great draw and attempts were made to reduce the numbers coming only for food by restricting the variety on offer. Similarly the data threw up the disproportionate numbers of women to men using the shop. In response the welcome notices were revised to specify men and women welcome and window displays were planned to attract men, with some success. Much of the Self-help Care Project depends upon enthusiastic, trained and supported volunteers to function effectively. The senior health shop plays a crucial role in recruiting volunteers and in addition is attractive to the media. Both the

Table 11.1 Comparison of senior health shop with more formal health services

	Male n%	Female n%	Total n%
More friendly: relaxed and informal	36 (29)	124 (25)	160 (26)
Easy to obtain info/leaflets	17 (14)	84 (17)	101 (16)
Have time to sit and talk	11 (9)	69 (14)	80 (13)
Can call in at any time	21 (17)	50 (10)	71 (11)
Unthreatening	11 (9)	55 (11)	66 (11)
Easier to talk here	–	35 (7)	35 (6)
It's women, not men	–	30 (6)	30 (5)
Food available	11 (9)	15 (3)	26 (4)
Other	36 (29)	139 (28)	175 (28)
Don't know/can't say	–	15 (3)	15 (2)
base (n)	123	496	619

BBC and Central TV have featured the senior health shop in programmes aimed at older viewers. Local radio and press know the shop very well and have featured it extensively over the years.

PEER HEALTH COUNSELLORS

In the context of this project, peer health counsellors are retired older people who have an interest in self-health and want to share their enthusiasm with their peer group in the form of satisfying voluntary work. The notion of peer health support amongst older people is gaining ground and is now part of the Ageing Well Initiative.

The Beth Johnson Foundation development occurred following the principal development officer's Churchill fellowship study tour of North America in 1981, where a peer health counsellor project was observed in Santa Monica. In this country, and in North America, a number of writers have described projects which are essentially part of a comprehensive self-help programme (Bernard and Ivers, 1986; Glendenning, 1985; Savo, 1984). Growing interest in the encouragement of self-health care amongst older people was demonstrated by the World Health Organization in 1981 and the US Department of Health in 1979 (WHO, 1981; US Department of Health, 1979).

The commitment demanded of peer health counsellors is substantial but the benefits to individual volunteers is identified by them in such comments as 'I've gained a greater insight into things which had never crossed my mind', 'I've certainly learned more about what can happen to people in old age and how to look after myself', 'I feel much more

Table 11.2 Health concerns of visitors

	1987				1988				Total
	March n%	June n%	Sept n%	Dec n%	March n%	June n%	Sept n%	Dec n%	n%
Nothing in particular	2 (4)	5 (13)	11 (20)	–	7 (8)	20 (18)	14 (13)	12 (11)	71 (11)
Generally interested	8 (17)	3 (8)	6 (11)	3 (6)	19 (21)	24 (21)	43 (39)	51 (46)	157 (25)
Diet and health food	15 (31)	14 (38)	30 (55)	22 (39)	54 (60)	56 (50)	52 (48)	52 (47)	295 (48)
Concern with weight	9 (19)	5 (14)	10 (18)	8 (14)	29 (32)	32 (29)	26 (24)	30 (27)	149 (24)
Exercising	14 (29)	6 (16)	5 (9)	6 (11)	22 (24)	13 (12)	24 (22)	16 (14)	106 (17)
A specific condition	7 (15)	9 (24)	7 (13)	18 (31)	5 (6)	12 (11)	14 (13)	9 (8)	81 (13)
Stress control and relaxation	7 (15)	6 (16)	6 (11)	5 (8)	15 (17)	11 (10)	17 (16)	10 (9)	77 (12)
Other	9 (19)	1 (3)	2 (4)	6 (11)	–	–	–	–	18 (3)
No response	–	–	–	–	2 (2)	3 (3)	4 (4)	7 (6)	16 (3)
base (n)	48	37	55	57	90	112	109	111	619

confident now whatever I'm doing'. Commitment includes training and ongoing contact with a project leader and fellow volunteers.

A training programme has been developed at the Foundation over a number of years (Ivers and Meade, 1990). Volunteers are asked to attend a three-day residential course which has proved to be effective in helping them to immerse themselves in what is often a new experience of learning. It is also useful in the purpose of agreeing which tasks will best suit the volunteer's skills, experience and personality. This basic course covers topics which are relevant to the volunteer's ability to take on the health counselling role. It does not attempt to train extensively in counselling techniques, but does include listening and communicating skills.

Staff members accompany volunteers on the course and contribute to sessions. Participants are also encouraged to share their own life experiences and demonstrate skills. The range of tasks available to trained peer health counsellors is discussed, and volunteers usually have a clear idea of where they would like to work. Placements arise as a result of these discussions and negotiations with staff who have the ultimate responsibility for ensuring that volunteers are appropriately placed. The range of tasks on offer is wide, and rarely is it impossible to place a volunteer although it might be necessary to offer something other than first choice. Volunteers are encouraged to consider their commitment throughout the process and where a volunteer has doubts they are encouraged to withdraw at any stage.

Following the basic training course peer health counsellors are asked to meet regularly with the leader of the project on which they are working and also to meet their fellow volunteers regularly. These meetings have a business and sharing element where aspects of the day-to-day management of a project is discussed, giving volunteers an opportunity to contribute. They also have a training element, which is determined by earlier discussion. An example would be the advocacy group which decided at a meeting that they needed to learn more about beginning relationships with vulnerable people who asked for advocacy. The staff group, which includes an experienced trainer, then devised an appropriate session.

Peer health counsellor training is offered to all volunteers with the Beth Johnson Foundation, and the range of projects on offer includes:

- working at the senior health shop,
- preparing and serving food at the senior centre, a drop-in facility offering social contact and educational opportunities,
- sharing skills by leading a special interest group,
- presenting self-health material to fairs, festivals, exhibitions, workshops, clubs, etc.,

- befriending and supporting individuals who wish to develop their own new health plan,
- leading gentle activity and discussion groups with older people in residential or sheltered housing situations,
- leading reminiscence sessions with people suffering from confusion or dementia,
- working on Care Line, a telephone help line described later in the chapter,
- becoming advocates, described in detail later in the chapter,
- helping with SCIPSHA (senior citizens involved in public services, health and advocacy), the Foundation's latest project, a roadshow visiting local neighbourhoods for a period of three months aiming to set up interest groups which will continue when the roadshow moves on.

Perhaps before leaving this section it would be worth noting that people who become peer health counsellors are a very typical group of the age range. Table 11.3 shows that they suffer a normal range of disabilities and conditions.

Table 11.3 Peer health counsellors – health status

Since retirement I am:	
More interested in health	6
Less interested	–
No difference	5
Total participants	11
Being retired has:	
Improved my health	5
Made my health worse	1
No difference	5
Total participants	11
Health difficulties in last six months:	
Arthritis/rheumatism	5
Indigestion	5
Sleeping	4
Since retirement I suffer:	
Always feeling tired	3
Shortness of breath	3
Spells of depression	3
Hearing difficulties	1
Total responses	24

CARE LINE

Peer health counsellors telephone frail housebound elderly people daily, to check on their health and well-being and to bring some contact with the outside world.

In planning self-health care we were conscious that it would not be possible for everyone to visit the senior health shop or to take advantage of other facilities. Care Line was an attempt to reach housebound elderly people. Referrals come from social workers, health visitors, doctors, nurses, carers and occasionally are self-referrals. An initial visit is made to the person and where possible in the company of the referrer. The purpose of this visit is to establish a number of things which will enable the daily call to be effective. Firstly, the visit goes some way to establishing the relationship between client and volunteers. Secondly, where the telephone is in relation to chair, bed, bathroom and kitchen will determine how long it takes the client to reply to the telephone. Occasionally it is necessary for volunteers and staff to seek the necessary funds to relocate the telephone. Thirdly, and perhaps the most vital task for the visitor, is to determine who are the significant people in the client's life. These are recorded as key persons who agree to being contacted by Care Line volunteers if there appears to be a problem during the daily call. The most worrying situation occurs when the telephone is not answered by a client who is known to be chair-bound or bed-bound. In many such events the client has gone to a doctor or hospital appointment or a friend has called to take them out for a drive. However, that has to be established by calling the key person or a list of people who may already know what is happening, but in any case will go immediately to check on the situation. The aim is to find a key person who lives nearby, but there may be a list of significant people including a social worker or community care worker, nurse, doctor, warden, etc. If a call is not answered volunteers will go through this list until they can establish their client's situation. As a last resort, if no key person can be contacted, Care Line has good contacts with community police officers who will gain entry if necessary.

This system has rescued a number of very vulnerable people who had collapsed, fallen or lapsed into unconsciousness. Very occasionally professional or police help has been enlisted only to find that the failure to respond to a call has an innocent explanation. Even so, it can reassure the person concerned that help will arrive if they are really in trouble. One woman actually telephoned to say 'I feel really safe, knowing that you don't let up until you find out what's wrong'.

Volunteers work in pairs on a rota system from an office, and at the end of each call record in the client's personal file a brief note about the call. Over a period of time, this record can point to changes in the person's condition, and is effective as a monitoring process. Care Line clients agree to this monitoring and to contact being made with their key persons. Volunteers involved in this project carry considerable responsibility for very vulnerable people and need to be able to enlist the help of someone who will take on the responsibility at the end of their session where a problem has not been resolved. A member of staff is responsible for the project and takes over from volunteers when necessary ensuring that volunteers do not return home feeling that someone is in serious trouble without help. The service is appreciated by the health and social service workers who refer, and is very popular with volunteers and clients. It is a low cost project: volunteers' expenses and the daily calls cost less than £1 per week per client, although the cost of professional support and office space would need to be included in a project without access to these facilities. It is possible for each pair of volunteers to make 40 calls during a period of two to three hours. At holiday times there is often a long period when offices are closed and services are restricted; for example, at Christmas 1993, the holiday period lasted for almost two weeks, a long time for an elderly person who has no family or friendly contact. In advance of such holidays, users of the service are asked if they will be at home alone. During the holiday referred to, 14 people out of a client group of 35 were going to be alone for the whole period. Volunteers offer to phone these clients from home each day and are recompensed for the cost of the calls. A back-up support person is always available.

A second Care Line office sited in a social service office is a new development and is being monitored by the department, which is also contributing to the cost by paying for four hours supervision time. The results of this experiment will be available in 1995.

HEALTH-RELATED ACTIVITIES

Early in the 1980s, two significant developments took place at the Beth Johnson Foundation. One was the setting up of a senior centre, a drop-in facility which was open to anyone over 50 years of age. There was, and is, no membership and every attempt is made to encourage users whatever their need.

Volunteers provide snacks and meals, and other volunteers lead craft or activity groups. People come to meet others, to eat or to take part in a class, and some 400 people make use of the centre over a three-day week. The centre has one paid worker who manages and co-ordinates, and activities on offer include music, crafts, painting, patchwork, dressmaking, crochet, dancing, yoga, popagility and a look after yourself class. A user committee organizes trips and holidays.

At the same time another group organized a variety of activities for older people. The Beth Johnson Leisure Association was initiated and developed within the Foundation but is an independent body in terms of finance, and with its own management committee. Regular activities on offer include five swimming sessions each week in different parts of the city, three rambling sessions catering for absolute beginners through to more experienced walkers, table tennis, bowls, badminton, fitness training and regular activity holidays. Occasional courses are also organized and have included sailing, abseiling, skiing and gliding. From this wide range of activities, it is usually possible to find one that will suit the needs of most people wishing to take up an active or creative pursuit in retirement. Through an extensive network across the area it is also possible to introduce enquirers to other agencies and activities perhaps closer to home, or catering for different interests. All of the Leisure Association's activities are led by experienced volunteers in their particular field. Most of the leaders have also taken advantage of peer health counsellor training. Ongoing training is regularly organized: for example, rambling leaders attend map reading and life saving courses. Swimming instructors are updated in safety measures.

The Leisure Association, through its management committee, contracts with a number of leisure centres and swimming pools for access to facilities and aims to recoup costs by charging a fee to users. The fees are kept intentionally low, to encourage as many people as possible to participate.

Both the senior centre and the Leisure Association have successes in attracting long term and loyal users while remaining open and friendly to newcomers. Peer health counsellors may introduce people to any of the activities, certain that they will be welcomed. An example taken from Bernard and Ivers (1986) follows: 'A recently retired man felt lonely and depressed, feeling that his physical and mental health might deteriorate through lack of activity. He was interested in painting and was encouraged to join the senior centre art group, and to go rambling, supported each step of the way by the peer health counsellor'.

ADVOCACY

As we became more confident about the range of tasks that trained and supported volunteers could and would undertake, it was possible to respond to other identified needs. In the late 1980s, the concept of citizen advocacy and the work of Wolf Wolfensberger (1977) in America and Sang and O'Brien (1984) in the UK was gaining interest. Earlier work had concentrated on finding advocates for people suffering from mental illness or learning difficulties, but interest was growing in extending advocacy to other vulnerable groups (see Rankin, 1989; Willis, 1990).

Peer health counsellors seemed to be suited to advocacy, and after some research a project was launched in 1989. In deciding where to target the new service, it became clear that there are certain times in an elderly person's life when they may experience increased feelings of disempowerment, disadvantage and vulnerability. One such period occurs when some trauma is suffered, requiring treatment in the acute stage. Following that stage many people will be ready to return home with the help of friends or family who may articulate the patient's wishes. Where there is no natural advocate, however, the patient is required to assert their own wishes, needs or preferences by entering the discussion and decision-making process being undertaken by professionals in the health and social services sectors. At such a time the older person may not feel able to make such a contribution, even though very important decisions may have to be made about living arrangements until the end of life. Indeed there is some evidence that when help is required with day-to-day living arrangements, older people often feel that they have no real choice and that decisions will be made by others whatever they may wish (Allen, Hogg and Peace, 1992).

With this in mind, negotiations were opened with a unit manager at the elderly care unit of the local health authority, and after a lengthy period where a great deal of discussion was necessary, agreement was reached on the operation of a pilot project (Ivers, 1994). Even so there was some anxiety and apprehension amongst staff, especially those with day-to-day responsibility for treatment and caring. The Foundation was able to employ an advocacy training and support worker with a grant under the Opportunities for Volunteering programme. During the pilot phase this worker visited wards and later, residential homes on a weekly basis. She would make contact with patients or clients who had read the Foundation's advocacy literature distributed by staff or whom staff referred because they recognized that the individual was unhappy with the situation and had observed that there was no effective natural advocate. The visits also served to familiarize staff with the concept of advocacy. During the first two years of the project a total of 35 people were introduced to advocates. At any one time there were approximately 20 partnerships in operation. Advocates were recruited following the same pattern as with all other Beth Johnson volunteers. People already involved with Beth Johnson projects heard about the new project through in-house discussions and a regular newsletter. Local radio and press were recruited to run publicity features, other organizations were contacted, including volunteer bureaux.

Advocates receive the programme of basic training, and continue with ongoing training as part of a monthly programme of meetings. Each volunteer is introduced to one partner and an effort is made to make a good or at least a viable match. Perhaps by the nature of the task, it was inevitable that the greatest number of volunteer advocates (17 from the first 20) came from middle-class backgrounds, with working experience of a professional or administrative nature. In direct contrast only one of the first 20 partners had a professional background, with 19 having worked in manual or low status jobs. The partners also exhibited a typical pattern of family or social contacts. Over a period of a month only six had contact with people other than the statutory service providers. The conclusion reached by Ivers (1994) is that few older people need an advocate in order to have their own needs, wishes or preferences heard. However, the minority have a desperate need for this type of help. Partnerships were mostly long term – lasting until the partner died, although in some instances they were ended after the presenting problems had been resolved. In particular, this project identified the need for longer term support and counselling for volunteers when partners who had become special friends died.

Tasks undertaken by advocates on behalf of their partners were very varied, but usually began with the collection of information. Examples include a partner who is being advised that residential care is the best option, but then wishes to consider a range of establishments as well as alternatives to residential care. It is often the case that introduction to an advocate slows down the rate at which a patient can be discharged from hospital and advocates frequently find themselves negotiating for time. It may be that the partner will eventually accept the advice of professionals, having considered options and implications but are not able to come to a decision at the same speed.

Since the implementation of the National Health Service and Community Care Act, from April 1993, regular requests are being made by health and social service staff for advocates to be involved with patients or clients who are subjects of multi-agency assessments. Indeed, the local social service department has recently decided that any funds that they allocate for advocacy must be spent primarily on this area of work. There is obviously some danger associated with such a decision, that other vulnerable people will be excluded from the service. Only by advocacy schemes maintaining complete independence from service-providing agencies will advocacy continue to serve vulnerable and disempowered people with a whole variety of needs and from different situations.

An example of a partner who was not subject to a multi-agency assessment and therefore under these restricted criteria would not be able to benefit from introduction to an advocate is given by Ivers (1994). A long term resident of a local authority home had been admitted after her last relation had died, even though she was only in her early forties. On admission, the residents were of mixed ages and abilities but over the years had become older and frailer. Many of the social and community activities that she had enjoyed were no longer available to her. The advocate took nearly a year to get to know her partner well and to establish some trust. She learned that her partner's wishes and needs concerned access to social events, to people of her own age, to updating her wardrobe and rebuilding her confidence so that she was able to take advantage of any social opportunity that presented. Advocate, partner and residential care staff agreed that the advocacy partnership had transformed the quality of life for this woman.

Advocates are required to meet with the advocacy training and support worker on a fortnightly basis for supervision and to attend monthly business, sharing and training meetings. However, they are quite clear that their sole loyalty is to their partner, and the code of conduct to which they agree requires them to help their partner become effective at self-advocacy and, where they need to be the advocate, to represent their wishes, needs and preferences as if they were their own.

REMINISCENCE

A very popular activity for peer health counsellors is reminiscence group work. Reminiscence is a natural everyday occurrence which most people engage in. It focuses on the personal way we experience and remember past events rather than on factual or historical accuracy. Over the past 25 years or so, the importance of this process for mental health and well-being has become appreciated. Peer health counsellors visit homes, often meeting people who suffer from confusion or dementia. The process of reminiscing helps their client to recall early events which are often remembered clearly even when recent memory is very poor. A particularly rewarding result of this development is the partnerships forged with agencies such as libraries and museums.

Although reminiscence is not acceptable to every resident of every establishment, it appears to bring pleasure to many. Where it is not welcome, volunteers quickly observe any unease, take the resident away from the group and spend some time with them.

The value of reminiscence to those people who are happy to take part is described in the Foundation's leaflet. 'Reminiscence is of benefit to elderly people themselves, to the staff and to volunteers.'

To elderly people because:

- It highlights their assets rather than their disabilities.
- It encourages feelings of self-worth and esteem.
- It enhances a sense of personal identity.
- It encourages and enriches social exchange.
- It is enjoyable and stimulating.

To the staff because:

- It can help to alter perception and understanding of elderly people by concentrating on past joys, achievements and pains rather than on present defects.
- It reverses the usual relationship in which elderly people receive from others by enabling them to give of their past experience and knowledge.
- It can open new and rewarding ways of communicating.

To volunteers because:

- The work is interesting, rewarding and very enjoyable.
- Volunteers work in groups enabling new and interesting contacts to be made.
- The Beth Johnson Foundation offers good training, support and social opportunities to its volunteers.

SUPPORT GROUPS FOR ALZHEIMER SUFFERERS

This area of development had first been pioneered by the Beth Johnson Foundation in 1980, resulting in a project which now has ten groups operating and is entirely independent. Some years later, and after the development of peer health counselling, the Foundation was approached by a community psychiatric nurse who wanted to see further developments particularly to serve a large rural area.

Peer health counsellors appeared to be suited to the type of small group work offered by this scheme, and currently work at three venues with a fourth planned in the near future.

Groups are deliberately kept small and are therefore suitable for small town or village developments. Venues are local to the users, all three taking place in church halls. The co-ordinator is a paid employee funded by a grant from the mental health section of the combined health care unit (North Staffordshire Health Authority). She is assisted by volunteers who have been trained as peer health counsellors. The user group is seldom more than ten and volunteers usually number around six, enabling each user to receive very personal attention. The groups are planned to be friendly, warm social events with users and volunteers taking part together in all activities, taking meals together and in the fact that volunteers also transport users to the group in their cars.

When volunteers and users arrive there is a short period where users can begin to feel safe. It is not certain that they will remember who the volunteers are or where they are being taken. The day begins with coffee followed by a short programme of gentle physical activity. After a meal, there are further activities of a quieter nature requiring some mental effort. Peer health counsellors who choose this type of work become skilled at developing each individual's potential performance, often to the amazement of carers who may then be persuaded to encourage more activity at home. Groups are held weekly at each venue and cannot be said to provide the extent of care which would enable a carer to remain at work, but have been found to help carers where traditional day care is found to be unsuitable or unacceptable. In the words of one spouse carer, 'I couldn't leave her with just anyone, but I'm happy to go and take a bit of time out because I know she is happy here and you will look after her as I would'. In addition to providing an acceptable service and a worthwhile voluntary task, the project helps to raise awareness of the condition and volunteers are able to present information about Alzheimer's disease informally or to local groups.

SENIOR CITIZENS INVOLVED IN PUBLIC SERVICES, HEALTH AND ADVOCACY

This latest development arises as a result of experience throughout the self-health care work and particularly advocacy. Often when an individual has been helped to challenge the system there emerges a problem which goes beyond the specific situation. It is not always appropriate for a volunteer or even a member of staff to challenge a department where a management or policy decision appears to be at the root of the problem that affects a service user so personally. The situation is recognized by service providers, many of whom declare their intention of involving users of services in planning so that services most nearly reach the perceived need of users. In practice this involvement is often difficult to achieve, although as a result of the National Health Service and Community Care Act 1990, health and social service departments have made attempts.

This project sets out to work alongside older people in small communities, encouraging them to consider the needs of older people in the locality and to decide which services could be made to be more user friendly.

As a result of interest and funding from the Department of Health and the European Commission, as part of the European Year of Elderly People and Solidarity between Generations (1993), it was possible to add on to the SCIPSHA initiative a roadshow approach to self-health care and advocacy. The SCIPSHA element is jointly funded by the Beth Johnson Foundation and charity projects.

In operational terms a SCIPSHA co-ordinator assisted by a self-health and advocacy worker visit small communities, such as housing estates, small town centres, villages. Visits will be for one day each week over a three-month period offering self-health advice and information including the blood pressure and weight checks, access to advocacy and an opportunity to discuss that neighbourhood in terms of older user friendliness.

At the end of the three-month period it is hoped that groups will continue, both as neighbourhood action and health maintenance. Colleagues in the various statutory authorities have been consulted during the planning stage of SCIPSHA and have been encouraging. There appears to be a general recognition that although many agencies are committed to user participation and consultation they have, as yet, not found a satisfactory formula. This new bottom-up approach is of interest and no doubt the development will be closely observed.

This chapter has attempted to describe a number of developments that have taken place in one small organization in the Midlands and also to highlight trends and interests which, given some encouragement, could have an influence on the process of empowering particular groups, in this case elderly people.

PRACTICAL EMPOWERMENT

In this chapter a number of projects have been described which show an underlying philosophy. The various areas of work highlight different concerns for elderly people but the common aim is to help those people to have some control over decisions which affect their daily lives. Elderly people who use the projects frequently feel totally disempowered. Examples of statements offered include:

> I can't go back to the doctor again, he is so busy and he has already told me what I should do (Self-health Care Project).

> It's no use complaining about this street, they take no notice at all (SCIPSHA Project).

> I don't like it here, but if you tell them that they could make it worse for me (Advocacy Project).

Such statements are frequently made to volunteers and staff.

The good news is that given sufficient information on which to base sound judgements and some encouragement, the elderly people concerned are able to gain the confidence needed to challenge professional decisions. This happens in all of the projects but is perhaps most easily observed through the advocacy partnerships. Elderly partners often feel anxious about their futures, perhaps after suffering a fall or a sudden illness.

Professional health and social service staff are concerned with efficient and rapid turnover of case loads and do not give the time necessary for the individual to work through the possible options and decide what suits their wishes, needs and preferences. Sufficient information for them to do this is often not offered. Once a group of professionals have agreed their decision it may not seem necessary to them to offer such information.

Many elderly people have decision making taken out of their control, even though they might have spent a lifetime making major decisions. Perhaps the most likely to experience disempowerments, however, are the poor elderly. Choices for them are restricted not only by professional judgements about what is best but also because of funding criteria and allocation of resources. Perhaps data collected from the SCIPSHA project will show how effectively the involvement and empowerment of older people can influence decisions to become more user friendly.

REFERENCES

Allen, I., Hogg, D. and Peace, S. (1992) *Elderly People – Choice, Participation and Satisfaction*, PSI Publishing, London.
Bernard, M. and Ivers, V. (1986) Peer health counselling – a way of countering dependency, in: *Dependency and Interdependency in Old Age*, (eds C. Phillipson, M. Bernard, P. Strang), Croom Helm, London.
Glendenning, F.J. (ed.) (1985) *New Initiatives in Self Health Care for Older People*, The Beth Johnson Foundation in association with the Department of Adult Education, University of Keele and the Health Education Council.
Ivers, V. (1994) *Advocacy in Action Working with Older People*, The Beth Johnson Foundation, Stoke-on-Trent.
Ivers, V., Meade, K. (1990) *Older Volunteers and Peer Health Counselling*, The Beth Johnson Foundation, Stoke-on-Trent.
Rankin, M. (1989) *Advocacy – A Case Study*, Volunteer Centre, Berkhamstead, Hertfordshire.
Savo, C. (1984) *Self Care and Self Help Programmes for Older Adults in the United States*, Health Education Council and Department of Adult Education, University of Keele.
Sang, J. and O'Brien, B. (1984) *Advocacy – the UK and American Experience*, King's Fund Project Paper No. 51, King's Fund Centre, London.
Sixsmith, A.J. (1986) Independence and home in later life, in: *Dependency and Interdependency in Old Age*, (eds C. Phillipson, M. Bernard, P. Strang), Croom Helm, London.
US Department of Health Education and Welfare (1979) *A Guide to Medical Self Care and Self Help Groups for the Elderly*, Government Office, Washington DC.
Willis, E. (1990) *Advocacy – Some Perspectives for the Nineties*, Volunteer Centre, Berkhampstead, Hertfordshire.
Wolfensberger, W. (1977) *A Multicomponent Advocacy and Protection Scheme*, Canadian Association of the Mentally Retarded, Toronto.
World Health Organization (1981) *Self-help and Health*, Report on a WHO Consultation, Copenhagen, 3–6 December 1980, WHO Regional Office for Europe.

12

Power and rights: the psychiatric system survivor movement

Vivien Lindow

BACKGROUND

Personal experience

I'm writing this chapter from personal experience. I lost my twenties to psychiatry. I first went into a mental hospital when I was 19. I spent my thirtieth birthday in my last mental hospital so far. It took me those 11 years of going in and out of big bins and psychiatric units in general hospitals to realize that psychiatry had nothing to offer me. The system did me more harm than good.

After a childhood that did not equip me to be an adult, left me terrified of other people, especially men, the last thing I needed was 'treatment' as a mental patient. My reaction to the whole world was one of fear, I had no idea how to tackle the most ordinary adult task or relationship. I was afraid to go and buy a newspaper. So what did they do in the psychiatric system?

They treated me as though I was ill, so I became more passive. Part of the deal of being a patient is to expect a cure. Since they kept filling me with pills, I thought they were trying to cure me. The drug companies keep bringing out new 'wonder drugs' so it is not surprising that people take on this state of mind, expecting the next drug to be a cure, thinking that doctors know best. It takes away one's initiative and the search for other, human action-based solutions.

They also treated me violently. I was a very compliant person, excruciatingly shy. Yet they gave me electric shocks to my head when I told them about my thoughts, calling it treatment. They legally and illegally prevented me from leaving the hospitals by using the Mental

Health Act and by taking my clothes away and forbidding me to leave. I had no idea I had any rights. Various members of mental health teams exploited me sexually.

All this to someone who was terrified of other people. No wonder I got worse, not better.

Some history

An early example of the patients' advocacy movement in the UK was in the last century. John Perceval was outraged by the treatment he received as a prisoner in the madhouse system of his day. When he managed to get out he became a lifelong writer and campaigner for the closing of the madhouses. He was a leading member of the Alleged Lunatics' Friend Society, started in 1846. Their focus was political action to attempt to gain law reform, also taking up the cases of individual patients.

The Alleged Lunatics' Friend Society was vehemently opposed by the Metropolitan Lunacy Commission and the rest of the 'lunacy' establishment that had vested interests in the control of mad people. Perceval once told a Select Committee of the House of Commons: 'I consider myself the attorney-general of all Her Majesty's madmen' (Podvoll, 1990). He was the forerunner of the modern psychiatric system survivor movement, which similarly opposes psychiatrists and other people with vested interests in controlling mentally distressed people.

The activities of the Alleged Lunatics' Friend Society were not very different from those of campaigning psychiatric system survivors today. Although there were individuals who protested as best they could about the treatment they received through the intervening years, an advocacy movement led by recipients of psychiatry did not re-form until the 1960s, when groups of protesting psychiatric patients and their allies started working together again.

We were fortunate to have R.D. Laing working and writing in Scotland and England from the 1960s, attempting to understand the meaning of the distress labelled as 'schizophrenia'. The psychiatric establishment successfully discredited this colleague, finally designating him 'mad' and therefore not to be heard. Since the 1960s psychiatric services have become even more bio-medical and oppressive.

The anti-psychiatry movement did not quite die as the psychiatric establishment trounced this example of humanity. The British Network for Alternatives to Psychiatry continued to meet, and was a forum for people who wanted to see change in the system throughout the 1970s. In the early 1980s, small groups of survivors were meeting, principally in Glasgow and London.

The year 1985 provided a turning-point. A World Congress of Mental

Health in Brighton, England, allowed different groups to hear about each other. Patients' rights activists from the USA, Holland, and Italy shared their experiences and gave a boost to the British survivor movement.

Survivors Speak Out was started soon afterwards to provide a national network for local groups, individual survivors and their allies. Survivors Speak Out had its first national conference of psychiatric system survivors in 1987, which produced a charter of demands (discussed later). Since then the mental health system user movement has expanded exponentially.

It is worth looking at the international setting, since one phenomenon of 'user involvement' in the UK is that survivors who say something unpopular are likely to be disempowered by being told they are not representative. There are many answers to this. How representative is the challenger? Was the point made a valid one? Since the stereotype of mad people is that we are inarticulate and irrational, nothing we say will count, since someone who is articulate cannot, according to this invalidation, be a genuine service user. But the most telling answer is that mental health service users who meet together in New Zealand, Japan, the USA, Ireland, Scotland, Wales and England say exactly the same kinds of things.

Since 1991 there has been a World Federation of Psychiatric Users (WFPU), meeting biennially at the World Congress for Mental Health and working in task groups in the interim. It is a brave enterprise; the poverty of most psychiatric survivors makes any world co-ordination difficult. This is why it meets at World Congress meetings: organizers fund some users from different countries to give papers. Mary O'Hagan, co-chair of the WFPU from New Zealand, said in her keynote address (unpublished) to the 1993 Congress in Tokyo:

> Movements like ours are a response from the oppressed to a situation that has become intolerable to them. The fact that the user movement exists indicates that society and the mental health system have done significant damage to us despite the good intentions of many people.

Before moving on to a description of the UK user movement, I will outline aspects of the mental health system being moved from the hospitals to our communities which make empowerment of service users such a challenge.

MARGINALIZATION AND DAMAGING SERVICES

A major difference between mental health service users and other community care users is that we can be legally detained without having committed an offence, on the say of mental health workers without any judicial process. There is no incentive for them to provide choice and attractive services if users can be compelled to receive them. Mental health service users are unlikely to complain to or about people who have such power over them.

The most frequent complaint among people who have received mental health services is that nobody listens. Traditional stereotypes combine with current ideas about mental distress, causing a situation in which mental health professionals are trained to ignore the content of what service users say.

In her pioneering book about user-managed alternative services, Judi Chamberlin (1988) identified this phenomenon as one aspect of 'mentalism'. Mentalism parallels sexism and racism in creating an oppressed underclass, in this case of people who have received psychiatric diagnosis and treatment. We are routinely discriminated against, both in the services that ostensibly exist to serve us and by members of wider society.

This prejudice hits us three ways in our lives:

- medical and scientific disempowerment and treatment
- psychoanalytic ideas
- historical stigma.

The alliance with science

The alliance of medicine with science has created an industry around mental distress. This industry includes the huge multinational drug companies and research departments within universities, and gives jobs to the wide variety of mental health professionals.

Mental health professionals are constantly expanding their empire. Ordinary, human reactions to troubles become 'illnesses', such as 'post-traumatic stress disorder'. These can be seen as either a wholly normal reaction to terrible circumstances, through which people need support or reactions to trauma can be defined as an illness and people enter the world of psychiatry, where they will be placed at the bottom of a hierarchy and exposed to the known dangers of psychiatric treatments.

I do not suggest that everything is wrong about calling emotional and mental distress an illness. Humans can categorize their experiences in any way they want. The problem comes when this categorization does more harm than good. Any help I have received within the system has never been medical. It is always a fellow human offering me respect and solidarity.

Scientists, including social scientists, tend to think about their fellow humans in a particular way. They have adopted a laboratory method more appropriate to stones and chemicals for studying people. Some difficulties about this are:

- Scientists count their view as more 'objective' and therefore more reliable than the view of the person most concerned. They earn their living from us, so their vested interest is large. Everyone is 'subjective'.
- The language of science disempowers. Scientists call the person they are researching the 'subject'. Monarchs have subjects.
- Science researchers accept the 'scientific' psychiatric colleague's definition of the situation rather than the person's own view. They usually also accept relatives' views as more valid than the person's (Rogers *et al.*, 1993).
- Because they cannot be studied by scientific method important factors are ignored or undervalued by research scientists. Examples of such factors are childhood experiences, current physical abuse and current emotional abuse such as the experience of racism and/or sexism.

The major expert is disempowered by all this.

As well as research, the training of all mental health workers suffers from both the dominance of psychiatry and the dehumanization of people's experience. One feature of this is discouragement of expression of emotion by either staff or service users (Johnstone, 1989). Any such expression is seen as not coping in workers and a further sign of mental illness in service users. Both professional people and service users are the poorer for this devaluation of emotional expression.

Another mechanism whereby the words of the patient are invalidated can be seen in the training needs of doctors and other mental health workers. Teaching demands the simplification of people's behaviour to allow teachers to illustrate the texts that students have read. This is one reason why a whole range of speech and behaviour gets categorized into diagnoses.

The medical habit of selective listening and observing to make a diagnosis is particularly relevant in psychiatry, where the words themselves are the symptoms rather than a means of describing them. If the psychiatrist is trying to identify illnesses, she or he is less likely to attend to the intrinsic meaning of what the patient says.

Arguments about the unscientific basis of psychiatry are particularly acute when it comes to diagnosis. There are well-articulated criticisms of the reliability and validity of psychiatric diagnoses (Warner, 1985; Boyle, 1990). That is, psychiatric diagnoses have no basis in physical science, however useful some mental health workers find them. The great tomes of diagnostic systems, such as the American Psychiatric Association's unfolding fiction in the various versions of the *Diagnostic and Statistic Manual of Mental Disorders*, are cultural products, not scientific findings.

Nor is the act of diagnosis morally neutral, even if it were an accurate and agreed process. It can lead to great harm, such as:

- the stigma of many psychiatric labels, and their adherence for life,
- the internalization of the idea that there is something wrong that only trained professional people can deal with, with the accompanying disempowerment,
- exposure to under-funded and disrespectful mental health services,
- above all, the toxic medical treatments that people receive.

There is no space here to go into all the harmful aspects of psychiatric treatments. Some few brave psychiatrists are willing to speak out about what is going on in the use of drugs and electro-convulsive therapy (ECT). If you only ever read one book about psychiatry, I suggest Peter Breggin's readable *Toxic Psychiatry* (1993). He is clear about the 'plague of brain damage' being caused by psychiatric procedures in the name of treatment.

As well as brain damage, and unexplained sudden deaths of people taking major tranquillizers (also known as neuroleptics and anti-psychotic drugs), these drugs frequently have permanent ill effects that enormously degrade the quality of life (Rogers *et al.*, 1993). I have taken these drugs over long periods, and I thought at the time that many of the effects were symptoms of my mental illness. Such effects are poor libido and impotence, debilitating sluggishness, dry saliva, constipation, inability to concentrate, skin rashes in sunshine, impaired eyesight and many others. Diagnosed people are depicted by psychiatrists and in the press as being irrational for not wanting to take these drugs. Believe me, not wanting to take these drugs is rational.

There is a double standard about drug testing for psychiatric medication. Derek Russell Davis (1991), a retired professor of psychiatry, points out the inadequacy of drug trials for all the major groups of drugs prescribed by psychiatrists, even when they are prescribed singly. He adds that 'there have been virtually no clinical trials of combinations of drugs; the adverse effects have not been evaluated'. Many, if not most, long-term mental health service users take completely untested combinations of drugs. Matthew Dumont (1990), another psychiatrist, observes that psychiatric trainees 'are no longer trained to observe and try to understand human behaviour, only to change it.' Detailing how dependent the psychiatric profession is on the drug industry for funding, and how toxic can be the products, he concludes: 'The difference between criminal drug abuse and legal medication is often as thin as the piece of paper on which the prescription is written, the law and the media treat one as a felony and the other as sacred'.

One reason why psychiatrists have aligned with the rest of science and medicine lies in preservation of their status and power in relation to fellow doctors. The discipline of psychiatry has so few real answers that it over-emphasizes its scientific basis and physical treatments. Without these, what would be left that non-medics cannot do?

Psychotherapy: talking down treatments

The psychoanalytic tradition has a similar disempowering effect to the medical one, and is often used alongside it. The labyrinth of interpretation makes sure that the person's words are never valued for their immediate meaning. Sometimes they are even held to mean the opposite of what the person says, through defence mechanisms or some other 'psychodynamic' process. The whole system can be a major put-down of the individual's own perceptions in deference to those of experts. If you have a complaint it's put down to your denial: another no-win situation for the client.

Many ideas used every day in mental health services are put-downs in the guise of therapeutic insight. Part of the stereotype held by many mental health workers is that their clients are manipulative and their behaviour is attention seeking. No thought is given to manipulation that everyone uses, as part of the way society works (writing a CV for a job, dressing up or down according to the event). Nor do these workers ask why a person behaves in a way they think is not appropriate to achieve a goal or get attention.

The power imbalance based on supposed expertise is probably the most pervasive feature of mental health services. Professional groupings vie to suggest that their remedy for emotional distress is the most valid. Most approaches to mental distress have a similar effect: the mental health worker claims to know better than the service user. Quite extraordinary, given the poor results.

There is also the question of sexual, physical and financial abuse of people in the mental health system. For a while this was generally thought to be mainly the province of the big mental hospitals, but recent revelations make it clear that the power imbalance in talking treatments is equally liable to lead to abuse (Masson, 1989).

Double and triple discrimination

Familiar and often quoted differences add to the imbalance of power in the system. The seats of psychiatry, psychology and social work are in the while, male middle class. More psychiatric service users are women than men (Showalter, 1985; Kitzinger and Perkins, 1993), and poor than rich. It seems that the less like a white male psychiatrist one is, the more likely one is to be bio-medicalized.

In Britain, black people are more often compulsorily detained, diagnosed as having 'schizophrenia' and drugged than white (Browne, 1990; Fernando, 1991). Asian people complain of the inappropriate nature of services for them (Webb-Johnson, 1991; Beliappa, 1991). Irish people are more often labelled according to the stereotype of drunk as alcoholic, whatever their troubles.

Gay people, people with physical and sensory impairments, people with learning difficulties, people diagnosed HIV positive: the list of groups who are badly served in the mental health system is enormous. These social dimensions show up another major disempowering feature of both medical and psychological approaches. Both bio-psychiatry and psychotherapy conveniently situate the problem and the remedy (if one is thought possible) in the person herself. Factors such as racism, sexism, poverty or mentalism do not then have to be addressed.

Fear and stigma

Mental health workers make sure that the division between themselves and the frightening 'others' is maintained, colluding with public stigmatization with oppression within services. Emotional distress is frightening not only to the person who experiences it, but to most other people. Panic and discrimination are still society's main responses to it. At least 90% of reports of mental illness in the popular media are connected with violence or unreliability.

We survivors are also prey to negative publicity about ex-patients living in cardboard boxes and other unsatisfactory places. This publicity suggests we are a national emergency; it does not suggest building more homes.

Discrimination and the law

It is perfectly legal to discriminate against people in housing, health and social services, employment, education, leisure facilities and any other public or private setting simply because they have used mental health services.

Employment is what most psychiatric system survivors mention first when this topic arises. Most job application forms have a question about health, sometimes even mental health, or the condition that the applicant must pass a medical examination. Our experience shows that health questions are there to screen us out.

There are many other settings, not least physical health care, where a 'record' of psychiatric treatment ensures inferior treatment or exclusion. People have heart attacks and end up in a mental hospital because of their psychiatric record. Serious symptoms are ignored because of the habit of doctors and nurses of regarding everything we say as symptoms of mental illness. Then we die.

Housing is another critical area for us. Supported housing and residential places are given on condition that we take toxic drugs to which we do not freely consent. Workers think they know better than us where we should live, and try to impose their will, by either threatening to withdraw other services or to section us under the Mental Health Act. Housing departments discriminate against us when awarding tenancies. In all of these ways we have fewer rights than other citizens. Most people would be deeply shocked if they faced such discrimination for the privilege of paying rent.

People who have committed criminal acts have a statute of limitation, after which they do not have to declare convictions for breaking the law. No such dispensations for those of us supposedly ill people. We have a life sentence of exclusion.

The failed attempts to get an effective Civil Rights Bill for disabled people through Parliament show how empty is government rhetoric about rights and a classless society. The USA government has had no such difficulty, and Americans with disabilities legislation have made a start in righting similar wrongs. Civil rights legislation to give us at least legal equality with other citizens is an urgent necessity.

Talk of citizens' rights and empowerment seems even more cynical when you realize that we can be locked away at the word of mental health workers without having done anything wrong. The fiction that such people know better than us and what is good for us has the force of law, without a judicial process.

Some people do have crises and later appreciate the help that was given, despite resistance at the time. Frequently, though, unhelpful things are repeated in crisis after crisis, alienating the person into non-compliance. These are measures that can be taken by people who have had more than one crisis. The crisis card, initially put together by Mike Lawson and now available through Survivors Speak Out (address at the end), enables people to state what has and has not helped them in previous crises, and to name an advocate who knows and can speak for their wishes. Mental health workers can empower people by giving long-term mental health service users copies of this card, consulting it in times of crisis, and acting on what it says.

The government is now enlarging the powers of psychiatrists and allied professionals to coerce us. Extension of the Mental Health Act is imminent, giving mental health workers powers under supervised discharge arrangements. Threats to section us under the Act have always been used to get people to do what workers want. Now the threats will have legal sanction. If the person in the community does not comply with conditions about where they will live, attend for treatment, what is put in their mouth or injected, then the person will be compulsorily confined in hospital.

The registers of non-compliant patients now authorized by the Department of Health are another outrage. We will not have to have committed an offence to be placed on one. Not that committing an offence is necessarily a predictor of future offences. These 'at risk' registers are now being compiled all over the country, and are reminiscent of the deeply degrading register of psychiatric patients in the USSR (Dispatches, 1989).

Instead of providing services that attract us, psychiatric professionals are finding new ways to control us now that their 'hospitals' are closing. Talk of empowerment in community care is insulting in the light of these developments of the 1990s.

THE PSYCHIATRIC SURVIVOR MOVEMENT

To counter all this oppression, the mental health system survivor movement is a fast-accelerating set of actions throughout the world, unlocking hitherto unimagined talents formerly suppressed by hospitals and drugs. Anything written is out of date in a month, so I hope that readers will regard this attempt at analysis with some charity.

There is no agreed terminology, except that most British survivors reject the term 'consumer', after the now-famous wit of an early member who proclaimed that we are consumers of psychiatry in the same way that a woodworm is a consumer of Rentokil (Barker and Peck, 1987). Here I use the words that sit most comfortably with me. The best way to find out what people like to be called is to ask them.

Survivors Speak Out remains an independent national survivor clearing-house for England and Wales, running an information service for psychiatric system survivors. Scotland has its own national network; so has Wales. Local groups meet in Northern Ireland. Various other national groups have entered the scene. To look at these developments I have categorized survivor action into three kinds:

- reactive: reacting to existing services (system advocacy, self-advocacy),
- alternative: user-controlled projects,
- creative: new ways of thinking about mental distress, and artistic activity.

There are no real divisions. A group involved in reacting to the system may also have a poetry section. This is simply a way to get a flavour of the great variety of service user self-empowerment activities.

Reactive: self-advocacy within the system

At the national conference at Edale Youth Hostel in 1987, members of Survivors Speak Out were able to agree a charter of needs and demands.

1. That mental health service providers recognize and use people's first hand experience of emotional distress for the good of others.
2. Provision of refuges, planned and under the control of survivors of psychiatry.
3. Provision of free counselling for all.
4. Choice of services, including self-help alternatives.
5. A government review of services, with recipients sharing their views.
6. Provision of resources to implement self-advocacy for all users.
7. Adequate funding for non-medical community services, especially crisis intervention.
8. Facility for representation of users and ex-users of services on statutory bodies, including Community Health Councils, Mental Health Tribunals and the Mental Health Act Commission.
9. Full and free access to all personal medical records.
10. Legal protection and means of redress for all psychiatric patients.
11. Establishment of the democratic right of staff to refuse to administer any treatment, without risk of sanction or prejudice.
12. The phasing out of electro-convulsive therapy and psycho-surgery.
13. Independent monitoring of drug use and its consequences.
14. Provision for all patients of full written and verbal information on treatments, including adverse research findings.
15. An end to discrimination against people who receive, or have received, psychiatric services, with particular regard to housing, employment, insurance, etc.

Many of these demands involve what has been by far the greatest level of activity in the UK survivor movement so far, self-advocacy within the existing system. As you can see, we have a very long way to go.

As well as national networking through Survivors Speak Out, a local product of the international conference in Brighton in 1985 was the action of Ingrid Barker and Edward Peck, a MIND worker and a manager, to facilitate the development of a Patients' Council in Nottingham on the model of the Netherlands system. This included financing a Dutch advocate to develop service user action in Nottingham, and in time a secure financial basis for the Patients' Council Support Group. This system involves a group of ex-hospital patients in the community supporting ward-level councils of in-patients, and helping to liaise with staff and managers to rectify complaints.

In Nottingham this model has been a great success in empowering service users and improving services, and has spread to community services and to the beginning of a relationship with the purchasers. The Patients' Council model has extended to places throughout the UK, in some being successful and in others, through lack of resources and commitment from managers, leaving individual service users feeling exploited and burnt out.

Although Patients' Councils are popular, they are by no means the only form of system advocacy. Users' forums set up by managers within and attached to particular services are now widespread, and independent user groups and survivor networks also engage in user consultation. The United Kingdom Advocacy Network has been started to service 'user-led' self-advocacy groups that choose to join.

Groups relating to purchasers are a more recent development. The Newcastle Mental Health Consumer Group is one model for these. Ingrid Barker, then a contracts manager in Newcastle, continued her empowering work with this idea. Consumer Group members are elected by service users, and paid for the work they do in planning and monitoring services. Members report that they often feel they have a real say in service improvement.

Though based on tremendously hard work by many system survivors individually and in groups, the development of the survivor movement owes a great deal to allies, mental health service workers in the statutory and voluntary sectors. The achievements in personal empowerment for service users can be seen everywhere, although there are very many service users who have not yet been reached by self-advocacy. Older people who use mental health services are often difficult for under-funded service user groups to reach, particularly when they are scattered in residential services. Black and Asian service users are now beginning to develop their own groups and voices, and this is likely to be a welcome expansion of the 1990s.

On the other hand, the tomato sauce approach to advocacy (a little bit on everything improves the flavour) sometimes has its drawbacks (Access to Health, 1992). Some service users are disillusioned, having worked hard for the services for no money, spent time giving their views with no change resulting. Announcing a new advocacy service or Patients' Council can salve a manager's conscience and give a public impression that all is well now, without tackling the real oppressions of mental health services.

Even when very real changes in quality of service occur as a result of self-advocacy, nothing seems to change what most psychiatrists do. There is real discontent among psychiatric system survivors in the Netherlands that after over 15 years of statutory Patients' Councils they have not changed psychiatrists' activities (Glasman, 1991).

The natural consequence of discontent with the sometimes poor results of advocacy within the system is a greater emphasis on campaigning activity. Campaigns associated with deaths in psychiatric institutions are an example. The community campaign about the death of Orville Blackwood in the Broadmoor institution in 1992, injected with three times the normal dose of major tranquillizers, was joined by survivors. York Survivors ran a media campaign about the death of Munir Yusuf Majothi (five injections in 40 minutes) who died in Clifton Hospital aged 26 in 1993. Other actions include joining with the wider disability movement over the campaign for a civil rights law to give us legal equality in society, and going to the press and media with personal experiences and campaigning points about psychoactive drugs and ECT.

Another important area of system advocacy is in the training being done by mental health system survivors. When this is a voyeuristic one-off session of personal history (sometimes even unpaid) then it can make little difference to the system, and the individual survivor may or may not benefit. Where a budget is provided to ensure that service users are involved in planning courses and providing a good critique of the system, allowing trainees to criticize what they are being taught in a constructive way, this can have a major effect (Craley, Nettle and Wallcraft, 1994).

Survivor leaders coming from the USA and New Zealand have been surprised at how much energy UK survivors put into the statutory systems, rather than providing our own alternatives. One reason for this, I think, is that we used to feel that we owned the NHS and that it should not harm us the way it does. However, the balance is beginning to be redressed by active survivors tiring of putting so much energy into the system to so little effect. Now more people are working to provide user-controlled alternatives, and creative activity is increasing enormously.

User-controlled alternatives

If the UK user movement has been slow in setting up alternative user-controlled services, in the 1990s things are changing fast. Here I am talking about projects more complex than the burgeoning self-help groups that have been giving mutual aid since at least the 1940s. I am talking about projects that provide a substitute or substantial supplement to traditional statutory and voluntary mental health services, and are controlled by the people who use them. My definition of user-controlled suggests that the people who use the alternative have control over the programmes, employment of workers and the total budget (Lindow, 1994a and 1994b).

One British trail-blazer is McMurphy's, started in 1986 in Sheffield.

This was the response of some young people living in a residential service who were dissatisfied with council day provision. They named their project after McMurphy in *One Flew Over the Cuckoo's Nest*, who made his own protest about state provision. This name gives a good flavour of user-controlled alternatives, based as they are on a conscious-ness that we are oppressed in society and disempowered by services supposed to help us. After a planning period, McMurphy's members took a long lease from the council on a near-derelict building, and the first three years activities focused on a skilful renovation into a smart but comfortable café atmosphere, complete with regulation-standard kitchen. Like all such projects, McMurphy's has been hampered by insecure and usually insufficient funding.

By far the most usual form of service is daytime support and activities, usually on a club model like McMurphy's. Sometimes the purpose is more specific, such as the Oakland Independent Support Centre in California, USA, which provides a multi-service centre aiming to serve homeless survivors. Reaching out to homeless survivors is a frequent theme in the USA, with psychiatric system survivors who have experienced homelessness providing the expertise.

Such day-support clubs and centres promote many activities. Some-times they focus mainly on survival needs: food, hot drinks, lockers, showers, washing machines, phones. They always include individual mutual support, sometimes running their own support groups and hosting outside groups. Of course, hanging in there, not necessarily doing anything else, is important, as are attending or holding various sporting or leisure activities. Creative activities flourish: more of this in the next section.

Survivor activities have focused on both emergency and permanent housing opportunities, for both shared and individual living arrange-ments, with mutual support and/or survivor-employed support workers. Employment schemes of many sorts are to be found. I have heard of messenger services, building co-ops, computer work, landscaping, gardening, training mental health professionals, paper processing (in Japan), printing, catering, TV production and various other business activities. These may provide training opportunities, for which grants are necessary, but they frequently attempt, and succeed in, being self-supporting. The co-operative structure is popular for both employment and housing self-help alternatives.

Mary O'Hagan (1993) has made an interesting analysis of the differences between user-controlled alternatives and traditional mental health services. As well as the more obvious advantages of smaller units and democratic decision making in survivor-operated alternatives, she points to the different values of choice as against removal of symptoms and the fact that people's roles are flexible, members being both helper and helped. Because they have (and want) no coercive powers, alternatives have to work hard to attract and keep new members.

One important activity in psychiatric survivor-controlled alternatives is the business of running the project. For one of the greatest challenges of these alternatives is to avoid what has been termed 'provideritus' (Yaskin, 1992). This is the tendency of user-controlled projects to become like traditional services, with one set of people, even if they have used mental health services, providing a service for others. Constant vigilance is exercised in these projects to prevent provideritus, starting with vision statements and a clearly democratic structure and, as with other oppressed groups, engaging in consciousness-raising activities. Experience shows that awareness of power issues needs to permeate the project, particularly the decision-making and conflict-resolution practices. Otherwise, it does not provide an alternative.

The fundamental notion of survivor-run projects is encapsulated in the title *Reaching Across*, a handbook edited by three USA survivors sharing much practical experience on the subject (Zinman, Harp and Budd, 1987). From our experiences of oppression within the system, we reach across to each other as equals. Su Budd writes:

> I wish us, as ex-patients, to strive to create a system of mutual support that is based on respect for each other's needs, contributions, strengths and limitations. I wish us to strive to perfect a system of support and nourishment, which is distinctly different from that of the mental health system, which emphasizes the medicalization of human feeling. (Zinman, Harp and Budd, 1987 p. 41.)

Creative activities

Concurrent with the development of other aspects of the survivor movement, two major forms of creative action have been taking place. These are:

- people joining together to come to new understandings of their experiences of mental and emotional distress,
- artistic activity.

Misunderstood people, traditionally robbed of their own meanings, have been getting together to create new understanding of our experiences. The early 1990s saw survivor-run conferences about self-injury, the experience of taking major tranquillizers and about eating distress. At these conferences, people met together to share experiences of what helped, and what did not. Mental health workers were invited to benefit from this shared wisdom. Publications from the conference about eating distress and self-harm are available (Pembroke, 1992 and 1994).

The hearing voices movement is making a major contribution to new thinking. The impetus for this came from two mental health workers in The Netherlands, Professor Marius Romme and Sandra Escher (1993). These two listened to what was being said by people who hear voices, and took it seriously. They became committed to finding a new response to these experiences, to replace the 'exterminate' professional attitudes to voices. In this country the challenge has been taken up mainly by voice hearers themselves; local groups have burgeoned and there is a national network with a newsletter. Sarah Bell (1994), founder member of Oxford Survivors, has published her own experiences and ideas, part of a growing literature of articles, chapters and books by mental health system survivors.

It is difficult to select from this growing literature, but I will mention two personal favourites. One is by Jimmy Laing (1992), a Scotsman who endured 50 years in the hands of psychiatry. The other is by the feminist Kate Millett (1990), who described her experience of incarceration by psychiatrists and enforced drug-taking. Both give moving factual accounts of their difficulty in gaining personal freedom from the power of psychiatry.

One of the few bright spots for people diagnosed by psychiatrists is the notion that genius is next to madness. There are numerous brilliantly creative people who have also been mad. I'm not artistic myself, my favourite is Vincent Van Gogh, and there have been stars in all forms of creative art. The contribution to literature, especially by women who have experienced severe emotional and mental distress, is vast.

As well as those of us who take our place in mainstream artistic activity, we can see the beginnings of our own culture of madness. The London-based Survivors' Poetry group published a successful volume (1992) which was shortlisted for the MIND/Allan Lane Book of the Year award in 1993. The group now has an office premises, gives professional poetry performances and is planning a further book. Survivors' Poetry groups are being established in many other places. Survivors' Poetry is the most visible creative endeavour so far, although local survivor groups have writing, painting and other activities. This will be an interesting area of development to watch. If society excludes us, we'll get on with it ourselves.

The section of this chapter on user-controlled alternatives is based on a research project I undertook supported by the Joseph Rowntree Foundation. The material presented here represents my findings, not necessarily reflecting the views of the Foundation.

APPENDIX: MENTAL HEALTH SYSTEMS SURVIVOR MOVEMENT
ADDRESSES

World Federation of Psychiatric Users
c/o Mary O'Hagan, PO Box 46018, Herne Bay, Auckland, New Zealand

European Network of Users and Ex-users in Mental Health
Rene van der Male, European Desk, PO Box 4006, 1009 BB Amsterdam,
The Netherlands

Survivors Speak Out
34 Osnaburgh Street, London NW1 3ND.
Tel: 0171 916 5472, Information service tel: 0171 916 6991.
Network of mental health system survivors, user groups and allies

Scottish Users' Network
40 Shandwyck Place, Edinburgh.
Network for mental health service users in Scotland

US Network, Wales
c/o Janet Cooke, Wales MIND, 23 St. Mary Street, Cardiff CF1 2AA.
National federation of service users in Wales

Hearing Voices Network
Creative Support, Fourways House, 16 Tariff Street, Manchester M1
2FN.
Tel: 0161 228 3896.
A network of people who hear voices

MINDLINK
Granta House, 15–19 Broadway, Stratford, London E15 4BQ.
Tel: 0181 519 2122.
MIND's consumer network

UK Advocacy Network
Suite 417, Premier House, 14 Cross Burgess Street, Sheffield S1 2HG.
Tel: 0114 275 3131.
Co-ordinating network for user-led system advocacy groups

Survivors' Poetry
34 Osnaburgh Street, London NW1 3ND.
Tel: 0171 916 5317

REFERENCES

Advocacy Information Pack (1992) Good Practices in Mental Health, London, tel.
    0171 289 2034.
Access to Health (1992) The tomato sauce of the health service: using advocates.
    Extract in *Advocacy Information Pack*, Good Practices in Mental Health, London.

220 *Power and rights: the psychiatric system survivor movement*

Barker, I. and Peck, E. (eds) (1987) *Power in Strange Places: User Empowerment in Mental Health Services*, Good Practices in Mental Health, London.
Beliappa, J. (1991) *Illness or Distress? Alternative Models of Mental Distress*, Confederation of Indian Organisations, 5 Westminster Bridge Road, London SW1 7XW.
Bell, S. (1994 edn) *Hearing Voices*. Send £3 to The Inner Bookshop, 111 Magdalen Road, Oxford OX4 1RQ.
Boyle, M. (1990) *Schizophrenia: A Scientific Delusion?* Routledge and Kegan Paul, London.
Breggin, P. (1993) *Toxic Psychiatry*, Fontana Paperback, London.
Browne, D. (1990) *Black People, Mental Health and the Courts*, Afro-Caribbean Mental Health Association, CRE and NACRO, 169 Clapham Road, London SW9 0PU.
Chamberlin, J. (1988) *On Our Own: Patient Controlled Alternatives to the Mental Health System*, MIND, Granta House, 15–19 Broadway, Stratford, London E15 4BQ.
Dispatches programme (1989) *Gorbachev's Asylums*, David Cohen, 11 January, Channel 4.
Dumont, M.P. (1990) In bed together at the market: psychiatry and the pharmaceutical industry. *American Journal of Orthopsychiatry*, 60 (4), pp. 484–485.
Fernando, S. (1991) *Mental Health, Race and Culture*, Macmillan/MIND, London.
Glasman, D. (1991) The challenge of patient power. *Health Service Journal*, **5**, September, pp. 16–17, and Divided opinions. *Health Service Journal*, **12**, September, p. 20.
Graley, R., Nettle, M. and Wallcraft, J. (eds) (1994) *Building on Experience: A training pack for mental health service users working as trainers, speakers and workshop facilitators*, Department of Health, London.
Johnstone, L. (1989) *Users and Abusers of Psychiatry*, Routledge and Kegan Paul, London.
Kitzinger, C. and Perkins, R. (1993) *Changing Our Minds: Lesbian Feminism and Psychology*, Only Women Press, London.
Laing, J. and McQuarrie, D. (1993) *Fifty Years in the System*, Corgi, London.
Lindow, V. (1994a) *Self-Help Alternatives to Mental Health Services*, MIND Publications, Granta House, 15–19 Broadway, Stratford, London E15 4BQ, tel: 0181 522 1746, when tone changes dial 223 or 224, concessionary rates for survivors from Survivors Speak Out.
Lindow, V. (1994b) *Purchasing Mental Health Services: Self-help Alternatives*, MIND Publications, London.
Masson, J. (1989) *Against Therapy*, Fontana/Collins, London.
Millett, K. (1990) *The Loony Bin Trip*, Virago, London.
O'Hagan, M. (1993) *Stopovers On My Way Home From Mars: A Winston Churchill Fellowship report on the psychiatric survivor movement in the USA, Britain and the Netherlands*, Survivors Speak Out.
Pembroke, L.R. (ed.) (1992) *Eating Distress: Perspectives from Personal Experience*, Survivors Speak Out.
Pembroke, L.R. (ed.) (1994) *Self-Harm: Perspectives from Personal Experience*, Survivors Speak Out.
Podvoll, E.M. (1990) *The Seduction of Madness: A Compassionate Approach to Recovery at Home*, Century, London.
Rogers, A., Pilgrim, D. and Lacey, R. (1993) *Experiencing Psychiatry: Users' Views of Services*, Macmillan/MIND, London.

Romme, M. and Escher, S. (1993) *Accepting Voices*, MIND, London.

Russell Davis, D. (1991) The debate on drugs: a personal view. *OPENMIND*, **49**, pp. 10–11.

Showalter, E. (1985) *The Female Malady: Women, Madness and Culture 1830–1980*, Virago, London.

Survivors' Poetry: From Dark to Light (1992) Survivors' Press, London.

Warner, R. (1985) *Recovery From Schizophrenia*, Routledge and Kegan Paul, London.

Webb-Johnson, A. (1991) *A Cry for Change: An Asian Perspective on Developing Quality Mental Health Care*, Confederation of Indian Organisations, 5 Westminster Bridge Road, London SW1 7XW.

Yaskin, Joseph C. (ed) (1992) *Nuts and Bolts: A Technical Assistance Guide for Mental Health Consumer/Survivor Self-Help Groups*, Project SHARE, Philadelphia, USA.

Zinman, S., Harp, H. and Budd, S. (eds) (1987) *Reaching Across: Mental Health Clients Helping Each Other*, California Network of Mental Health Clients, 1722 J Street, Suite 324, Sacramento, CA 95814, USA (send $25).

13

Citizen advocacy and people with learning disabilities in Wales

Paul Ramcharan

INTRODUCTION

It has been argued that the relationship between the State and its citizens, or subjects in the case of Britain as a constitutional monarchy, is structured as a mutually beneficial contract. Plato saw the Athenians and the Athenian State as having made this contract to give protection to its citizens through national defence and the universal application of law. Hobbes, in contrast, argued that without the State selfish and self-seeking humans would create his oft-cited 'war of all against all'. Humans had therefore made a contract with each other to invest representatives with the power and authority to make rules, or laws, by which citizens would abide.

A series of rights and privileges are conferred upon citizens and, theoretically at least, redress is possible where these are infringed. Moreover, whilst the common and criminal law are available to all for seeking redress for such infringement, the State also recognizes the special needs or interests of specific groups, who may require added or specialist protection and rights. Examples of legislation which reflect this latter interest include the Disabled Persons Act 1986, the NHS and Community Care Act 1990, and the Mental Health Acts 1959 and 1983. Stated in this way the relationship between the State and the individual would seem to be a fair and just contract. However, this claim remains problematic in a number of ways, and for a number of reasons.

Excluding for the purposes of this chapter that view which calls for a revolution or an alternative State apparatus, there remains within the above contract the necessity for the State to confer sufficient privilege on its citizens/subjects to prevent civil unrest and disobedience. However, it remains difficult in an elected representative democracy for minority groups to elect members to represent their interests. (In a system of proportional representation minority group parties such as the new Grey parties in Germany have, with their weight in numbers, been able to elect representatives to government.) Moreover, it is unlikely, given this lack of a voice and their special interests, that the electorate as a whole would either (get to) know of these special interests, or see the State's reneging on such interests as contravening the ideal of the conferment of sufficient privilege upon themselves. In short such groups can lack an empowered voice in the legislative process.

One dimension of Lukes' (1974) definition of power is being able to strike off the agenda issues identified as not being in the interests of the powerful. One way of placing these interests back on the agenda is to organize as a group, thus increasing the power base and the ability to place pressure on relevant others to change; such groups may make interests more widely known to the public or speak out on areas of common or group interests such as those outlined above. We might term the use of such pressure, social or interest group activity as 'group advocacy'. The term 'advocacy' here is used loosely to describe speaking 'for' or 'on behalf of' oneself or other(s). It is in this way that groups seek changes to the system, to the nature of the rights accorded to the group and to legitimation for their views.

However, as well as changing the rights accorded in legislation, it is also necessary to ensure that the individual's rights are met within the presently existing legislation. But this too is highly problematic. Take, for example, the Mental Health Act 1983 which includes rules about compulsory admission to hospital. Under each section of the Act are specific rules about categories of persons who are eligible to sanction admission and about treatments that are possible. It is also the case that the sections are only implemented where admission represents 'the least restrictive alternative'. Admission under section also confers rights to a Mental Health Review Tribunal (MHRT) hearing after three weeks and then six monthly, to review the veracity of the involuntary admission.

However, since 90% of hospital patients are voluntary residents, these rights do not apply to them. Moreover, and as Gostin (1983) points out, only 20% of those eligible for MHRT hearings have used this opportunity. In addition, even if such rights were accorded to all in-patients they remain specified rights, i.e. the Mental Health Act does not cover all the possible rights issues for every single individual. There are therefore problems which relate to the extent of coverage of specified rights as well as the content of those rights in relation to both people and issues.

The point here is that the availability of rights is not the same as accessibility to those rights. Inaccessibility might be due to their limited

224 Citizen advocacy and people with learning disabilities in Wales

coverage; to economic circumstances where access to personal lawyers, for example, is expensive and beyond the means of an already socio-economically deprived group or individual; by virtue of lack of information or indeed cognitive ability to recognize infringements to one's rights.

One way of overcoming inaccessibility to rights and entitlements is by encouraging participation in decision making. Indeed Biehal (1993) goes so far as to suggest that this should be a right in itself, namely that the:

> rights of users of social services to be treated as equal citizens rather than as passive recipients of professional decisions must be founded on the right to participate fully in decisions about the services they receive. (Biehal, 1993 p. 456.)

However, Biehal also points out that the rights embodied in policy statements do not automatically lead to rights in practice. This is significant given the present community care reforms which make a number of recommendations in relation to such participation. For example, the reforms variously state, '. . . the statutory requirement on LAs to consult in the planning process' (DoH, 1990 para 2.2); that 'major providers of care services, service users and their carers, all need to be involved during the planning process' (DoH, 1990 para 2.4); that in terms of needs the assessor should take '. . . account of the user's and carers' own preferences' (DoH, 1990 para 3.25) and so forth. Extending Biehal's argument to the recent community care legislation, there are clear difficulties in protecting the rights and entitlements of individuals, even where rights are apparently enshrined in statute. The difference between what is possible for the individual to do for themselves, and ensuring that their rights and entitlements are met, marks the territory of the different forms of independent advocacy.

THE PLACE OF CITIZEN ADVOCACY

A key figure in the development of citizen advocacy in the United States and Canada, Wolfensberger proposes limitless possible forms of advocacy which might be delineated by asking a series of questions as adopted in Figure 13.1. Some examples of organizations or individuals who may fill particular advocacy roles are shown in Table 13.1.

Most forms of advocacy are either 'issue' or 'crisis' oriented. For example, a union will organize strikes for groups of employees or else represent an individual at a disciplinary hearing, i.e. after a problem has become a crisis. The Mental Health Act Commission or Age Concern might deal with issues which affect large numbers of individuals about such matters as clothing or seclusion policies in hospital or the writing of

Figure 13.1 Categories of advocacy.

For whom?	Individual, group, self, class (e.g. elderly)
For what?	Services, service inclusion, service quality, legal rights, life and health, a valued life and image, extension of community connectedness
Towards or against whom?	Institutions, other agencies, functionaries, families, other individuals
By whom?	Paid profession (e.g. lawyer), citizen collectives (voluntary organizations e.g. Age Concern), service workers, pressure groups (Grey Panthers), unpaid citizens
How done?	Persuasion, education, confrontation, litigation, demonstration, modelling, whistle-blowing

Table 13.1 Forms of advocacy for individuals and/or groups.

		The 'by whom' dimension of advocacy	
		Individual	*Collectivity or its representative*
The 'for whom' dimension of advocacy	Individual	• Welfare rights officer* • Personal self-advocacy • Personal citizen advocacy (Paid individual advocacies) • Lawyer • Ombudsman	• Mental Health Review Tribunal* • Social/health service* • Paid collective (e.g. union for individual dispute with employer) • Voluntary organization (e.g. Age Concern or Citizen Advice Bureau)
	Collectivity/class	• Legislative representative • Class advocates • Most cases of whistle-blowing • Lawyer	• Collective self-advocacy (e.g. Grey Panthers, VIA) • Advocacy orientated voluntary organizations (e.g. Age Concern) • Mental Health Act Commission*

This table is an edited version of an unpublished teaching aide designed by Prof. Wolf Wolfensberger of Syracuse University, New York, and reprinted here with his permission. Prof. Wolfensberger has asked me to point out that those items marked with an asterisk did not occur in the original training materials. Excluded from the diagram are Wolfensberger's references to: Scandinavian-type ombudsman, many in-house advocacy forms, most forms of agency advocacy for individuals, empowered public or quasi-public protective services, certain public interest advocates, certain in-house advocates, some kinds of advocacy-oriented voluntary agencies and some public interest advocates. The changes reflect my wish to make the table reflect the subject matter of this chapter and make its contents culturally relevant.

wills. A lawyer advocating for an individual will do so after a problem has reached such a crisis that recourse to the law is required. However, such 'advocacy for collectives' or single 'problem/crisis based advocacy' may 'lose the individual'. Such forms of advocacy cannot take into account the mundane, everyday needs of individuals, their preferences, desires and wishes as they move about in their everyday environments. Moreover, and referring to my initial discussion in relation to the contract between the State and citizen or subject, it is exceptionally difficult for the fingers of the State to reach this far into people's everyday lives. Most of us would not want the State to dictate our everyday lives in this way, to be involved in our mundane choices and interactions, in making friends, choosing what to eat, to wear or what to do during the day, for example.

Yet for many vulnerable and disadvantaged people who are economically deprived, and placed at the hands of substitute choices made by service providers within service contexts and others, their lives are very much confined within parameters set by others. It can be argued then that it is not (only) the extraordinary features of the rights of vulnerable individuals that need guarding, but rather (also) the choices they should be afforded as rights in their everyday lives. Citizen advocacy which involves a one-to-one relationship between the advocate and partner has much potential in ensuring that the choices of people with learning disabilities and their rights are respected. Although it is the citizen advocate's role to seek to make choices on the basis of their partner's wishes, there are likely to be some cases where substitute decisions will be required to be made. This is a difficult issue which has recently been addressed by the Law Commission (1995). Where there is a need to go beyond advocacy in everyday life to deal with problems in relation to specified rights, or through legal process, the citizen advocate may have to rely largely on the other forms of advocacy to ensure redress. Citizen advocacy, then, is by no means meant to be a replacement for all the other forms, but a way of making sure that individuals who might not otherwise have had access to these other advocacies, do so.

Whilst it may be argued that service personnel have a similar input into the everyday rights and choices of individuals in their care, this differs from citizen advocacy in a number of key ways. Service professionals are socialized to apply universalistic principles (Parsons, 1952) to their clients, to remain detached, and not to get emotionally involved. In contrast citizen advocates become involved in the person's life, speaking for, with and on their behalf as if their partner's problems were their own. Moreover, it has been argued that professionals are socialized into a professional culture in which their methods of assessment may obfuscate the personal choice of clients (Dowson, 1990) or where their interests are better served by conformity with their profession or their work organization (Wilding, 1982), at the expense of the client's interests. In contrast, the citizen advocate avoids these conflicts of interest by maintaining an independence from the service sector and as maintained in principles set out by the National Citizen Advocacy (NCA) (Butler *et al.*, 1988) by ensuring that the advocate is not rewarded, monetarily or otherwise, for their role.

Up to this point citizen advocacy has been described in terms of the practical help and support citizen advocates can harness in maintaining and promoting the rights of individuals. This has been termed the 'instrumental dimension' of citizen advocacy. But there is also a second dimension, the expressive dimension, in which the advocate befriends their partner, gives them moral and emotional support and, furthermore, contributes (at least for persons with a learning disability) in seeking to extend their community connectedness and integration. Given this role, citizen advocacy theory proposes that the relationships should be a 'long-term' commitment.

Whilst service workers and others may seek to maintain an individual's rights they do not befriend. Whilst befrienders befriend, they do not systematically or formally undertake an advocacy role. National Citizen Advocacy defines citizen advocacy as:

. . . the persuasive and supportive activities of trained, selected volunteers and coordinating staff working on behalf of those who are disabled, disadvantaged and not in a good position to exercise or defend their rights as citizens. Citizen advocates are persons who are independent of those providing direct services to people with disabilities. Working on a one-to-one basis, they attempt to foster respect for the rights and dignity of those whose interests they represent. This may involve helping to express the individual's concerns and aspirations, obtaining day-to-day social, recreational, health and related services, and providing other practical and emotional support. (Butler *et al.*, 1988. p. 2)

National Citizen Advocacy was an organization which sought to support citizen advocacy and its development in Britain, and to seek to ensure the maintenance of the principles of citizen advocacy. It has now changed its name to Citizen Advocacy Information and Training (CAIT).

It was at least some of the thinking outlined above which led those who wrote the All-Wales Strategy to recognize the need for the development of advocacy services in Wales:

The voluntary organisations in Wales should establish advocacy schemes for mentally handicapped people . . . They should be organised so as to be completely independent of the service providing agencies. (Welsh Office, 1983 para 4.3, xi.)

Following this proposal a number of self-advocacy and citizen advocacy initiatives have been launched in Wales. The remainder of this chapter is devoted to a consideration of aspects of the citizen advocacy experience as encountered in Wales under the All-Wales Strategy.

PARTICIPATION AND EMPOWERMENT UNDER THE ALL-WALES STRATEGY

The difficulties of putting policy into practice in relation to the participatory processes outlined above are exemplified in the experience of the All-Wales Strategy for the Development of Services for Mentally Handicapped People (Welsh Office, 1983), referred to as 'AWS' for brevity. This policy initiative was far more systematic than the present community care reforms in relation to participatory processes. It set out the principles that persons with a learning disability should have the '. . . right to normal patterns of life in the community', the '. . . right to be treated as individuals' and the right to '. . . additional help from the communities in which they live and from professional services if they are to develop their maximum potential as individuals' (Welsh Office, 1983). With these principles were allocated ring-fenced monies for the development of relevant services to meet these aims.

Two categories of participation were envisaged in this strategy. Firstly it was proposed that each person with a learning disability should have an individual programme plan (IPP) in which they would be involved with family carers and professionals in setting future goals and meeting needs. These plans were to be 'the engine of change' in that following an assessment of individual needs, plans could then be made to provide the relevant services to meet these needs. Secondly, it was envisaged that carer and user representatives should be involved in service planning at the area level (area work groups, AWGs), at the community mental handicap team, i.e. CMHT (local planning groups, LPGs) level and at the county level. But there have been problems. In terms of participation in planning, for example, it was found that not all CMHTs had instituted a local planning group (Welsh Office, 1989) and that where they existed they were dominated by family carers, with little evidence that change had been effected by people with learning disabilities themselves. Moreover, these planning forums remained a part of the service culture, which as Abrams (1984) points out, could lead (at county level especially) to 'domination' by statutory service members; to possible 'conflicts' between key stakeholders such as service users and carers in terms of their own respective values and interests; or to 'integration' of participants into the service culture and hence the loss of an independent and critical voice.

More problematic perhaps was evidence on the individual planning side. Humphreys (1986), for example, found that parents and key workers tended to make the majority of contributions at individual planning meetings, and users least. Moreover, with an average of nine people invited and seven attending, the process was exceptionally time-consuming, particularly given the large case loads of professionals.

Further evidence on individual planning (McGrath *et al.*, 1991) casts some doubt on the efficiency of the individual planning mechanism. It shows that whilst 48% of the study sample ($n = 743$) reported that they had been involved in a meeting with professionals, only 21% talked of having an agreed plan for future services and only 11% stated that they had an individual plan. This implies that meeting people's wishes and needs via participatory practices does not necessarily ensure the rights and entitlements of individuals. So has citizen advocacy, which seeks to ensure such rights and entitlements, as well as to empower the person in their everyday lives, helped?

A PROBLEM OF LEGITIMACY?

The experience of citizen advocacy (i.e. those projects providing a citizen advocacy partnership input for persons with learning disabilities) under the AWS highlights one of the most oft-cited problems reported by citizen advocacy projects and their advocates, i.e. in seeking legitimacy from others, particularly service personnel, and in speaking up, for and with their partner. This problem works at a number of levels, in terms of project funding, in terms of the practical tasks of running a citizen advocacy office, and in terms of the work of the partnerships. Some of these experiences, together with some of the important gains made for individuals under the All-Wales Strategy, are outlined in the section below.

Independent funding

To avoid conflicts of interest, citizen advocacy projects should be funded independently of the statutory sector. Indeed, as outlined earlier, the AWS document makes it clear that the projects should be supported by the voluntary sector. Despite this, only one of the projects in Wales is funded wholly independently (by Charity Projects Ltd, the 'Red Nose' fund). The rest are funded from AWS monies, the funding being directed through the county planning groups. The arrangements have not been entirely without problems.

For example, one project, jointly funded by two counties has had problems in convincing one of the county planning groups of both the equity of provision between clients from their county and the other, as well as the efficacy of their work. The threat to withdraw funding has occurred on a number of occasions. There is now a county observer at the management meetings, and some of the project's work practices and systems of accountability have been tied more closely to the county's interests.

In another case, funds originally directed through the country planning group were redirected through the county resettlement grant. This led to claims that the project should be providing a citizen advocacy input for all those persons in the county who were being resettled. But the rate of advocate recruitment was too slow to make such provision. One solution used by the project was the idea of the 'house advocate' who would provide advocacy for all persons resettled to one house. As well as losing the benefits of a one-to-one citizen advocacy (CA) relationship the advocates were also, theoretically at least, in a position of having to advocate for one of their partners over another, were such a need to arise. The functioning of the project was therefore compromised in that the statutory sector had taken hold of the agenda in relation to some aspects of the project's functioning.

Up until recently another project had worked without too much intervention from the county planning forum through which its money had been directed. However, a number of elements of the recent community care legislation have convinced the county of the need for an overall advocacy strategy which might incorporate a number of forms of advocacy for all specialisms, including learning disability. Were the present overall funding for advocacy not to be increased, then the level of funding for the project, given its present learning disability and citizen advocacy remit, might be seriously compromised.

For a number of reasons, and after the county had set targets for advocate recruitment, two unfilled posts were frozen by another county planning group whilst a review was undertaken of the project. Since the review, a new management and operational structure have been implemented to improve the project's functioning. However, the review group's findings were numerous, some of their observations summing up quite well the difficulties the Welsh citizen advocacy projects have faced in seeking to work independently of the statutory sector:

> The independence of the project was compromised by a lack of clarity over its relationship with its funder and this undermined its working relationship with other statutory bodies.

and, if the county's purpose is:

> . . . to promote citizen advocacy, then it needs to give up any claim to ownership and develop appropriate funding mechanisms to ensure accountability without compromising independence.

This was an internal report to a county planning forum to inform their decisions regarding the project and its functioning. The quotes have been used with their permission.

The above problems certainly back up the claim for the need for independence of funding from the statutory sector, but given the present economic climate the projects in Wales have been unable to secure funding from other sources. There would seem to be a need to go back to the strategy to examine the possibilities of funding through the voluntary sector, particularly given the emphasis of recent legislation regarding the 'mixed economy of welfare'. Despite these problems, the citizen advocacy projects in Wales have carried on functioning. Some further aspects of this functioning are now considered.

Organization and recruitment

Citizen advocates are recruited by co-ordinators working in citizen advocacy offices. There are six projects in Wales which provide citizen advocacy for persons with a learning disability. One of these also provides self and formal (i.e. co-ordinator's) advocacy and two further projects provide citizen advocacy, one for persons with disabilities, the other for any person deemed to require an advocacy input. For those offices providing citizen advocacy there are a number of functions required to bring the advocate and partner together. These are summarized in Figure 13.2.

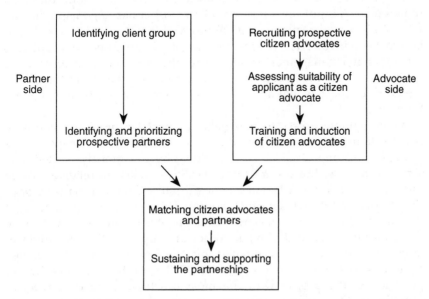

Figure 13.2 Co-ordinator's work in forming citizen advocacy partnerships.

Given the limitations of space I intend to proceed by making some comments regarding the 'identification and prioritization of prospective partners', and the 'recruiting of advocates'.

The citizen advocacy projects in Wales do not cover the whole country. Each project has its own identified catchment area. For example, whilst one project covers an area of about 14 miles by 7 miles, another covers a large rural area and another a large metropolitan county. The need to maintain as much independence of the projects from the statutory sector has meant that the projects do not accept referrals from the local CMHTs (community mental handicap teams) nor from hospitals. Questions therefore arise as to how co-ordinators find, identify and prioritize prospective partners.

For persons still living in the mental hospitals, access has had to be negotiated by the projects. These negotiations have often been difficult. One approach, premised on the idea that residents had the right to visitors and hence advocates also, led to a series of gate-keeping measures by the hospital. The lack of negotiation, misunderstandings by hospital staff about the nature and goals of citizen advocacy, and difficulties in interpreting the rights of advocates led to a breakdown of the relations necessary to sustain the citizen advocates in their role within the hospital.

In contrast, some projects have sought to negotiate access to hospitals. Hospital staff were taken on as advisors to the management committee of one project and helped to negotiate access to the hospital villas. The co-ordinators then prioritized persons whom they felt required a CA input. In contrast another project has negotiated directly with the hospital management themselves for access to villas. It has latterly been involved in writing a Resident's Charter and contributed to other hospital management groups. The latter approach has raised some questions as to the extent of incorporation of the project into the structure of the hospital and the possible effect upon its independent functioning.

Whilst gaining access to hospitals has posed a problem, recruiting persons living dispersed within the community has posed an even more serious challenge. Project co-ordinators have variously visited day services, hostels, houses and other facilities, talked to relatives where they have been known, and in one case discussed possible partners with service personnel 'outside office hours'. This serendipitous method of identifying prospective partners means that it is not necessarily the case that those most in need of an advocacy are targeted. The difficulties in targeting are further exacerbated by the small number of citizen advocates so far recruited in Wales, i.e. 57. To put this into some kind of perspective, the project with the most functioning citizen advocates ($n = 27$) and the smallest catchment area of all the projects in Wales has a coterminous catchment with a CMHT which has over 300 adults registered with a learning disability, together with a hospital with a population still over 100.

The recruitment of advocates has been a hugely difficult process for the schemes in Wales. A visit to citizen advocacy projects in Victoria, Australia, showed that their co-ordinators expect to recruit on average one advocate per month (Ramcharan and Grant, 1993). At a time when the numbers of persons volunteering seem to be decreasing, citizen advocacy, with its principle of not paying advocates even their expenses, is likely to be less attractive to volunteers, particularly those dependent upon social security benefits or those on low incomes.

One effect of the low advocate recruitment rate is that co-ordinators have invested huge amounts of time and resources into recruitment with few dividends in terms of successful advocate recruitment. This has led recently to consideration of how advocacy projects might broaden both their remit and their volunteering base. For example, two projects have made bids to local authorities for the handling of complaints procedures under the new NHS and Community Care Act. Others have sought to use the volunteers for befriending purposes in the hope that the relationship might grow into a citizen advocacy partnership; others propose using volunteers to network friends and others as potential advocates for the projects; and, as already reported, yet others have developed an advocacy scheme for all the residents of a single house. In each instance these changes may fundamentally affect the nature of the citizen advocacy partnerships. Citizen advocacy as a principled pursuit may be at risk of being diluted, losing its primary focus and its cutting edge.

The partnerships

Some problems have now been considered in relation to bringing the citizen advocacy partnerships together. The present research, whilst looking at the operation of the citizen advocacy office and its management, has also examined relationships between advocates and their partners. In the final analysis it must be the outcomes of these relationships by which citizen advocacy initiatives must be judged.

Tyne's (1991) evaluative findings in relation to the Sheffield Citizen Advocacy Project showed significant improvements in the social contacts and emotional support dimension (i.e. the expressive dimension) of the partnerships, but a perhaps less than successful input by advocates on the instrumental or practical problem-solving side. Analysis of the AWS data which is ongoing has yielded the following provisional findings which to some extent stand in contrast to those of Tyne.

The 23 interviews with citizen advocates so far conducted indicate a significant increase in the participation of partners in socializing, social events and a growth in their network of acquaintances (although no independent friendships have yet been formed out of the partnerships). The meetings between advocates and partners have more of the cadence and character of everyday life, of going shopping, eating out, visiting relatives, going to the pub, or chatting, listening to music or watching TV. These meetings differ substantially from the everyday nuances of life experienced by partners in their care settings. Without exception, those partners able to communicate their likes have registered positive feelings towards their citizen advocate.

However, interpretation of these social and supportive activities as falling wholly into the expressive dimension of advocacy is misleading. Figure 13.3 may help in demonstrating this. It shows that to achieve rights and entitlements (Box D) it is first necessary for the person to recognize their needs and interests (Box A) and then to make them known (Box B) and heard by others (Box C).

By pressing interviewees it soon became clear that activities which are expressive usually incorporate elements of the instrumental. The two are by no means mutually exclusive. The simple act of giving partners new experiences widened the choices available to them in making informed decisions about their wishes, needs and entitlements (Box A). Moreover, there are a number of interpersonal interactions involved in advocates and partners communing together. Amongst other things some of those advocating for partners unable to communicate verbally

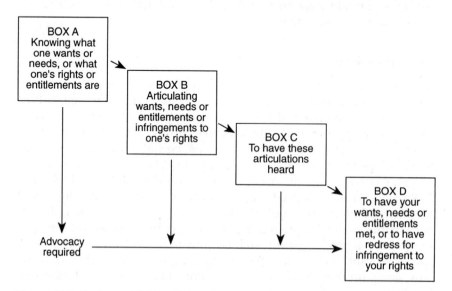

Figure 13.3 Basic model identifying the need for advocacy.

have, over time, developed what may be termed a 'private language' in which they can interpret the person's wishes from their non-verbal communications, the pitch and intensity of any sounds that they make, and so forth. In this way, the person otherwise unable to make their views known or heard can do so through their advocate (Boxes B and C). The growth of the expressive dimensions of citizen advocacy has therefore had spin-offs on the instrumental side in terms of the extension of everyday choice making for partners.

On the largely instrumental or practical help side citizen advocates have succeeded in securing services for their partners; initiated and been involved in case reviews and individual plans; helped sort out partners' wills; fought for reductions in and changes to drug regimes; secured aids and adaptations such as wheel chairs, spectacles, handrails; ensured full entitlement to welfare benefits; contacted (lost) relatives; been involved with resettlement for their partner and changed some practices in their partners' places of residence. These are the outcomes of advocacy (Box D). Citizen advocates also describe establishing the procedural precursors to these outcomes as set out in Boxes A–C. For example, one advocate felt that professionals in an individual planning meeting were speaking too esoterically for his partner to understand. He describes stopping them several times and asking 'Now, what are you *actually* trying to say?'. By doing so his partner might thereby be able to make an informed choice (Box A) about his wishes and needs in relation to what was being proposed. Another advocate describes his main role as '. . . sharing information of what [partner's name] wants . . . At IP meetings when his parents are there he's very worried about upsetting them . . . whereas because I'm not in that situation I can raise the issues' (Boxes B and C).

Despite these positive outcomes, there have been problems, and in particular one specific problem. The difficulties referred to earlier in terms of the project negotiating access to hospitals has been experienced at the interpersonal level by advocates in contact with statutory sector personnel. Of the 23 citizen advocates so far interviewed, 17 have had some contact with the statutory services, whether CMHT, hospital, hostel, or group home staff. Of these, four report no problems with staff, for example 'I can't speak too highly of the hostel staff. What I do, they do a million times over', and 'the staff are excellent over there'.

However, 13 advocates expressed problems in their advocacy role when this role meant some contact with statutory sector personnel. Some examples of citizen advocates' comments in this regard are set out below.

1. 'I think because the people on the ward have known her for so long
   . . . that I feel that, well, who the hell am I? . . . If she was in her own
   home I could be much more involved.'

2. 'I think they [hostel staff] felt it was a threat . . . Although being advocate I should be able to say "yes, I will go down and knock on door", I couldn't. I'm not that strong.'

3. 'There's a general atmosphere up there that they just can't be bothered . . . I mean if I was a lot more confident in what I was doing I'd think, I'll say something about that.'

4. 'Well the thing is, I don't really know what goes on in the house . . . I don't want to feel nosey or awkward by asking.'

5. 'I periodically ask them [group home staff] what they're doing. They like it. I think they looked on advocates as being a bit of nosey parkers.'

6. 'I would go down and look at goals set and speak to staff, but what would happen was that staff would say "I don't know". It was so difficult to push for things.'

7. 'We were going into the hospital blind. They didn't want us in. They wanted us as someone just to take them out . . . No interference . . . Not doing anything at all.'

8. 'I did go slowly . . so that I didn't tread on anyone's corns or anything. Could have upset them quite a few times with the manner of his.'

But why should the relationship between citizen advocates and service personnel be so problematic? As Simons (1993) points out, citizen advocates are not anti-service sector. But looking back to Abrams' work cited earlier, neither do they want to become integrated and incorporated into that sector. They need to maintain their distance so that they can speak independently. Moreover, the gate-keeping role (quote 6 for example) of service personnel is very effective, particularly in residential settings. Given that both 'incorporation' and 'conflict' are ruled out, it is Abrams' last category, i.e. that of domination, that may be at the heart of the problem.

As Crawley (1990) has pointed out, and as intimated in quotes (5) and (7) above, professionals may construe citizen advocates' challenges as threats to their professional practice. Indeed as these quotes show, some advocates are aware of the professionals' caring role (quote 1), or given differences in professionals' input in comparison to their own preferences, are unsure of the veracity of their claims (quote 3), or simply feel that they do not have the right to challenge professionals (quotes 1 and 8). Simply put, the issue is one of 'domination', or from another perspective, the issue of legitimation and authority.

For service personnel, the statutory responsibility to care for their clients/patients gives their actions some recognition, or authority of action, as well as a series of rights, duties and obligations accruing to these actions. No such statutory authority is held by the citizen advocate. Neither of the two recent opportunities to accord such authority through appointeeship and guardianship in the Mental Health Act 1983 and The Disabled Persons Act 1986 have been implemented. This has been a bitter blow for the citizen advocacy movement.

What the research data seem to indicate is that where there are clear and recognizable infringements to rights or entitlements such as in relation to complaints and welfare benefits, once picked up, these are dealt with well. However, where the issues or rights and entitlements are not so easily identified, for example in relation to access to case notes, to group homes and hostels, in relation to standards of dress or the nature of staff-client interactions, then there are likely to be problems. It is very difficult to legislate at this level of the individual's life and there therefore remains some interpretation involved in deciding what is acceptable for the individual in these terms.

In summary, where there remains some interpretation involved in deciding what is acceptable for an individual, the authority (as in 'right') to make these interpretations rests with service personnel. As the interviewee in quote 1 suggests, if only their partner was living independently, there would be a lot more that she would have the authority to do in terms of improving their general quality of life. But of course, this does nothing regarding the partner's rights in their present situation.

CONCLUSIONS

It has been argued in this chapter that the All-Wales Strategy was more systematically geared to the participation of people with learning disabilities in individual planning than the present White Paper which suggests, in comparison that:

> Assessments should **take account of** the wishes of the individual and his or her carer . . . and where possible should include their active participation. (DoH, 1989.) [Bold my emphasis.]

To the extent that the care manager may carry the authority to define need, even having taken account of the user's or citizen advocate's wishes; to the extent that the sale of services as goods is made by proxy by care managers, rather than by the user as in a service brokerage model; to the extent that we start with a set level of funding for overall provision rather than with a set of rights that should be accorded to each citizen. To this extent will the rights of individuals be set largely by the cash nexus and systems of professional hegemony rather than by the rights to citizenship that should be accorded each individual.

One is led to ask whether, in such a system of limited resources and zero-growth in funding, changing the outcomes for one person through citizen advocacy thereby denies another. Citizen advocacy does not, after all, seek to change the system of privilege accorded by government to its disabled citizens. Changing this system is an important and complementary task of other advocacies. This of course leads us back to the introductory notes to this chapter and to the question as to how much the State owes its disabled and disadvantaged citizens/subjects.

REFERENCES

Abrams, P. (1984) Realities of neighbourhood care: the inter-actions between statutory, voluntary and informal sectors. *Policy and Politics*, **12** (4), pp. 414–428.

Biehal, N. (1993) Changing practice: participation, rights and community care. *British Journal of Social Work*, **23**, pp. 443–458.

Butler, K., Carr, S. and Sullivan, F. (1988) *Citizen Advocacy: A Powerful Partnership*, National Citizen Advocacy, London.

Consumer Involvement Sub-Group (1991) *Consumer Involvement and the All Wales Strategy*, Cardiff, Welsh Office, October.

Crawley, B. (1990) Advocacy as a threat or ally to professional practice?, in *The Roles and Tasks of CMHTs*, (eds G. Brown and G. Wistow), Avebury, Aldershot.

DoH (1989) *Caring for People: Community Care in the Next Decade and Beyond*, HMSO, London.

DoH (1990) *Community Care in the Next Decade and Beyond: Policy Guidance*, HMSO, London.

DoH/SSI (1991) *Caring for People: Community Care in the Next Decade and Beyond. Policy Guidance*, HMSO, London.

Dowson, S. (1990) *Who Does What? The Process of Enabling People with Learning Difficulties to Achieve What They Need and Want*, Values into Action, London.

Gostin, L. (1983) *A Practical Guide to Mental Health Law*, MIND, London.

Humphrey, S. (1986) Individual planning in Nimrod: results of an evaluation of the system four years on, in *CMHTs: Theory and Practice*, (eds G. Grant, S. Humphrey and M. McGrath), BIMH Publications, Kidderminster, pp. 78–92.

Law Commission (1995) *Mental Incapacity. Item 9 of the Fourth Programme of Law Reform: Mentally Incapacitated Adults*, Law Commission No 231, HMSO, London.

Lukes, S. (1974) *Power: A Radical View*, Macmillan, London.

McGrath, M., Grant, G. and Ramcharan, P. (1991) *Service Packages: Factors Affecting Carers' Appraisals of Intermediate Outcomes*, September, Centre for Social Policy Research and Development, Bangor.

Parsons, T. (1952) *The Social System*, Tavistock Publications, London.

Ramcharan, P. and Grant, G. (1993) *Individual Planning and Citizen Advocacy in the State of Victoria Australia: Report of a Brief Study Visit*, Centre for Social Policy Research and Development, Bangor.

Simons, K. (1993) *Citizen Advocacy: The Inside View*, Norah Fry Research Centre, Bristol.

Tyne, A. (1991) *A Report of an Evaluation of Sheffield Citizen Advocacy*, Sheffield Citizen Advocacy and National Development Team, Sheffield.

Welsh Office (1983) *All Wales Strategy for the Development of Services for Mentally Handicapped People*, March, Welsh Office, Cardiff.

Welsh Office (1989) *Still a Small Voice: Consumer Involvement in the All Wales Strategy*, December, Welsh Office, Cardiff.

Wilding, P. (1982) *Professional Power and Social Welfare*, Routledge and Kegan Paul, London.

Wolfensberger, W. (1977) *A Multi-component Advocacy/Protection Schema*, Canadian Association for the Mentally Retarded, Law and Mental Retardation Monograph Series, Toronto.

Wolfensberger, W. and Thomas, S. (1991) *Social Advocacies on Behalf of Disadvantaged People*, August, Conference Notes, Newcastle.

Part Three

Empowerment – Professional Practice: Challenges and Opportunities

14

Effective support for self-help: some lessons from the experience of the Self-Help Alliance

Eric Miller, Fiddy Abraham, Dione Hills, Elizabeth Sommerlad, Elliot Stern and Barbara Webb

INTRODUCTION

'Support for self-help' could seem a contradiction. For Samuel Smiles, of course, self-help meant individual self-sufficiency – a philosophy that implied that every man is an island. Even in today's world of self-help groups providing mutual aid, there is often an idealized image of a set of like-minded people spontaneously getting together with a common purpose and managing themselves independently of any external resources. For a few groups that may indeed be the reality. Most, however, have needed outside help at some point in their history, whether in the form of advice on how to organize themselves or of a rent-free room to meet in. Some would not have formed at all or not have survived if that help had not been available.

The Self-Help Alliance (SHA), set up in the 1980s, was a large-scale, government-funded experiment in identifying and meeting such support needs. The authors of this chapter were members of a Tavistock Institute research team (led by Stern and Miller) which was commissioned to evaluate the programme. The first part of the chapter describes the origins of the SHA and the processes – including political negotiations – involved in establishing its role (Miller, 1988). The second part of the chapter explores the experience of the consortium in funding and overseeing local self-help support projects in different parts of the country. The outcome was a set of development workers, each with a distinctive approach, operating in a variety of local conditions – for example, urban and rural – and relating to hundreds of self-help groups of different kinds (Miller, 1988; Abraham, 1989). This was a rare research opportunity and some of the lessons learnt from it are distilled in the final section of the chapter.

FORMATION OF THE SELF-HELP ALLIANCE

The Self-Help Alliance (SHA) was one element in the 'Helping the community to care' initiative, which was launched by the then Department of Health and Social Security (DHSS) in July 1984. The initiative was designed to enhance the role of the voluntary sector in developing approaches to community care.

During the 1970s the self-help movement had been burgeoning, nationally and internationally. Of particular interest to the Department was the 'Nottingham experiment'. The Nottingham Self-help Team owed its origins to development work in the voluntary sector, by workers based at Nottingham Council for Voluntary Service. The team was set up in 1982 to encourage and support new groups, to provide practical services and to provide information to professional workers and voluntary organizations. Its ethos was very much a community development approach (Wilson, 1989). In addition the Department was influenced by research that suggested that, whilst national voluntary bodies fostering self-help – some of which, such as Gingerbread and Mencap, were receiving DHSS funding – were providing a **vertical** supportive network for local groups, there was also a recognizable need for **horizontal** support structures at local level (Richardson and Goodman, 1983). This became the focus. Although social service departments (SSDs) might have seemed to be well placed to identify and respond to such needs, local authorities were traditionally resistant to accepting central government funding earmarked for specific purposes. Consequently the Department opted for a strategy of creating local infrastructures using the voluntary sector. In contrast to the specialist interests of the national bodies, the local projects were to be generalist, addressing a range of different needs and concerns, though these were limited to the DHSS field of health and social welfare. Campaigning groups were also excluded, so that the government would not find that it was indirectly funding protests against its own policies. The DHSS emphasized that the programme was experimental and time-limited: there was to be no expectation of long-term funding from central government.

Use of a consortium of national voluntary organizations to run the programme was the key element in the strategy. The Department lacked the capability to do so itself, and there was a precedent in a previous programme, Opportunities for Volunteering. Some of these national bodies had the requisite knowledge of the local voluntary sector; they also offered a vehicle for distilling and disseminating lessons from local experience which might otherwise be lost. The role of the Department was therefore to allocate a budget and define a brief; to reach agreement with the consortium on how the brief was to be implemented; and to establish timescales, funding limits and control mechanisms (including monitoring and evaluation). The consortium would then have the task of selecting local projects, allocating funds to them and overseeing their performance.

The Department invited two bodies to form the nucleus of the consortium: the National Council for Voluntary Organizations (NCVO) and the Volunteer Centre (VC). Both had been engaged in administering the Opportunities for Volunteering funds; NCVO had strong links with the national voluntary associations and VC, through its network of voluntary bureaux, was tied into local development activities alongside statutory and non-statutory health and social service agencies. The opportunity to disburse £1.75 million was tempting but they were cautious. The two bodies were at that time jointly planning a National Self-Help Support Centre (which in fact took another two years to come to fruition) and they were explicitly seeking non-governmental sources of funds for this, because they did not want the centre to be tainted by the belief that it was implementing a government policy to promote self-help as a means of cutting costs in the statutory sector. In the event they accepted the Department's assurances that the new initiative was intended to enlarge the effectiveness of existing statutory functions, not to reduce them, and more generally to enhance quality of life.

Since there were no other agencies suitable for the task, NCVO and VC were in quite a strong bargaining position. They used this to produce significant changes in the Department's initial proposal: the timescale was increased from two years to three; instead of 40 local projects, the number was scaled down to 15–20, which could then be better resourced (including reasonable salaries for development workers); and a larger proportion of the total budget was earmarked for central activities, which were to be extended beyond administration to cover development, training and consultancy. DHSS had intended that the local projects would be based in councils for voluntary service (CsVS); now other types of local intermediary bodies were added: rural community councils (RCCs), voluntary bureaux (VBx), community relations councils (CRCs), and settlements and social action centres. The Department wanted a single model of self-help support to be adopted, based on the Nottingham experience; NCVO in particular argued, successfully, for more than one approach.

NCVO and VC also pressed to widen the consortium. Five bodies were invited: the CVS National Association (CVSNA), the Standing

Committee of RCCs, VBx National Voice, the National Association of CRCs (NACRC), and the British Association of Settlements and Social Action Centres (BASSAC). The first four accepted; BASSAC was less amenable. Some of its local affiliates were politically radical and active in campaigning, and it was dubious about the government's motives; also it resented not having had a voice in shaping the scheme. BASSAC therefore took up an observer role, which it maintained for a year before becoming a full member of the consortium.

Other interest groups too had objections or were seen as potentially threatened. Some national voluntary associations argued that the funding should have been routed through them. The Association of County Councils formally protested to the Secretary of State at yet another short-term funding initiative, which would put a further burden on local authority resources at the end of the funding period. As for health authorities, which were seen as an important potential resource, so far untapped, the SHA was concerned that health professionals might regard self-help as subversive: empowering patients and encouraging consumer feedback represented a challenge to professional perspectives and to paternalistic service provision. Objections from trade unions were also foreseen, and the SHA found it necessary to state that the scheme was 'not intended . . . to develop the opportunities for voluntary work as if this were a substitute for paid employment, nor to encourage groups as a way of replacing professional care'. The political (with both a small and a capital P) sensitivity of the scheme is reflected in the following statement by the director of VC, which attempted to define the place of self-help within the wider networks of care provision:

> The NCVO and the Volunteer Centre . . . , in responding to the DHSS, recognize the potential of self-help as one strand in the complex interweaving of family care, informal help, voluntary agency and statutory services . . . Both agencies are on record about the need to maintain resources for welfare provision while recognizing that pluralistic approaches to provision, whatever the resource provision, are vital. So whilst re-affirming that self-help is not a substitute for statutory resources, NCVO and VC join with others in an Alliance to further this modest programme . . . as an example of partnership, of mixed provision, at a time when major changes in policy for SSDs are forecast and major challenges for resources in both the NHS and social services exist.

One 'political' problem, never fully resolved, was participation of ethnic minorities. The Department's implicit classification of self-help groups was by shared issue or need – for example, single parenthood or depression – and although the SHA quickly recognized that 'black self-help' might need separate attention and indeed it obliged local projects with substantial ethnic minorities to involve their representatives, representation on the SHA itself was missing. The initial SHA committee members were all white. A year later a black body – the National Federation of Self-Help Organizations (NFSHO) – was invited to join the Alliance, but it understandably said 'no', arguing that only through involvement of the black community in the initial design of the programme and its criteria for implementation could the distinctive needs of that community have been properly addressed. The SHA's response was to recommend the DHSS to mount a separate scheme to support black self-help. Eventually the Alliance did recruit one black body, the Standing Conference on Ethnic Minority Senior Citizens (SCEMSC), and later co-opted black individuals onto the committee, but the programme remained vulnerable to accusations of institutional racism.

THE SELF-HELP ALLIANCE IN ACTION

The Secretary of State had announced the programme in July 1984; the committee of the newly formed Alliance met for the first time early in November, and the next tasks were to define more closely the brief for the local projects and to appoint agencies to run them.

The scope of both 'self-help' and 'support' needed definition. It was decided to focus on self-help groups formed around a specific health or social problem and accepted that campaigning groups should be excluded. There were criticisms that this definition was too narrow. For example, the emphasis on groups disqualified some mutual support systems in rural areas, and multipurpose associations important among ethnic minorities would also be off-limits. As for support, the local project was to be a source of advice for people starting new groups, to publicize self-help and to encourage partnership and understanding between professional workers and self-help groups. It was to be 'enabling rather than proactive: backing up groups rather than organizing them; building networks between groups rather than co-ordinating; facilitating rather than promoting; and seeing educational processes as important as specific outcomes'. Setting the boundaries in this way was, despite criticisms, seen as necessary to provide a basis for coherent development and learning from the experiment. However, the guidelines were not presented as an inflexible blueprint: 'schemes should be built on local resources and needs'. Ultimately, in fact, local conditions, combined with the individual stances of the development workers, generated quite a wide range of approaches.

Potential sponsoring agencies were required to have some experience of self-help support and the demonstrable competence to manage a local project with at least one development worker and a back-up person. Of the 65 who applied, 48 were deemed eligible and 18 were approved. Two-thirds of these were CsVS, others were diverse, and the geographical spread was wide. That was in the late summer of 1985; during the autumn and winter the new project managers began to recruit and activate their teams.

Meanwhile, the SHA had been forming its own central team: a national development officer (NDO), an administrative assistant, and a secretary. Treasury pressures squeezed out a specific budget for consultancy; the NDO would partly fill the gap, though with the constraint that she would also be overseeing the projects in a managerial role. The SHA was also making plans for training, though here too the budget was less than they had wished. Training was seen as a means of helping the local workers to acquire a shared identity as part of a national programme and to maximize the learning from it. They would therefore come together fairly regularly. Project managers would gather, say, twice a year for the same purpose. The first induction sessions for development workers were held in 1986.

Another key element of the programme was research and evaluation. On this, both the DHSS and SHA were agreed. However, their priorities differed. The SHA favoured an approach that would emphasize self-evaluation by the local development workers; while the department was more interested in outcomes: the value or otherwise of funding such workers for promotion and support of self-help groups. Both wanted an overview of the scheme as a whole, including the mechanism of central funding of local voluntary agencies through a national consortium. The selection of the Tavistock Institute to take the research/evaluation role was on the basis of a developmental approach to evaluation, in line with the Institute's tradition of action research. It would encourage self-evaluation by local projects and ongoing learning from experience whilst retaining more conventional research methods, such as surveys. The research would contribute to the task of the development workers and they, reciprocally, would be contributing to the research task. This role was funded directly by the Department, which provided the chair of a Research Steering Group with Alliance representation. The Tavistock Institute team also started work at the beginning of 1986.

Thus the organizational arrangements for the programme were somewhat complex. Local 'host agencies' had prepared proposals and applied for funding of the projects; they managed the funds and each had appointed an agency member as project manager (unpaid): in some this was the overall director of the agency but usually not. However, both the project managers and the local development workers had accountabilities to the SHA: the former for the spending of money and periodic reporting, and both for participation in the national training and also in the evaluation; but the workers were drawn more closely into the orbit of the SHA and also of the research/evaluation team, which in turn related to all levels in the system, from the workers to the Department.

Predictably, it took several months to 'run in' this machinery and make it work. At local level, for example, there were tensions to be resolved between the original conception of the project and the orientation of the incoming workers, who, if they did not always initially have greater knowledge of self-help, rapidly acquired it through experience and through the shared SHA training. Relations between the projects and the SHA were marked by similar tensions and implicit or explicit negotiations. Partly intentionally, the SHA was taking a relatively reactive stance towards the projects. There was uncertainty on both sides of the boundary about the SHA's managerial role and authority. Project workers attributed to the committee, which they had never met, much more power and cohesion than it either had or aspired to. Workers met together on the training events, and their real complaints about the felt unresponsiveness of the training consultants to their needs were magnified by displaced frustrations about the absent and invisible 'management'.

By the end of the first year this running-in phase was over. Nearly all the projects had settled down and were hard at work, though one or two crises required intervention from the centre. The roles of the SHA committee and the central management team had become relatively clear and settled. The NDO and some committee members were paying rostered visits to projects, while some projects hosted meetings of the committee. The research team had established effective collaboration at all levels. Development workers had organized themselves, nationally and regionally, to a point where they could manage their own training – they had become a self-help group – and appoint regional representatives to the SHA committee. The chair of the committee convened periodic one-day review meetings with project managers collectively.

From the second year onwards, the more settled internal relations enabled the SHA, particularly through the NDO, to become more outward-looking, in terms of spreading the self-help message, including the accumulating experiences of the projects themselves, at national level and also through participation in European conferences. Many project workers too were taking part in conferences and workshops, some abroad, and a few were publishing material. The National Self-Help Support Centre was finally launched and as the three years of the programme drew towards a close, the SHA became increasingly active in dissemination. By then, of course, there was progressively more to disseminate. Some of this is now outlined.

OUTCOMES AND LESSONS

The programme succeeded in a number of ways in demonstrating that local, 'horizontal' support could be useful and effective. For example:

- Between them, the 18 projects contributed to setting up about 500 new groups, of which about 85% continued for at least a year.
- They provided support, of various kinds and degrees of intensity, to about 1000 pre-existing groups.
- Within the overall 'health and welfare' definition, a very wide range of groups were supported. (Among new groups formed in 1987–88, the five most common themes were: tranquillizer withdrawal, menopause, cancer support, depression, and single parents.)
- They achieved constructive networking: first, among different self-help groups in the same locality; and second, between groups (and group members) and relevant workers in the statutory and voluntary sectors.
- Using a variety of means, they raised the profile of self-help in the locality, among both potential users and professionals.

However, as indicated earlier, the local project workers were not simply doing a development job; they were also being helped by the research team to undertake an ongoing self-evaluation of what they were doing. Consequently they were constantly checking the effects of their actions against their intentions and learning from that experience in quite a systematic way – an application of the scientific method. Beyond that, almost every development worker became a member of at least one of the research groups formed by the Tavistock team to explore self-help support in different contexts; for example, specific issues that arise in working in rural areas or with ethnic minority groups (Abraham *et al.*, 1988; Abraham and Webb, 1989; Hills *et al.*, 1988; Miller *et al.*, 1988; Sommerlad and Hills, 1990).

The project workers provided various different types of support, ranging from the practical to the developmental:

- **Information**: Local health and social services and policy, statutory entitlements, other local groups, national associations, reference material, constitution, fundraising, group work.
- **Advice**: Publicity, fundraising, running events, group structure and process.
- **Practical help**: On meeting rooms, speakers, publicity (e.g. design and placement of posters and other materials).
- **Office assistance**: Typing, photocopying, mailing, stationery.
- **Brokering**: Increasing links to professionals; advocacy; gaining access for groups to services.

- **Skills development**: Training workshops, modelling roles in groups, group-work exercises and games.
- **Emotional support**: Counselling, enabling, facilitating, encouraging, energizing.
- **Leadership**: Initiating, co-ordinating, undertaking group management tasks.

Additionally, local projects were engaged in more general promotional activities, through fairs, study days, articles in the press and so on, to disseminate the idea of self-help among both professionals and the public at large.

For any one project to engage effectively in all these different kinds of activities was plainly impossible. Choices had to be made. Implicitly or explicitly therefore the projects were formulating strategies which gave some approaches and activities priority over others. The choice of strategy and of the particular intervention in any one case was a product of many variables: characteristics of the development worker herself; characteristics of the individual group; and the influences of their environments.

A development worker brings with her a conception of self-help together with an ideology and a preferred way of working. For example, she may attach great importance to empowerment, which will shape her relation to groups. In this programme, some workers preferred to concentrate on practical support external to the group, while others, though not neglecting practical aspects, were more comfortable in taking a developmental role within groups. The worker's gender and ethnicity were also significant variables: an ethnic minority worker has a potential advantage in relating to groups with the same ethnicity.

The kinds of support appropriate to a group will depend on its stage and development and its purposes. The development worker is often involved at the embryonic stage: one or two people with a particular problem or interest may seek help in setting up a group; or she may identify a need and take an initiative in attracting potential members. The new group may benefit from both practical help, for example, publicity and a meeting-place, and more 'internal' forms of support, for example, a facilitator in the early stages of group formation and organization. The purposes for which members join groups and which shape their collective character fall into four clusters:

- **empowerment**, which could be personal (increased confidence and self-esteem) or collective, as in campaigning for better services on behalf of all, and often a mix of both;
- **therapy**, with the aim of treating and curing a condition, such as an eating disorder;

- **coping and improving the quality of life** for people with an incurable or stigmatizing condition;
- **respite**, being able to relax in a way only possible among people with a shared problem.

These are not mutually exclusive; some groups serve more than one function and often there is an educational strand running through them. Plainly, any intervention must be consistent with the purpose. Emphasis on empowerment is unlikely to be welcomed by a group whose members are seeking respite from day-to-day struggles.

We found that the roles that the workers took up in relation to groups were also influenced in a number of ways by the wider set of relationships in which they operated. The characteristics of the host agency were an important factor. An agency with a traditional welfare ideology was not a comfortable base for a worker with a more modern ideology of community development. *Laissez-faire* management could give the worker ample discretion, but she would need to look elsewhere for support and supervision. The slow, gradual process of developing effective self-help among some ethnic minority communities and other populations lacking resources and developed skills is not attainable within an agency that is judging performance of the project by the number of new groups formed. It is difficult for a black worker to relate to black groups if she is operating from a predominantly white agency which lacks credibility with local black communities, and so on. Obviously important too was the relationship to the overall SHA programme. As we have seen, the SHA, in its initial brief, communicated a particular approach to selp-help support, which tended to be accepted somewhat uncritically by project managers in the host agencies, but which was often not consistent with either the ethos of the individual practitioners themselves or with the needs and opportunities they actually encountered in the field. Thus in practice some campaigning groups did receive support. The research team, for its part, was receptive to diversity, innovation and experimentation as and when they emerged. Development workers also learned from and were influenced by each other's experiences, both indirectly through the research team and, increasingly as time went on, directly through the self-help groupings that they formed amongst themselves.

Many of the local groups that were the 'clients' of the project also had other relationships that influenced the ways in which they defined their needs and related to the development workers. Most ongoing groups had received support at start-up from other local sources (such as voluntary agencies or health professionals) or from a national association to which they were affiliated, and some from both. Sometimes development workers were able to make useful links with such national bodies: for example, getting information about a particular condition or actually collaborating in the formation of a group. But it could also prove difficult for a worker espousing participative and democratic values to provide effective 'horizontal' support if the 'vertical' support from a national body prescribed a hierarchical committee structure and formal rules of procedure.

The nature of work with groups was also affected by two other types of enviromental factors: demographic and institutional. The main demographic variables were geography (urban *v.* rural), ethnicity, and social class. The experiences of the programme showed that both in rural populations and among many ethnic minorities effective self-help was achieved not through transplanting conventional models but by building on existing social forms, such as affiliation to a church. Both ethnic minorities and segregated working-class estates were more likely to produce generalist groups, orientated to mutual aid and campaigning. Single-issue groups linked to national organizations were more likely to have a middle-class membership; non-affiliated groups could attract both classes provided that they met in a location perceived as socially 'neutral'. When referring individuals as potential members, development workers needed to take these cultural variables into account, to ensure 'goodness of fit'. It was notable that the membership of self-help groups was preponderantly female – as were the SHA development workers.

As for the local institutional environment, three elements were particularly relevant: the strength of the local voluntary sector; voluntary/ statutory relations; and the local tradition of self-help. Where these were strong, the worker could more easily take up her brokering role in mediating between groups (and individuals) and institutional resources: for example, to influence service provision or to obtain an appropriate referral for an individual. It was also relevant to her other role, of promoting self-help as such. If the worker already had local knowledge and/or was employed by an agency with strong local links, these tasks were obviously easier. The relationships she made, however, were also affected by her ideology and conception of self-help – in particular whether self-help was seen as complementary to existing services or as an alternative to them. Our research showed a strong tendency for contacts with local statutory and voluntary agencies to become more numerous over the three years of the programme. This suggested that development workers had succeeded in gaining increased institutional acceptance and legitimation of self-help, though some professionals (including most GPs) proved difficult to mobilize.

Whilst we have been emphasizing the variety in types of groups, types of intervention and so forth and the choices that have to be made – a point we shall come back to in our concluding section – it would be a mistake to overlook some underlying commonalities. Probably all self-help support workers would agree that the desired output of their activities is a group that is self-managing and that meets the needs of its members.

A viable self-managing group is likely to have such characteristics as these:

- It has a shared sense of purpose. (In most cases this is explicit; in generalist self-help groups it may be less so.)
- It has a shared culture, e.g. there is at least tacit agreement on acceptable/unacceptable behaviour.
- It has reasonably clear criteria for inclusion/exclusion of prospective members.
- It has sufficient structure – whether formal or informal – to get things done.
- Decision making and responsibilities are shared, so that whilst the group is likely to have a core of key members who play a more prominent role than others, it is not so dependent on these that it will collapse should one such member leave.
- It experiences effectiveness in relation to its environment (e.g. legitimating a stigmatized condition; raising funds; influencing statutory service provision) or at least it experiences some external recognition to reinforce its sense of identity and self-worth.
- It is effective at the individual level; its members value the group experience and feel they benefit from being able to share a common problem.
- It is also able to identify its own limitations and has the self-confidence and security to seek external help (e.g. from professionals) without being taken over. Its dependence is mature and realistic.
- It can make space for new members and allow old ones to leave without threat to its identity.
- It can make the decision to disband if it is no longer meeting a need or (as in a campaigning group) if its purposes have been fulfilled.

The group will meet members' needs if:

- It enables new members to feel that there is space for them.
- It provides new contacts and potential friendships with others sharing the same condition.
- There is sufficient congruence between the member's self-perception and the identity that the group confers upon the member.
- It builds members' self-esteem and self-confidence; it gives them the experience of being valued and effective.
- It provides for dependency needs – it is a safe place to be – while . . .
- . . . it also promotes their independence – their capacity to control their own lives.

These lists do not pretend to be the last word: the items might be modified and extended. However, they offer useful criteria for thinking about what forms of support with what intensity are appropriate – and these vary at different stages of a group's life cycle – and also how to provide it. The issue of 'how' is important. The self-managing group is likely to enable its members to be or become self-managing. Consequently, the interventions of the support worker should reinforce the group's capacity for self-management. She therefore attempts to meet the group's needs in a way that models or reflects the way in which an effective group meets its members' needs. (The research team, recognizing this, consciously tried to relate to the development workers in a manner that would enhance their capacity for self-management, and thus to provide a model. Correspondingly, it appeared that this was how the project managers related to the development workers in the most effective projects.)

Whilst these principles may have general validity, their application in practice will obviously depend on the particular situation. The nature of the shared condition tends to affect the ability to move towards self-management:

- People with conditions that are socially stigmatized are likely to have lower self-esteem.
- Some conditions in themselves predispose to greater dependency and less capacity for individual self-management.

Both these propositions may apply, for example, to mental illness. However, appropriate support for such groups is not different in kind. The desired outcome is the same: a self-managing group that meets members' needs. The difference is in the length and intensity of support required. It may involve a pre-self-help phase, working with individuals, as well as a more extended period of dependency of the group itself before it becomes 'weaned' as it were.

In the SHA programme, some development workers were anxious about dependency: they feared that if they allowed a group to become at all dependent on them it might never become independent. Certainly, a group that can survive only through continuing outside support can hardly be called a self-help group. On the other hand, there is an element of dependence in almost every approach that the worker receives. For a worker who chooses to operate within a group, strategies and approaches are available which will help in managing dependency in the relationship and in taking up an enabling and empowering role – acquiring, in other words, a sense of 'appropriate dependency' in relation to groups at different stages of their lifecycle:

- She avoids uninvited interventions, though her availability needs to be known.

- She does not avoid dependency; nor does she respond to it by taking a 'parental' role. She works with it and through it by maintaining an 'adult' relationship. (Note that it is the group members, not the worker, who are the experts on their condition.)
- She negotiates (and periodically renegotiates as necessary) an explicit definition of the nature and degree of her involvement. One strategy is to contract to work with the group for a limited period.
- She reduces the dependency by avoiding being the unique resource. Linking the group with other self-help groups and with suitable professionals is a way of doing this.
- She devises ways of helping the group to experience effectiveness in setting and reaching attainable goals.

To quote one project manager: 'A support worker knows she has been successful if the group is pleased and excited about itself and thinks it has done all the work itself. That is the mark of good support work – getting the group to think that the successes are all their own'.

CONCLUSIONS

Our evaluation addressed various policy issues relating to the SHA programme as a whole: for example, the appropriate mechanisms for overall management of such a scheme by the Department of Health; the distinctive needs of ethnic minority groups; and the implications of time-limited funding. (Only half the local projects secured resources to continue – generally on a reduced scale – after the three years. Follow-up funding from local social services was small and from health authorities minimal.) Here, however, we confine ourselves to lessons for self-help support as such.

Our evidence showed that local 'horizontal' support can make a significant and positive contribution to self-help. Support strategies can be specific to the local population and conditions and can target particular local needs. For example, a local project can introduce self-help as part of a package of mental health services in planned discharge of psychiatric patients from a hospital; or it can contribute to community building by giving backing to a women's group on a housing estate. Thus through independent assessment of local needs workers can promote or support groups not covered by national organizations, while also providing specific local support for groups that do have national affiliation. Moreover, through participating in, and indeed developing local networks of voluntary and statutory workers they are able to link groups to agencies, services and individual workers relevant to a group's needs.

As illustrated above, from the experience of the programme it proved possible to put forward some broad propositions about the characteristics of effective self-help groups and about the nature of effective intervention by support workers. The research did not, however, lead to advocacy of a particular model of self-help support. On the contrary, it illuminated the variety of activities and approaches that support workers adopt, while it also showed that choices have to be made. The worker cannot be all things to all people. The selected strategy and method of working will be contingent on a number of specific variables: the skills and orientation of the worker herself, the presenting needs of existing and potential groups and the local environment, institutional and demographic. But a decision to invest resources in one strategy – for example, to operate only externally to the groups themselves, or conversely to opt for intensive work with groups with mentally ill members – means that the other support needs, unless resources come from elsewhere, will not be met. Whatever the choice, the experience of the programme underlined the value of conscious self-evaluation in helping the development workers to be explicit about what they were trying to do, why and how; to monitor the outcomes against their expectations; and then, if necessary, to modify the approach or try something different and to evaluate that too.

One final point: self-help support is a mentally and often emotionally demanding task. Attention therefore has to be given to support for the support workers.

REFERENCES

Abraham, F. (1989) Delivering self-help support: the first year in operating the Self-Help Alliance Scheme. *COVAS Occasional Paper*, No 6, The Tavistock Institute, London.

Abraham, F., Sommerlad, E. *et al.* (1988) Self-help support and black people: start-up strategies in four Self-Help Alliance projects. *COVAS Occasional Paper*, No 4, The Tavistock Institute, London.

Abraham, F. and Webb, B. (1989) Mental health and self-help support. *COVAS Occasional Paper*, No 5, The Tavistock Institute, London.

Hills, N., Stern, E., Staines, M. *et al.* (1989) Self-help in rural areas: is it different? *COVAS Occasional Paper*, No 3, The Tavistock Institute, London.

Miller, E. (1988) Support for self-help: the origins and development of the Self-Help Alliance. *COVAS Occasional Paper*, No 1, The Tavistock Institute, London.

Miller, E., Webb, B. *et al.* (1988) The nature of effective self-help support in different contexts. *COVAS Occasional Paper*, No 2, The Tavistock Institute, London.

Richardson, A. and Goodman, M. (1983) *Self-help and Social Care: Mutual Aid Organizations in Practice*, Policy Studies Institute, London.

Sommerlad, E. and Hills, D. (1990) Managing an innovative project: issues in the relationship between host organizations and projects. *COVAS Occasional paper*, No 7, The Tavistock Institute, London.

Wilson, J. (1989) Supporting self-help: six years of work in an English city. *Health Promotion*, **4** (3), pp. 215–224.

15

User first –
implications for management

Mervyn Eastman

INTRODUCTION

Social services and health care professionals work within organizations that frequently proclaim the centrality of the user and patient. The 'vision thing' represents a potentially powerful framework of rhetoric shared by managers in local government and NHS trusts and provider units. If the NHS and Community Care Act (1990) did nothing else, it at least gave a legislative structure in placing users and their carers somewhere on the agenda, if not at the core.

This chapter invites the reader to explore the implications for management if organizations are to take seriously the notion of empowerment and what a user first approach means if rhetoric is to become reality in the daily experience of individual users and their carers (Jowell, 1991). To do this effectively I make some basic assumptions: that the reader shares the philosophy of a user first approach; and believes, as I do, that traditional power bases – client *v.* professional, worker *v.* management – have to fundamentally shift if needs-led assessment processes and care planning systems are to be translated into practical and meaningful services for users and carers and become the norm, rather than the exception.

The discussion will be focused on social work given that it is my field of experience and has always as a profession claimed to have at its core a set of values that place the client first.

THE VALUE BASE OF SOCIAL WORK

Social work training in the late 1960s and 1970s made much of the values held by the profession (Biestek, 1961; Hollis, 1972; Younghusband,

1978). Respect for persons; self-determination; equality and fairness continue to have particular significance for social work managers within both statutory and independent sector care organizations. These values, it could be argued, underpin their very existence.

In contrast to individualistic and liberal values is the recognition that social work exists within a political framework and is itself a political activity (Jordan and Parton, 1983). Thus social work must also be understood within the context of political and organizational processes.

This inherent tension between these values and the sometimes coercive functions of social work (Raynor, 1985) is enshrined in legislation such as the Mental Health Act 1983 and Children Act 1989 that give local authorities powers and duties both to protect vulnerable people and control them.

If empowerment means that the user and their carers set the service agenda (what is provided and how) we need to recognize these inherent tensions and the limitations imposed by the organizational and political framework as to how far users can determine what is or is not provided. For example, resource shortfall may prevent the client/user living where they would like, or with whom. Choices may be overriden for their own protection or somebody else's, i.e. their children. Again, the user may be incapable of making an informed choice. Nonetheless the values of respect for persons and self-determination impose a duty on workers to explain as fully as is practicable the whys and the wherefores at every stage in the decision-making process.

Community care legislation was welcomed by most professionals if only for its rhetoric in encouraging the statutory services to include users in deciding their own needs via assessment and determining the content, style and delivery of services via the care planning process. The tensions, however, between the user's wishes and preferences and the service provider's professional judgement about appropriateness cannot be casually noted then ignored. User participation in decision making about what service ought to be provided and at what cost are sharp nettles needing to be grasped by social services' managers and elected local councillors.

The Barclay Report (1982) examining the role and task of social workers appears very dated a decade after its publication. In re-reading Chapter 10, which concentrated on values, methods, skills and knowledge, I was struck by the suggestion that social workers determine whether the client can participate and whether the client can control. The implicit message appears to be that power lies in the knowledge and skill base of the professional. A very different emphasis from that of the Community Care Act.

Managers within social services have, by and large, been drawn from the rank and file of the profession (my own route) and whilst accepting the social work task and the value base on which it rests, little attention traditionally has been paid to the task and function of managing staff generally or mangement specifically. Poorly managed staff and resources are not only wasteful but can be abusive to users and their carers. What, then, are the implications of these shifting values and inherent tensions for today's manager? In the non-user first organization I would say very few! Service managers, team leaders, care plan co-ordinators and the myriad others who make up 'gatekeepers of service' can still claim to put the user first in exactly the same way as we did in the 1970s and early 1980s. But, in reality, there need to be some very definite transitions; firstly from the user being a passive recipient of services, designed and delivered by professionals who decide what is in the user's best interests, to the user setting the service menu, purchasing their own care plan from direct grants based on their own assessment of need. Secondly, a transition from power in the hands of professionals and managers of the organization being held by users. Such transitions challenge not only social services departments but directors of finance, district auditors and even the Department of Health and Social Services Inspectorate.

DISEMPOWERMENT AND ORGANIZATIONAL ABUSE

Thus, for over 40 years social work has been claiming to represent and defend the user, advocate for and support the user yet throughout this period there has been a succession of scandals in children's homes, elderly person's homes and hostels for vulnerable adults. Are these simply 'bad apple' incidents? By no means. As Wardhaugh and Wilding (1993) argue management and professional attitudes and practice play a significant part in what they call the 'corruption of care'. Whilst that corruption has been frequently in residential provision, I would argue corruption, coerciveness and intimidation are evident in field work, day and home care practice and in managerial decision making at both a policy and strategic level.

Wardhaugh and Wilding (1993) suggest that this corruption of care stems from a 'betrayal of the basic values on which the organization is supposedly based' but what does this mean in the context of a user first organization?

There is firstly the issue of the absolute corruption of both power and powerlessness (Peters, 1989). The vulnerability of social services users with little, if any, influence on or knowledge of the systems and processes within local government renders them dependent on the professional worker. However the relationship between powerless users and powerful staff can be reflected in organizations by that between powerless workers and powerful managers. If those with managerial responsibility take their staff for granted, give them little support and do not allow appropriate consultation, the worker can feel worthless. Wardhaugh and Wilding compellingly argue that this 'creates a dangerous ambivalence'.

Thus, the 'bicycle manager' is created (Wagner, 1981) – the one who, like riding a bicycle, kowtows to those above and stamps on those below. Staff who abuse often feel abused themselves by their managers. The investigations into abuse in residential homes, including Nye Bevan Lodge (1981), Pindown (Levy and Kahan, 1991) and the Normansfield Inquiry (HMSO, 1978), all demonstrated the extent of management failure. There was total disregard of effective monitoring and evaluation, control and accountability. As staff were thus 'abused', users were simultaneously depersonalized, marginalized and discounted throughout the particular units involved and the worker organizations. There was a collusion with bad practice because the emphasis and focus were not on the individual user but the surface 'smooth running' of the organization. Keeping within cash limited budgets, obsession with processes and procedures and not causing political or organizational embarrassment can mask abusive practice. Professional autonomy focusing on outcomes can allow managers to abdicate their managerial responsibilities in ensuring, as Goffman (1961) says, 'humane standards of treatment'. Cultures of subcare can develop where the standard becomes acceptable throughout the organization.

If users are unable to assert themselves; staff are allowed to simply get on with it; managers are told to 'keep the lid down', we have a cocktail of disempowerment which explodes into the physical, emotional and organizational abuse of users, where nobody is accountable.

These various examples of institutionalized abuse suggest that where professional 'expertise' is believed to define needs and determine the most appropriate services regardless of the level of user participation there will be an undermining of the value base of the profession whereby these values became a ritualized rhetoric seldom challenged despite the experience of the user.

Before leaving this notion of professional or staff disempowerment, a brief word about fear. In discussion with users and their carers over many years one theme has constantly struck me about why people do not complain or assert their rights. The response is frequently: 'I'm afraid'. Of what? They will take the service away, or I may not even get a service. Fear is an invisible, yet powerful barrier to empowerment (Ryan and Oestreich, 1991). Little has been written in either social work or management texts on how distrust and indifference by staff and organizations can lead to service users becoming caught up in a culture of depersonalization. If I am devalued by my managers how can I sustain my regard of the client or carer's rights to be at the very centre of my practice? Staff and their managers who feel under siege cannot, in my view, sustain an approach to users that focuses on high quality responses or 'humane standards' in service provision. Staff who are disempowered by silence, brevity, snubbery, insults, blaming, discrediting, yelling and screaming from managers exist in an organizational culture of corruption which inevitably leads to dysfunction and further discounting and disempowerment of the service user.

ARE SOCIAL SERVICE DEPARTMENTS AND
CARE AGENCIES CUSTOMER-ORIENTED?

There are at least three key principles that determine whether an organization is customer-oriented. First, managers at executive and senior level have an active, even intensive involvement with users. Second, staff in both frontline operational and support administrative roles have an approach to their tasks that is classed as 'people-oriented'. Last, the organization has simple though intensive measurements of performance in which the user is integral to feeding back to the organization at all levels their experience and views.

Put another way, the challenge for care agencies is to develop obsessions for service; quality; tailored responses to individual needs and listening to the user. Managers, whether directorate, senior, middle or supervisory, are increasingly required to have not only a clear intellectual grasp of their function within the total organization, but a firm belief in its aims and values and actively work towards a user orientation through involvement and performance measurement.

Some doubt that this will be facilitated by the community care legislation. Bob Holman in his book *A New Deal for Social Welfare* (1993) argues that this legislation, imposing as it does internal and external markets, is likely, in the context of central government spending restrictions and 'the doctrine of management superiority', to have devastating effects through 'managerial social work'. He alleges that the task of enabling social workers and staff to do their jobs has been hijacked by New Right management theory and philosophy. Social work, Holman claims, is becoming less creative and tied down by procedures and centralized headquarter decision making. This emphasis is responsible for undermining the values of social work and practice. Holman chooses to ignore the paternalism of the traditional Left but his argument cannot be brushed aside as it demonstrates the tensions that exist between autonomy and decision making of frontline staff and the management task. However, I see nothing in the legislation which requires social services departments to maintain (and certainly not increase) managerial levels within the organization. Those departments which have genuinely adopted the user first ethos advocated in the NHS and Community Care Act have characteristics that would please Holman as they will possess structures which challenge and confront managers as they have never done before or since the Seebohm Report (1968).

Until the Community Care Act changed the agenda, the fundamental question 'what does the customer want?' (Druker, 1989) was seldom asked. It was the professional who defined needs and wants on the basis of their discipline, be it social work, occupational therapy, medicine or a mishmash of pseudopsychology, sociology and psychoanalysis. Here the customer was classified and labelled in stereotyped groupings – disabled, elderly, blind, black, poor, offender or psychiatric. The manager of today is asking what do clients and potential clients need, not what box can we put them in most conveniently for the organization?

However, needs-led assessment means very little if the user is not central in determining those needs. The care planning process is irrelevant if it does not genuinely address the wants, and the preference of the user or their carer. Social services staff have to address and confront the conflict between a needs-led assessment that determines the service provision and the user knowing exactly what services they need. The danger here is that the process and procedure of the new assessments become the focus leaving the user as disempowered by the bureaucracy as he or she was before the Community Care Act.

IMPLICATIONS FOR MANAGEMENT AND ORGANIZATIONS

Providing services that users want requires that organizations have mechanisms in place to ascertain what their wants are. Peters and Austin (1986) examined several key areas of such organizational competence through an analysis of how hundreds of American and international organizations viewed and treated their customers. Management theories and approaches, like most, undergo criticism and revision and some are finally discredited. The work of Tom Peters (Peters and Waterman, 1982; Peters, 1989; Peters, 1992), Robert Waterman and Nancy Austin is no different. In recent years their approach and doctrine have been severely attacked (Solomon, 1993) and strenuously defended (Jarstall, 1994; Wooller, 1994). It is perhaps too early to evaluate the longer term influence of Peters' work specifically but nevertheless the emphasis they placed on customer satisfaction, care or obsession, remains a constant theme of management gurus (Heller, 1994a). What, therefore, can we take from their understanding of client first organizations in relation to community care agencies?

Based on the work of Peters and Austin and Heller, I propose several performance indicators for user first care agencies which should be then made public and incorporated into the community care plans of social services departments.

- All printed matter, bulletins, reports should focus on the user and their carers. All development, strategic and resource reports would benefit from supporting data from users as to the value of what is being proposed or argued. This ensures that professional experts and their managers have at least asked the question – what does the customer want?
- Frontline staff should be given unique respect. This is given expression at least in part through conditions of service and pay. Traditionally managers have been paid more than the frontline staff. Why? Each worker needs to experience conditions that clearly demonstrate their value to the organization.
- Staff who support operational workers should be given equal consideration. Receptionists at area offices, domestic staff in provider units (old people's homes, hostels) are adequately trained. They too are given adequate monetary reward and a satisfactory working environment.
- Frontline staff and those who deal directly with users and carers should be regularly consulted about policies and procedures. They are closest to the users and have most knowledge of what they want.
- All levels of management support staff in finance, administration, personnel, training and staff development, purchasing officers should be required to meet users in their job descriptions. Separation of purchaser and provider functions does not preclude the active involvement of so-called purchasers in meeting and dealing with the users of the service that have been purchased.
- Language and terminology associated with the user should be neither degrading or contemptuous. Terms that are derogatory to users are not permitted. Staff using such terms in written notes, telephone conversations or staff meetings should be severely censored.
- The user/carer should be treated as a unique person, not a 'case' or a statistic. Every member of staff, whatever their task or function in the organization, should behave in such a way that demonstrates the high regard they have for the user. This includes informal interactions in staff rooms, coffee areas, as well as formal forums.
- Case reviews, reports, even meetings should begin with an analysis of the direct impact of any proposed action or policy on the client. Better still, the user or carer should be, if possible, at the review or jointly prepare the report. If the user or carer is not involved in the meeting or review this should be agreed by senior managers. As such, it is considered a significant exception.

- User satisfaction should be measured as closely as budget control. User feedback mechanisms and systems should be an integral part of the management function. Each unit of operation and support should engage users in feeding back on performance. Regular surveys (even over the telephone) and other systems should be designed to actively seek out views and act on them. Community development has an important role to play in this activity given the assumption that local people should determine their own needs and organizations, in partnership with those communities, should work out strategies to meet those needs.

- The evaluation and appraisal of staff (especially managers) should be based on what users and carers think of them although users and workers can be in conflict over needs and wants; for instance, workers taking a child into care or sectioning under the Mental Health Act may be perceived as perverse, dangerous, or even unprofessional. Resource restrictions could prevent meeting the user's needs/wants which in turn is seen as an individual worker's failure rather than that of their managers or elected councillors, proprietors or managing directors. These realities can be used to excuse not involving users in staff appraisal but they must be incorporated into responsive systems.

- Complaints response mechanisms. Under the Community Care Act, social services departments have to have in place appropriate systems to investigate user/carer complaints. They ought to focus on both immediacy and personalization of response. Managers have an important role in monitoring complaints but as important is the introduction of changes that result from specific complaints. Any analysis of complaints may demonstrate that most complaints are about the attitude of both staff and managers rather than resource shortfalls. Where resources are a factor, management information systems can effectively provide data for elected councillors to help their decision making about future funding.

- Keeping promises and agreements to users and their carers. Many users complain that promised telephone calls, letters and appointments are not kept. Organizations that take seriously the user first ethos adopt heavy sanctions against managers whose workers fail to have basic courtesy. How many users of social services feel they have been ignored or discounted because a worker has failed to return a telephone call or taken an age to reply to a letter?

- Executive and senior managers should spend time with users and carers. A director or senior manager who does not allow for direct face to face time with users soon becomes alienated and distanced from the very people they are there to serve. Regular time to meet users ensures they remain the focus of their attention and thinking. Some local authorities have adopted user forums, quality circles and quarterly feedback sessions which allow that interface necessary in a user first organization.

These performance indicators for user first organizations are not exhaustive. Indeed, Peters and Austin (1986) highlight others but I have only emphasized those which have a direct impact on care agencies. What is significant is that user first is not simply a set of principles but must translate into everyday practice. The actual experience of users having been consistently evaluated will inform the organization if those ideals are being met.

That transition, however, will not happen overnight and there are a number of pre-conditions necessary before users can experience a genuine user first organization. The final part of this chapter seeks to identify those prerequisites if the corruption of care is to be avoided and replaced by user focused departments or agencies. Empowerment through line management requires a significant change in the traditional structures and lines of accountability in most local authorities or large care organizations. The traditional culture of command and control management has to give way to staff teams working with delegated cash limited budgets and resources. Headquarter staff should have no role in decision making and should have no resources on which to draw, since all such decisions have been transferred to frontline operational staff. Examples in industry abound (National Power, Kimberly-Clark, Vauxhall Motors, Campaa Computers Manufacturing).

The key change is in accountability. The heavier the hierarchy the less accountability there is. Between directors or managing directors and users there should exist only three or four tiers but only two between user and a decision to release resources and prioritization. I have experienced over the years between six to eight levels of decision making before a resource was released to meet a client's needs.

What does such an organization look like? It is extremely flat (a matrix), virtually totally decentralized in terms of decision making and resources; everybody in the organization is responsible for not only their own performance but that of their peers (self-managed managers). Users and carers are an integral part of that decision making and there are systems of feedback, evaluation and monitoring (Heller, 1994b). It has been a surprise to many external bodies when they have discovered that Enfield Social Services operates within a matrix structure.

Accountability is made transparent to users and we constantly strive towards a goal whereby individual managers hold personal and corporate responsibility for frontline failure, poor performance or even discourtesy to users or their carers.

There is no room in a user first organization for 'it's somebody else's

responsibility' mentality. The implications are not only for the organization but each individual manager. Supervision, consultation and
appraisal mechanisms relate not only to the outcome but how that
outcome is achieved.

Professional care workers, support staff and managers at all levels are
required to regard the user and carer as experts on their own needs and
wants. The skill now required in an empowering user first organization
is to provide, within the context of local policies and priorities, services
that the user values and understands. Community care will only be
considered successful if, in a few years time, the type of service
provided and the style of its delivery have dramatically changed.
Empowered users and carers will challenge the expertise of professionals
and if they are to foster this and develop their skills professionals will
need to improve their managerial skills too.

It is fitting to conclude this contribution on 'user first' by reporting to
the words of a service user:

> We approached the Social Services and received a visit from a
> social worker, but we were told that because mother was not 60 she
> was basically a hospital case and they could not help us. The doctor
> seemed to pass the buck to Social Services and they passed the
> buck back to the doctor who passed it back to us . . . (Cleveland,
> 1984).

REFERENCES

Barclay, P.M. (1982) *Social Workers, their Roles and Tasks*. The report of a working
    party set up in October 1980, at the request of the Secretary of State for Social
    Services, by the National Institute for Social Work, under the chairmanship of
    Peter Barclay. National Institute for Social Work, Bedford Square Press,
    London.
Biestek, F.E. (1961) *The Casework Relationship*, Allen and Unwin, London.
Cleveland, R.P. (1984) in *Old Age Abuse: A New Perspective*, (ed. M. Eastman),
    Chapman & Hall, London.
Druker, P.F. (1985) *The Practice of Management*, Heinemann Professional
    Publishing, Oxford.
Goffman, E. (1961) *Asylums*, Anchor Books, New York.
Heller, R. (1994a) Customer focus means commitment to constant change.
    Management Today, January, pp. 19–22.
Heller, R. (1994b) The manager's dilemma. *Management Today*, January,
    pp. 42–44.
HMSO (1978) *Report of the Committee of Inquiry into Normansfield Hospital*, Cmnd.
    7397, London.
Hollis, F. (1972) *Casework: A Psychosocial Therapy*, 2nd edn, Random House,
    London.
Holman, B. (1993) *A New Deal for Social Welfare*, Lion Publishing, Oxford.
Jartstall, M. (1994) The Tom Peters affair. *Business Age*, (40) January.

Jordan, B. and Parton, N. (1983) *The Political Dimensions of Social Work*, Basil Blackwell, Oxford.

Jowell, T. (1991) Challenges and opportunities. Paper to five Ministerial 'Policy into Practice' Conferences held during January 1991. HMSO *Policy into Practice: Caring for People* 1991, No. 4. London.

Levy, A. and Kahan, B. (1991) *The Pindown Experience and the Protection of Children: The Report of the Staffordshire Child Care Inquiry 1990*, Staffordshire County Council.

Nye Bevan Lodge (1981) Report of London Borough of Southwark.

Peters, T. (1989) *Thriving on Chaos*, Pan Books, London.

Peters, T. (1992) *Liberation Management: Necessary Disorganisation for the Neosecond Nineties*, Macmillan, London.

Peters, T. and Austin, N. (1986) *A Passion for Excellence: The Leadership Difference*, Warner Books, New York.

Peters, T. and Waterman, R.H. Jr (1982) *In Search of Excellence: Lessons from America's Best Run Companies*, Warner Books, New York.

Raynor, P. (1985) *Social Work, Justice and Control*, Basil Blackwell, Oxford.

Ryan, K.D. and Oestreich, D.K. (1991) *Driving Fear out of the Workplace: How to Overcome the Invisible Barriers to Quality, Productivity and Innovation*, Jossey-Bass Publishers, San Francisco and Oxford.

Seebohm Report (1968) *Report of the Committee on Local Authority and Allied Personal Social Services*, HMSO (1968).

Solomon, A. (1993) Buyer beware. *Business Age*, (38) November.

Wardhaugh, H. and Wilding, P. (1993) Towards an explanation of the corruption of care. *Journal of Critical Social Policy*, **13** (1), pp. 4–31.

Wooller, J. (1994) The Tom Peters affair. *Business Age*, January.

Younghusband, E. (1978) *Social Work in Britain: 1950–1975*, George Allen and Unwin, London.

16

From 'elder protection' to 'adult empowerment': critical reflections on a UK campaign

Phil Slater

> This is not the time for such help, nor is it the time for those defenders.
>
> (Virgil, *Aeneid*)

INTRODUCTION

In 1990s Britain, welfare services to adults are being developed under the auspices of 'community care', a policy which finds its clearest expression in the White Paper, *Caring for People: Community Care in the Next Decade and Beyond* (DoH, 1989). Statutory enactment of the policy was effected via the National Health Service and Community Care Act 1990, and overall *Policy Guidance* was issued the same year (DoH, 1990).

A year later, the various strands of the *Policy Guidance* were elaborated in a series of individual documents, including complementary guides on care management and assessment for managers and practitioners respectively. The 'Summary of practice guidance' common to both these publications makes the bold claim that behind the new service delivery strategy lies an unequivocal policy of 'empowerment':

> The rationale for this reorganisation is the empowerment of users and carers. Instead of users and carers being subordinate to the wishes of service-providers, the roles will be progressively adjusted. In this way, users and carers will be enabled to exercise the same power as consumers of other services. (DoH, 1991a p. 11; DoH, 1991b p. 90)

Hence, in the estimation of the Department of Health, it is legitimate to speak of a fundamental 'redressing of the balance of power'.

This claim has not, of course, gone unchallenged. One well-known academic-*cum*-activist cites the government's record on the Disabled Persons Act 1986, antidiscriminatory legislation generally, and the vexed question of direct payment of monies to disabled people and their organizations, as evidence that while the government 'may want a market in social welfare, it does not want a market where users (as they are now euphemistically being called) have any power' (Oliver, 1991 p. 15). In the estimation of somewhat more differentiating critics, by contrast, the 'heterogeneous meanings' of 'community care' have meant that it can actually be exploited 'as a vehicle for user empowerment and the demystification of professionalism' (Levick, 1992 p. 79).

But one progressive feature of the policy seems to have passed completely unnoticed: namely, the significantly (though by no means comprehensively) destigmatizing, and thereby potentially empowering effect of the assessment dimension's 'generic' force. While community care services themselves continue to be provided under the auspices of fragmented legislation based on a variety of stigmatizing client group labels ('elderly', 'mentally disordered', etc.), assessment should transcend this constraining horizon and be genuinely 'needs-led'. Thus, for example, two parallel assessments of an elderly disabled person on the one hand and a non-elderly adult with learning difficulties on the other would differ solely by explicit reference to their differing individual needs, rather than by reference to distinct stereotypes of 'old age' and 'mental handicap' respectively. This implies a common title of 'adult', which, as will be demonstrated in due course, has a particular affinity for the concept of 'empowerment'.

Meanwhile, however, the implementation of this 'generic' community care policy in 1990s Britain has been closely shadowed by a parallel, and in many ways inverse phenomenon: namely, the campaign to promote public awareness, political recognition and professional action in respect of a phenomenon by the title of 'elder abuse'. As the present chapter will demonstrate, this campaign is characterized by an unwitting, but unremitting **disempowerment** of the objects of its concern. First, older adults are segregated from other adults as a social group *sui generis*. Second, despite the apparently deferential label of 'elders', they are portrayed as an intrinsically vulnerable group. Third, they are subjected to the paternalistic concern of professionals and civil servants; and fourth, they are threatened with legislative incursions into their adult liberties.

By way of contrast, a 'generic' focus on adults and adulthood will be seen not only to avoid the worst pitfalls of paternalistic 'protection', but also to offer a strategic opening for the empowerment philosophy propounded by the growing users' movement.

THE 'ELDER ABUSE' CAMPAIGN

Known in the 1980s as 'old age abuse', as per the title of the sole UK book on the subject at that time (Eastman, 1984), the revamped phenomenon of 'elder abuse' has witnessed a major renaissance in the 1990s. Articles and monographs mushroomed to the point where it became meaningful for one author to produce an overview (Penhale, 1992). The same year saw the production of a training manual (Biggs and Phillipson, 1992), and a 'handbook for professionals' (Pritchard, 1992), rapidly followed by two new books (Bennett and Kingston, 1993; Decalmer and Glendenning, 1993), a second edition of *Old Age Abuse* (Eastman, 1994), and the published proceedings of a relevant conference (McCreadie, 1993).

The year 1993 witnessed the launch of a pressure group under the title of 'Action on Elder Abuse', issuing a bi-monthly *Bulletin*, and launching a series of Working Papers with the publication of the proceedings of an international conference (Action on Elder Abuse, 1994). This development was shadowed by a related, but independent campaign in the trade press (*Community Care*, 1993). The latter opened with a deliberately alarming scenario: 'hundreds of thousands of elderly people are being abused in their own homes – physically and emotionally neglected; sexually abused; and financially abused' (*Community Care* 6 May 1993 p. 17). And the penultimate week's contribution claimed with great satisfaction that 'since our campaign started, elder abuse has shot to the top of the agenda' (*Community Care* 22 July 1993 p. 22).

While something of an exaggeration, this claim is not wholly without foundation. Earlier in the decade, Age Concern Institute of Gerontology had published the results of an exploratory study commissioned by the Department of Health (McCreadie, 1991). This in turn was followed by a Social Services Inspectorate London Region Survey (DoH, 1992), and draft Department of Health Practice Guidelines, the final version of which was finally published (DoH, 1993), circulated to local authorities, and thereby propelled into the headlines in the midst of *Community Care's* campaign.

It would be churlish to impugn the genuine humanitarian motivation behind these initiatives. Indeed, the reader could scarcely fail to be moved by the eloquence of the closing words of two major books on the subject: one ends with the hope that this research 'will contribute to a radical change in the perception of old age, a change that will allow later life to be enjoyed free from all forms of abuse' (Bennett and Kingston, 1993 p. 155), while the other concludes with the related hope that 'we may, as a result of what we learn, find ways in which we may increase the quality of life of all older people' (Glendenning and Decalmer, 1993 p. 168).

But while the personal and professional integrity of the campaigners is not in question, the strategic vision of contributing to an enhanced perception and quality of later life by focusing on elder abuse needs to be subjected to critical scrutiny. One might well recall the forceful contribution of an American commentator in the previous decade, who, while not disputing that some older people do experience abuse, nonetheless challenged the developing orthodoxy by posing a funda-mental question: 'to what extent will the well-being of older persons be protected and enhanced by conceptualizing the above-described behaviour as elder abuse for which special programming is required?' (Callahan, 1988 p. 453.)

The position of Callahan himself, working at the time in a Massachusetts-based Policy Centre on Ageing, was that such program-ming should be resisted, and that action on elder abuse should be integrated within the work of specialist social services teams dedicated to working with elderly people generally. But critical examination of the elder abuse phenomenon demands that the questioning goes even deeper. Ultimately, one has to ask: to what extent will the well-being of older people be enhanced by a specialist reference to age at all?

The question can be reframed in several ways. At a time when community care assessment and care management processes are beginning to integrate older people into a generic framework appropriate to adults in general, what arguments can be adduced for re-focusing on older people as a distinct subgroup in their own right? More importantly, what is the actual effect of this renewed age focus on the perception of the needs of older adults? What alternative terminology might be employed, and with what consequences? And last but certainly not least, how does this entire discussion interact with the concept of empowerment, which, as noted earlier, enjoys something of a contro-versial existence on the margins of social policy?

THE 'ELDER' FOCUS

For many elder abuse campaigners and commentators, the question of the age focus simply does not arise: rather, elder abuse is a given phenomenon, and while detailed consideration is often devoted to the meaning and even legitimacy of the 'abuse' component, the 'elder' dimension does not appear to warrant further reflection.

To the extent that this position involves any explicit statement on the age focus at all, it is the following argument reported (but not subscribed to in that form) in an important article on research methodology: 'the fact that health and social care provision categorises the elderly as a distinct group means that prevention and intervention should take place within the existing framework of those who work with or represent elderly people' (Ogg and Munn-Giddings, 1993 p. 394). Such a position implicitly accepts the 'social construction of old age' (Phillipson, 1982) as given and unproblematical, rather than regarding it as a subject for enquiry and critical debate.

Among those who do offer a substantive argument for the specialist age focus, the least popular (but possibly most candid) view is the one that holds old age to be some sort of disability in its own right. One British author has noted that this particular view is actually enshrined in statutory law in the state of Florida (Glendenning, 1993 p. 29), while an American commentator claims to detect double-figure instances of states enacting laws implying 'a presumption of less than full competency purely on the basis of age' (Crystal, 1986 p. 338).

Writing in a wholly different context (unrelated to elder abuse as such), a particularly insightful critic has detected a similar current in British social policy as a whole:

> The use of the word 'age' in legislation has helped to create age discrimination. Age was put alongside grave chronic disease, infirmity or physical incapacity as a qualifier in the 1948 National Assistance Act, and to this day the word continues to be used in legislation as a blanket term to imply dependence. This practice encourages the belief that old age is a condition similar to disability. (Scrutton, 1990 p. 26)

At the very least, this sobering thought ought to give pause for critical reflection on the social, and in particular ideological 'construction' of old age.

Sadly, no such effect can be detected in the case of the Law Commission's work on mental incapacitation. Even their first report (Law Commission, 1991) postdated Scrutton, yet two years later their publications were still confirming the stigmatizing pattern he pinpointed so clearly. Broadening out their original brief to include 'vulnerability' generally, they currently offer the following provisional definition: 'a person is vulnerable if **by reason of old age**, infirmity or disability (including mental disorder within the meaning of the Mental Health Act 1983) he is unable to take care of himself or to protect himself from others' (Law Commission, 1993 p. 28 and p. 78 – emphasis added).

However, by and large the grounds for specifying age in the elder abuse campaign are not bound up with a direct identification of later life as a disability in its own right, but with an empirically verified higher prevalence of disabling conditions affecting some but by no means all older adults. This can be traced back to the very first book on the subject in Britain:

> Certainly the myth of increasing senility with ageing must be countered, but it should also be remembered that one in seven of those over 75 suffer to a greater or lesser extent from some mental disorder. Certainly the myth of loneliness must be countered but it should also be remembered that many elderly people feel isolated, whether they live at home or with their families . . . The fact is that many of the ten million people over the age of 60 are frail, are handicapped, are facing disabilities either alone or with the support of sons, daughters, nieces, neighbours or even spouses. (Eastman, 1984 p. 12f.)

Demographic developments since the mid 1980s would, if anything, reinforce this picture, which is reiterated, though somewhat more tentatively, in the second edition of this pioneering work (Eastman, 1994).

But the argument itself, while seemingly convincing, is by no means conclusive. Examined with dispassionate logic, the increased prevalence of disabling conditions in later life might just as easily suggest a non-age specific focus on the common conditions themselves (for example, diabetes), rather than on the chronological age of the majority of the people affected. This alternative line of thought will be examined in due course. For the moment, however, Eastman's quantitative considerations serve as a useful bridge to the elder abuse campaign's final and most forceful argument for the specialist age focus.

In this account, a perverse situation emerges where, on the one hand elderly people share disproportionately in a broad range of generic disabling conditions, and yet on the other hand they are less likely than their non-elderly counterparts to receive an equitable level or quality of service. For confirmation that this is so, one need look no further than the Department of Health, whose Practice Guidelines on elder abuse proceed from the premise that 'ageism is widespread in society and there is a tendency to give attention to the problems of young people when all are considered together' (DoH, 1993 p. 1). The context makes clear that 'young people' here refers to non-elderly adults, as opposed to children.

This argument too can be traced to the mid 1980s, in particular to the efforts of Age Concern:

> In theory a combination of good practice and adequate resources would ensure that vulnerable elderly people have their needs and those of their carers met. However, in the real world there is intense competition for very limited resources and some form of legislation is needed, designed to meet the needs of this vulnerable group of people and giving them and their carers access to

consideration and an assessment of their needs for support and care. (Age Concern, 1986 p. 130.)

While not subscribed to in this form by the Department of Health, Age Concern's elaboration of the equitability argument into a demand for age-specific legislation has remained fundamental to the subsequent elder abuse campaign.

The detailed legislative provisions proposed by the elder abuse campaign will be examined directly. For the moment, it is essential to recognize that the campaign's age-specific focus does not follow with the force of a strictly logical deduction from the equitability argument, any more than it did from the prevalence argument examined earlier. From the apparent fact of the inequitable level and quality of service extended to older adults, one can argue equally cogently for the assimilation of demographic (including age-based) data into quality assurance and control systems. Ethnic monitoring of the take-up of generic services provides something of a model in this regard. Extended and adapted to the question of differential age take-up, such an approach could focus attention on ensuring older adults' equitable access to services, without requiring that the services themselves should be demarcated along the lines of age as such.

THE CASE FOR 'PROTECTION'

It would appear that while the elder abuse campaign can adduce substantial arguments for its age-specific focus, none of these arguments is conclusive. Be that as it may, however, the campaigners themselves appear to be satisfied with their stated case, for the moment at least. This being so, it is necessary to move on to an examination of the consequences of that position in terms of stated objectives.

Legislative reform, as already noted, is at the heart of these objectives. The exploratory study commissioned by the Department of Health identifies the following starting point for the debate:

Situations are arising involving elderly people about which professionals are extremely unhappy, yet they are not sure how to deal with them. Some involve violence, some neglect, some the exploitation of an older person's assets. In this country professionals find existing legislation unsatisfactory. In the vast majority of areas there are no guidelines in the form of policies or procedures. (McCreadie, 1991 p. 57.)

As a summary of the existing debate, this is a fair statement, no doubt. In passing, however, the reader might well take issue with the idea that 'professional unhappiness', 'uncertainty' and 'dissatisfaction', which are doubtless relevant to the discussion, should actually form the starting point for considerations of major legislative reforms affecting the lives of millions of non-professionals.

The author of a *Handbook for Professionals* confesses that 'one of the most frustrating things in working with elderly abuse is the fact that there is little legislation to protect vulnerable elderly people', and cites in particular the absence of 'any sort of Place of Safety Order when there are suspicions that a person is being abused' (Pritchard, 1992 p. 50). Once again, the lineage of this theme is traceable to Age Concern's *The Law and Vulnerable Elderly People*. As indicated by the title, this pursued a relatively broad theme, but the legislative proposals made in this text were to form the backbone of the subsequent elder abuse campaign, including the most controversial proposal of an Emergency Intervention Order, equivalent to the Place of Safety Order whose absence is bemoaned by Pritchard.

As proposed, an Emergency Intervention Order, made by a justice 'upon the application of any party who would satisfy the court of having a proper interest in the welfare of the old person', could make the following directions: first, that specific help be brought to the old person where he/she resides, subject to the availability of such help; second, that the old person be 'removed to a place of safety'; and/or thirdly, that named individuals be restrained from assaulting, molesting or otherwise interfering with the old person, or be excluded from the old person's home (Age Concern, 1986 p. 136).

While there remains a certain equivocation in terms of the elderly person's right 'as an adult' to refuse any intervention (Age Concern, 1986 p. 137), a subsequent publication by the same organization nails its colours firmly to the mast in favour of paternalistic compulsion:

> It seems clear that, with certain safeguards, we need some legal machinery, similar to the provision of Place of Safety Orders for children, by which an old person could be received into residential care for their own protection, at least for a limited period of time, which would afford a breathing space for all concerned and enable a proper assessment to be made of the situation – including the wishes of the old person **once they were out of the violent or neglectful environment**. (Stevenson, 1989 p. 27 – emphasis added.)

This, according to the author, is totally distinct from 'unwarrantable intrusion'.

By calling for enhanced legal powers for professionals to 'intervene in abusive situations' (*Community Care*, 6 May 1993 p. 17), the current trade press campaign has demonstrated the abiding attraction of Age Concern's legalistic remedies. And when the Law Commission Paper on public law protection of mentally incapacitated and other vulnerable adults followed suit by advocating the enactment of what it terms an Emergency Protection Order (Law Commission, 1993 p. 47ff.), campaigners pressing for the introduction of statutory powers of intervention in elder abuse cases were cock-a-hoop: 'with the Law Commission blueprint on the table, the bandwagon of legislative change starts to look unstoppable' (*Community Care*, 1 July 1993 p. 16f.).

In reality, the elder abuse campaign's invocation of the Law Commission's initiative is somewhat misleading, to say the least. While the Commission's proposed Emergency Protection Order might well **apply** in some situations involving older adults, it is certainly not **characterized** by any exclusive age reference: on the contrary, elder abuse is actually recast in a broader category of 'adult vulnerability' in general. The inclusion of elderly vulnerable people with their non-elderly counterparts means that the former can share in an adult right to protection from statutory powers. Thus, the granting of an order in respect of a person who is vulnerable but not mentally incapacitated or mentally disordered should be dependent on reasonable grounds to believe that the victim would not object to the order being made.

This is restated as a general principle in the overall argument:

> The authorities may not know whether a person is incapacitated or only vulnerable until they have gained access to him and made some inquiries. Once the position has become clear, however, our present view is that a person who is capable of making his own decisions has the right to decline the authorities' help and protection, even if this means that he is left in an environment which is harmful to him. If he is capable of making the choice, that is a choice he must be allowed to make. It follows that longer term decision-making powers will not be justified. (Law Commission, 1993 p. 7.)

From this, it would appear that freedom, independence and autonomy are valued more highly when older adults are not labelled according to their age, but given individual consideration with reference to the actual circumstances in which they find themselves, circumstances whch they may well share with other, non-elderly adults.

THE 'ADULT' ALTERNATIVE

This state of affairs confirms Scrutton's suggestion of 'a single measure, brilliant in its simplicity, which would guard against old-age discrimination more effectively than any other':

This would be to outlaw general references to age in all current and
future legislation where it is used to imply frailty or the need for
services . . . To ban the use of the word in legislation would
encourage awareness that age is not an illness or a disability. It
would encourage the idea that to be old and disabled is not so
different from being young and disabled; that dementia is a mental
illness, not an inevitable feature of old age. It would stress that it is
the circumstances and condition of individuals, not their age, that
is significant. (Scrutton, 1990 p. 26f. – original emphasis.)

The corollary of this proposition is tentatively stated in a more recent
publication, which points out that while the current paucity of law
specifically aimed at elders is generally interpreted as a sign of 'ageist
neglect', it might just as reasonably be attributed to 'a non-ageist
attitude that what is needed is general law that applies to all people'
(Open Learning Foundation, 1993 p. 23).

The Law Commission's work on vulnerable adults has already been
cited as an example of this strategy in operation. The other major
example is the unjustly neglected work of the Association of Directors of
Social Services on 'adults at risk', prompted by the much-publicized fate
of Beverley Lewis, a multiply disabled young woman who died in
conditions of almost total neglect. This case preceded the mushrooming
of interest in elder abuse, and the ADSS's initiative proceeded on largely
pragmatic, *ad hoc* lines, rather than exerting great academic efforts in
defence of its generic adults focus.

Even so, the resulting circulation of *Guidance for Directors of Social
Services* revealed a keen awareness of the need to maintain appropriate
boundaries between paternalistic protection and adult autonomy.
Indeed, the document actually identifies one of the risks to which
adults are exposed as 'excessive and unwarranted restriction of freedom'
(ADSS, 1991 para. 2.1). In the subsequent section on the 'policy and
practice context', this gives rise to a salutary note of caution against
paternalistic zeal:

While the management of situations in which risk occurs is an
inherent part of the work of social services departments, it must be
remembered that departments are not charged with responsibility
for universal protection . . . Given that a significant part of the
responsibility of social services departments is to enable people to
maintain their independence and capacity for self-direction, there
is a very fine line to be drawn between intervention which is
inadequate and intervention which is excessive and intrusive.
(ADSS, 1991 para. 3.2)

This commitment to individual autonomy does not, however, warrant a devil-may-care response when professionals are confronted with clients refusing to accept help. On the contrary, a crucial part of the professional task is 'actively to encourage users to express views and to consider the implications of their actions or choices' (ADSS, 1991 para. 4.4). The overall duty of care demands that 'where an adult at risk refuses to accept or to follow advice for his or her own safety or welfare the utmost care must be taken to ascertain, as far as possible, his or her reasons for refusing' (ADSS, 1991 para. 7.1.10). This might well involve a family/networking strategy: where, for example, the risk is located in a care relationship, 'the attempt should be made to enable both user and carer (assuming they are capable of doing so) to face and explore the difficulties and any possible means of overcoming them' (ADSS, 1991 para. 7.2.3).

In the overwhelming majority of cases, the individuals about whom the professionals are concerned retain an absolute right to refuse such help; they are after all adults! Only a tiny minority of cases will permit and/or demand the exercise of compulsory powers (Slater, 1994); in such instances, 'the greatest possible effort must be made to ensure that the client understands what is proposed, and the authority's reasons for invoking compulsory powers' (ADSS, 1991 para. 7.1.11). More importantly, and in direct contrast to the elder abuse campaign, this guidance contents itself with operating within the existing law and makes no proposals for an extension of statutory powers.

In what might variously be interpreted as an act either of liberal-minded magnanimity or of muddle-headed illogicality, the editors of *Community Care* opened the pages of their elder abuse campaign to proponents of the ADSS-style 'adults' focus, which was thereby deservedly brought back to the public's attention. Even a co-ordinator of elderly services questioned the wisdom of the specialist age reference:

> In Birmingham we have moved away from 'elder abuse' to 'adult protection', and this is for two main reasons. We feel that elder abuse is much too emotive, and why pick out elders when you can apply the same protective principles, for example, to a woman in her twenties with learning difficulties. (*Community Care*, 1993, **22**, July, p. 22.)

Another contribution reported that 'the ADSS supports a review of the law but opposes piecemeal reform on elder abuse only', while one particular director, who at the time doubled up as chairman of the ADSS's Elderly Persons' Committee, specifically repudiated the nascent 'elder abuse industry' (*Community Care*, 10 June 1993 p. 18f.).

By and large, however, the generic 'adults at risk' initiative remains sorely underdeveloped, not only in terms of the sheer quantity of publications propounding its particular position, but equally with regards to the explicit theoretical sophistication thereof. Not that substantive arguments in favour of a generic adults focus are not available: on the contrary, chapters and articles have been published on both sides of the Atlantic over several years (Crystal, 1986; Slater, 1993; Ashton, 1994). Nonetheless, the ADSS's own efforts on this front have remained remarkably modest, which might in part explain the relative neglect experienced by its valuable 'adults at risk' initiative.

THE 'ELDER' FOCUS REASSERTED

The elder abuse campaign, by contrast, is characterized not only by a greater volume of published output, but also by a greater readiness to pursue the theoretical ramifications of its position. At its best, this includes a commendable attempt to give some consideration to the possible and actual counter-arguments of the 'adults' lobby, which at the very least helps to broaden the terms of reference of the debate as a whole.

Bennett and Kingston, for example, cite a particularly powerful expression of the 'adults' lobby (Crystal, 1986), and inform the reader of the latter's contention that 'elder abuse and neglect should not be defined as a distinct form of abuse and may be classified under the more generic term "adult abuse", which encompasses all adults 18 years and above'. Disappointingly, however, the authors do not actually engage with the argument as such, and rapidly reassert their own favoured 'philosophical position' of a model 'unique to elder abuse and neglect' (Bennett and Kingston, 1993 p. 47). Thereby, the authors dogmatically endorse, rather than convincingly argue the best-known counter-argument to Crystal, according to which 'older persons are especially vulnerable to certain kinds of maltreatment at the hands of family members, . . . this maltreatment can be defined and measured, and . . . the success of various interventions can be evaluated' (Wolf and Pillemer, 1989 p. 15).

Another book published the same year as Bennett and Kingston (Decalmer and Glendenning, 1993) appears somewhat more open. In an introductory chapter entitled 'What is elder abuse and neglect?', one of the editors presents the issue of whether or not 'elder abuse has characteristics which distinguish it from the abuse of other adults' as an 'unresolved question' (Glendenning, 1993 p. 11). But once again, Wolf and Pillemer's argument for specific elder abuse programmes emerges victorious (Glendenning 1993, p. 33f.). Furthermore, the preference for age-specific terminology is in many ways a foregone conclusion given the title not only of the particular chapter in question, but of the whole book, namely, *The Mistreatment of Elderly People*.

The concluding chapter of that book even goes on the offensive: 'having guidelines for "adults" makes the assumption that elderly people are no more at risk than members of the general population and could well lead to a failure of local authorities to address the special needs of elderly people who are at risk' (Glendenning and Decalmer, 1993 p. 162). But this position is wholly confused. First, as a matter of empirical fact, the 'adults' model makes no such assumption, nor indeed any assumption, about comparative incidence across age boundaries. Second, in terms of pure logic, this means that the sentence is itself guilty of an assumption amounting to a simple *non sequitur*. Third, on the methodological front, the authors fail to substantiate their own premise that elderly people at risk have 'special needs' by demonstrating what those 'special needs' actually are.

Precisely the same state of affairs is apparent in the Department of Health's Practice Guidelines, which explicitly take the view that 'abuse to older people should be considered separately from other forms of abuse', so as to 'take account of the **particular issues** relating to the abuse of older people' (DoH, 1993 p. 1 – emphasis added). Nowhere is the reader enlightened as to the nature of the supposed 'particular issues' demarcating elders from younger adults; instead, the reader is treated to a reminder of the differences between elders and children (DoH, 1993 p. 10 and p. 29f.). The latter differences constitute an important consideration in their own right, of course; but they are strictly irrelevant to the question of the age-specific differentiation among adults.

Finally, a loyal inspector at the Department of Health bravely seizes the occasion of an address to an elder abuse conference (McCreadie, 1993) to offer at least one example of the 'particular issues that arise in elder abuse', namely, 'the changing burden for the carer having a parent, on whom they used to depend, now so heavily dependent on them' (Shawcross, 1993 p. 27). Unfortunately for the inspector, the assumption that the perpetrator is the victim's adult child had already been qualified by empirical research findings, even as reported in the Department of Health's own publication of the previous year. This cited the phenomenon of marital violence in old age, such that the elder abuse in question could equally be labelled 'marital abuse' or 'domestic violence' (DoH, 1992 p. 6).

Interestingly, another speaker at the same conference shared the results of her research into local authority guidelines and procedures, reporting 'an equal division between those departments focusing on elder abuse and those concentrating on the abuse of vulnerable adults (which obviously also incorporates issues of elder abuse)'. This division appears to have resulted from *ad hoc* promptings, rather than funda- mental considerations of a conscious nature: in other words, 'no clear pattern of preference in this respect emerged' (Penhale, 1993a p. 14). It would appear therefore that little has changed since 1991, when Age Concern's exploratory study argued that it would be 'futile' to continue a lengthy debate on the definition of elder abuse: 'a decision is first needed on whether to refer to *adult* abuse of which elder abuse is a part' (McCreadie, 1991 p. 58 – original emphasis).

If the decision on terminology were left to the activists and commentators within the elder abuse field itself, the result would be a foregone conclusion, of course. As the 'exploratory study' itself notes in passing, when the participants at a US research conference agreed the appropriateness of a specialist age focus, they did so 'not unnaturally', given that they were all employed 'in the field of elder abuse' to begin with (McCreadie, 1991 p. 9). Similarly, but more forcefully, a review of Bennett and Kingston's important book asks how the latter's reliance on the politically neutral model of 'social problem construction' (Blumer, 1971) can be reconciled with 'professional power struggles and our roles in perhaps manufacturing an "elder abuse enterprise" '. Crucially, this model 'neglects the voices of older people themselves and reminds us that their voices still have to contribute to the "legitimacy" of concepts such as abuse and neglect' (Manthorpe, 1993 p. 4).

THE PERTINENCE OF 'EMPOWERMENT'

This invocation of the 'users' voice' provides a convenient cue for a resumed consideration of the concept of empowerment, which was earlier shown to enjoy a rather precarious existence on the margins of current social policy.

By and large, the concept is absent from elder abuse literature, even in contexts where it would seem to be most relevant (Penhale, 1993b). Very occasionally, the word empowerment pops up (Phillipson, 1992 p. 3; Bennett and Kingston, 1993 p. 47), but this is usually in the form of a profession of faith, rather than a substantive dimension of the argument as a whole. Certainly, the elder abuse campaign does not attempt any detailed exposition of the concept, and stakes no coherent claim to an empowerment strategy as such.

Given this situation, it is necessary to fall back on general discussions originating in totally different contexts. One early contributor, wryly observing that empowerment was becoming the buzz word of the late 1980s, defines it as 'the process by which individuals, groups and/or communities become able to take control of their circumstances and achieve their own goals, thereby being able to work towards maximising the quality of their lives' (Adams, 1990 p. 42f.). The authors of a subsequent book on care management define it as 'the process by which clients (users, consumers) begin to take, or are helped to take, greater responsibility for their own lives and services' (Orme and Glastonbury, 1993 p. 189).

In the estimation of a further commentator, an empowering model of professional practice pursues two related objectives: first, 'to overcome responses among clients that arise from negative valuations so that they see themselves as able to have some impact on their problem', and second, 'to locate and remove blocks and find and reinforce supports to effective problem-solving'. This involves, among other things, helping clients to see professionals as 'having knowledge and skills that clients can use' (Payne, 1991 p. 230). It implies a three-fold role definition for the professionals concerned: first, as 'resources consultant', linking clients to resources in ways which improve their self-esteem and problem-solving abilities; second, as 'sensitizer', assisting clients to gain self-knowledge; and third, as 'teacher/trainer', imparting skills which enable the client to complete specific tasks (Payne, 1991 p. 232).

Viewed from the vantage point of professional bodies, this is a fair statement of the parameters within which an empowerment strategy might be conceived. Viewed in general socio-political terms, however, it is open to challenge on the grounds that it presupposes the constitution of relevant 'knowledge and skills' prior to 'client' involvment. As such, the very notion of client power is curtailed *a priori*. Worse still, by accepting professional knowledge and skills as socially neutral, the underlying power dimension is actually concealed. A justly famous book on power in the caring professions sums up more than a decade's work on this front by displacing the scenario of an 'open association between the expert and the needy' in favour of a critical perspective which argues that 'professionals seek to control the patient/client, not only in the form of power exercised over individuals, but also to the extent of the capacity to define who and what a client/patient is and should be' (Hugman, 1991 p. 113).

In line with this radical critique of professional power relations, the user movement's understanding of empowerment as 'self-empowerment' involves, in the words of two prominent activists, a 'journey from our own personal needs to influencing and changing attitudes, values, policy and practices that affect them'. This entails concerted action on three complementary fronts: first, 'developing our own accounts', which means users defining the appropriate terms for expressing their needs in an empowering way; second, 'forming our own judgements', which means users devising their own strategy for empowering action; and third, 'negotiating with others', which means user organizations relating to professional and other bodies with the status of primary actors as opposed to passive recipients (Beresford and Croft, 1993 p. 131ff.).

As reported earlier, some activists have formed the judgement that negotiating with others can be productively pursued under the auspices of community care, whose stated commitment to user involvement can be exploited for the promotion of genuine user power. Judging by the words of the initial Department of Health report on elder abuse, the latter debate would appear to offer similar openings:

> The NHS and Community Care Act 1990 has a strong commitment to the notion of choice and independence for users of social services. A core philosophy is that the user has a role to play in determining what services are provided. In the context of elder abuse, this viewpoint means that both the abused person and the abuser have a key part in determining guidelines for intervention and what resources should be available to deal with abuse. (DoH, 1992 p. 19f.)

This is developed and extended in the subsequent Practice Guidelines, which emphasize that overall policy should be shaped in collaboration with relevant voluntary organizations, 'some of which will include older people themselves' (DoH, 1992 p. 9).

Taking this a step further, a 'senior father' on the elder abuse circuit used the occasion of summing up and concluding a major conference to relocate the elder abuse phenomenon within an overall community care framework that has user power at its heart: by creating a situation where the entire 'agenda for services' was set by those at whom such services were aimed, it would be possible to achieve 'outcomes determined by users, not professionals' (Eastman 1993 p. 32).

This would not immediately address the deeper problems identified in the radical critique of 'care', 'caring' and 'carers' as general concepts of **disempowerment** (Morris, 1993 p. 149ff.); but it would at least ensure a level playing field, where older adults could realize 'user involvement' in community services on an equal footing with their younger counterparts. By contrast, the social construction of elders as a separate category reinforces the ideology of old age as a peculiar vulnerability *per se*: 'this approach, far from empowering the few, may disable the many' (Ashton, 1994 p. 2).

User involvement along generic, non-age specific lines could promote the empowerment both of older adults, as well as of adults generally (all of whom are ageing in the strictly chronological sense) by enabling them to determine their own preferences in terms of constitutive terminology. As part of this process, McCreadie's question of whether to refer to adult abuse in general as opposed to elder abuse in particular could then be decided by the very people directly affected, whether currently or potentially, by that decision and the policy and practice that flowed from it. This would confirm the user movement's view that 'developing our own accounts' actually constitutes 'the starting point for our empowerment' (Beresford and Croft, 1993 p. 131).

Interestingly, the radical empowerment opportunities offered by a critical engagement with the elder abuse industry have not been seized on by the activists and commentators of the user movement. This is disappointing, but not wholly surprising. The fact is that the user movement has been spearheaded by a predominantly non-elderly disability movement, whose social model of disability (Oliver, 1990) unwittingly reproduced social policy's segregation of older disabled people as a separate elderly group *sui generis*. As one commendably self-critical activist has conceded, the disadvantage of this preoccupation with youth was that 'when disability started to be defined as a civil rights issue during the 1980s, older disabled people were excluded' (Morris, 1993 p. 9). And yet, so the argument continues, one can scarcely deny that 'the human and civil rights that younger, fitter, more articulate disabled people are claiming for themselves should also be accorded to those who are older and/or less articulate' (Morris, 1993 p. 151).

To date, attempts to dismantle the artificial distinction between 'young' and 'old' disabled adults have tended to focus on 'people who are ageing with a disability' (Zarb, 1991), as opposed to including people who become disabled in old age as equal constituents of the disability movement. Regrettably, this continuing neglect unconsciously reinforces the stereotype of disablement in later life as pertaining to old age as such, and gives virtually free rein to the professional construction of an elder abuse industry where empowerment is supplanted by paternalism.

CONCLUSION

In conclusion, it would appear that the status of disabled elders could be significantly enhanced by their formal acknowledgement as *bona fide* adults within the user movement. But the benefits would by no means be exclusively one way. By extending the social model of disability to challenge the social construction of old age, the user movement would be advancing its own cause at the sharp end of the professional construction of individual vulnerability. Similarly, a critique of the paternalistic legal reforms advocated by the developing elder abuse industry could be marshalled to bolster the user movement's own campaign for anti-discrimination legislation (Bynoe *et al.*, 1991), and *vice versa*.

At the end of the day, an empowerment strategy for elders, and an empowerment strategy for adults, could be articulated as one and the same thing, to the mutual and enhanced benefit of all concerned.

REFERENCES

Action on Elder Abuse (1994) *A Report On The Proceedings Of The First International Symposium On Elder Abuse*, Working Papers No. 1. Action on Elder Abuse, London.

Adams, R. (1990) *Self-Help, Social Work and Empowerment*, Macmillan, Basingstoke.

Age Concern (1986) *The Law And Vulnerable Elderly People*, Age Concern, Mitcham.

Ashton, G. (1994) Action on elder abuse: has it got its focus right? *Action On Elder Abuse Bulletin*, **6**.

Association of Directors of Social Services (1991) *Adults At Risk: Guidance For Directors Of Social Services*, ADSS, Stockport.

Bennett, G. and Kingston, P. (1993) *Elder Abuse: Concepts, Theories And Interventions*, Chapman & Hall, London.

Beresford, P. and Croft, S. (1993) *Citizen Involvement: A Practical Guide For Change*, Macmillan, Basingstoke.

Biggs, S. and Phillipson, C. (1992) *Understanding Elder Abuse: A Training Manual For Helping Professionals*, Longman, Harlow.

Blumer, H. (1971) Social problems as collective behavior. *Social Problems*, **18**(3).

Bynoe, I., Oliver, M. and Barnes, C. (1991) *Equal Rights For Disabled People: The Case For A New Law*, Institute for Public Policy Research, London.

Callahan, J. (1988) Elder abuse: some questions for policy makers. *The Gerontologists*, **28** (4).

Crystal, S. (1986) Social policy and elder abuse, in *Elder Abuse: Conflict In The Family*, (eds K. Pillemer and R. Wolf), Auburn House, Dover.

Community Care (1993) Campaign: elder abuse. 6 May to 29 July.

Decalmer, P. and Glendenning, F. (eds) (1993) *The Mistreatment Of Elderly People*, Sage, London.

Department of Health (1989) *Caring For People: Community Care In The Next Decade And Beyond*, HMSO, London.

Department of Health (1990) *Community Care in the Next Decade and Beyond: Policy Guidance*, HMSO, London.

Department of Health (1991a) *Care Management And Assessment: Managers' Guide*, HMSO, London.

Department of Health (1991b) *Care Management And Assessment: Practitioners' Guide*, HMSO, London.

Department of Health (1992) *Confronting Elder Abuse: An SSI London Region Survey*, HMSO, London.

Department of Health (1993) *No Longer Afraid: The Safeguard Of Older People In Domestic Settings*, Practice Guidelines, HMSO, London.

Eastman, M. (1984) *Old Age Abuse*, Age Concern, Mitcham.

Eastman, M. (1993) Summing up and conclusions, in *Elder Abuse: New Findings And Policy Guidelines*, (ed. C. McCreadie), Age Concern Institute of Gerontology, London.

Eastman, M. (ed.) (1994) *Old Age Abuse: A New Perspective*, 2nd edn, Chapman & Hall, London.

Glendenning, F. (1993) What is elder abuse and neglect, in *The Mistreatment Of Elderly People*, (eds P. Decalmer and F. Glendenning), Sage, London.

Glendenning, F. and Decalmer, P. (1993) Looking to the future, in *The Mistreatment Of Elderly People*, (eds P. Decalmer and F. Glendenning), Sage, London.

Hugman, R. (1991) *Power In Caring Professions*, Macmillan, Basingstoke.

Law Commission (1991) *Mentally Incapacitated Adults And Decision-Making: An Overview*, HMSO, London.

Law Commission (1993) *Mentally Incapacitated And Other Vulnerable Adults: Public Law Protection*, HMSO, London.

Levick, P. (1992) The Janus face of community care legislation: an opportunity for radical possibilities? *Critical Social Policy*, **12** (1).

Manthorpe, J. (1993) Review of Bennett and Kingston (see above), *Action On Elder Abuse Bulletin*, **2**.

McCreadie, C. (1991) *Elder Abuse: An Exploratory Study*, Age Concern Institute of Gerontology, London.

McCreadie, C. (ed.) (1993) *Elder Abuse: New Findings And Policy Guidelines*, Age Concern Institute of Gerontology, London.

Morris, J. (1993) *Independent Lives? Community Care And Disabled People*, Macmillan, Basingstoke.

Ogg, J. and Munn-Giddings, C. (1993) Researching elder abuse. *Ageing And Society*, **13** (3).

Oliver, M. (1990) *The Politics Of Disablement*, Macmillan, Basingstoke.

Oliver, M. (1991) From disabling to supportive environments, in *Social Work, Disabled People And Disabling Environments*, (ed. M. Oliver), Jessica Kingsley, London.

Open Learning Foundation (1993) *Disabled People, Older People, Criminal Violence In The Home*, Unit Workbook, BASW, Birmingham.

Orme, J. and Glastonbury, B. (1993) *Care Management: Tasks And Workloads*, Macmillan, Basingstoke.

Payne, M. (1991) *Modern Social Work Theory: A Critical Introduction*, Macmillan, Basingstoke.

Penhale, B. (1992) Elder abuse: an overview. *Elders*, **1** (3).

Penhale, B. (1993a) Local authority guidelines and procedures, in *Elder Abuse: New Findings And Policy Guidelines*, (ed. C. McCreadie), Age Concern Institute of Gerontology, London.

Penhale, B. (1993b) The abuse of elderly people: considerations for practice. *British Journal Of Social Work*, **23** (2).

Phillipson, C. (1982) *Capitalism And The Construction Of Old Age*, Macmillan, London.

Phillipson, C. (1992) Confronting elder abuse: fact and fiction. *Generations Review*, **2** (3).

Pritchard, J. (1992) *The Abuse Of Elderly People: A Handbook For Professionals*, Jessica Kingsley, London.

Scrutton, S. (1990) Ageism: the foundation of age discrimination, in *Age: The Unrecognised Discrimination*, (ed. E. McEwen), Age Concern, London.

Shawcross, C. (1993) Elder abuse policy: developments in the Social Services

Inspectorate of the Department of Health, in *Elder Abuse: New Findings And Policy Guidelines*, (ed. C. McCreadie), Age Concern Institute of Gerontology, London.

Slater, P. (1993) Elder abuse and legal reform, *Elders*, **2** (3).

Slater, P. (1994) Social work and old age abuse: laying down the law, in *Old Age Abuse: A New Perspective*, 2nd edn, (ed. M. Eastman), Chapman & Hall, London.

Stevenson, O. (1989) *Age And Vulnerability: A Guide To Better Care*, Edward Arnold, London.

Wolf, R. and Pillemer, K. (1989) *Helping Elderly Victims: The Reality Of Elder Abuse*, Columbia University, New York.

Zarb, G. (1991) Creating a supportive environment: meeting the needs of people who are ageing with a disability, in *Social Work, Disabled People And Disabling Environments*, (ed. M. Oliver), Jessica Kingsley, London.

17

Professional fantasies, consumer realities: a carer's view of empowerment

Gillian Hughes

INTRODUCTION

Nine year old Julia is our middle child, with an older sister Laura (11) and a younger sister Alexandra (3). Julia had neurosurgery to remove a 'minor lesion' in her brain when she was 19 months old. Although she had developed well as a baby, she unexpectedly emerged from the operation with severe learning difficulties as well as autistic, disinhibited behaviour. She was therefore referred to many specialists in epilepsy, paediatric neurology and neurosurgery. A second neurosurgical operation when she was four years old successfully treated her epilepsy, but her developmental difficulties remain to this day.

The 'disinhibition' has caused us more problems as a family than any other aspect of Julia's difficulties, as she needs to be watched constantly to prevent her harming herself and others. If she notices a lapse in supervision she may attempt such things as running away, penetrating electric sockets, breaking glass, diving in front of traffic or plunging into open water, depending on the opportunity. She can also be aggressive to strangers and loved ones alike.

As Julia needs unblinking supervision to protect herself and those around her, our family has received home-based support as well as day care and respite care. These services have been provided by the local social services department for whom her father also works as a social work team leader. I worked before having children as a social worker for a child development team in London and have worked since as a group worker, area team social worker and lecturer.

In the last few years Julia has received the education she needs and our family has received the level of help we all need to get the best out of our lives.

Eighteen months ago she was placed by our LEA at a residential school for children with complex communication disorders where she has clearly benefited from daily speech therapy, one-to-one classroom support and a totally safe educational environment. Significantly, she has recently been able to make friends in her own peer group for the first time since toddlerhood. With the right level of supervision Julia feels safe enough to express herself in many ways. Although her speech is very disordered she can read, and enjoys newspapers and books, music and horseriding, a hug and a good laugh.

Julia is at home frequently, and we continue to use home-based support. All of our struggles (including Julia's) since the first operation eight years ago would take several volumes to describe. This chapter simply focuses on our ambiguous dealings with other social services department (SSD) employees, illustrating our different perspectives of 'empowerment'. Missing from the account which follows is the sense which Julia has made of the encounters described. The story from her point of view remains to be told, since the only story I can tell is my own.

'EMPOWERMENT' – WHOSE REVOLUTION?

As liberalizing concepts like empowerment are absorbed into professional academic discourse, the distance between the would-be transformers of human services and those whose lives they seek to transform is not necessarily reduced. Referring to public perceptions of psychiatry in 1975, Pearson observed:

> . . . if psychiatry can be said to have captured a hold on the liberal imagination, it does not drive away our common language which embodies quite different sentiments: 'nut doctor', 'funny farm', 'trick cyclist', 'loony bin', 'shrink'. The tenacity of this common-sense jargon alerts us to the danger and falsity of accepting a professional world view . . . as the only possible view of that profession's activities . . . Insiders to professional codes and practices see revolutions in thought and humanisation in practice where Everyman sees problems of morality, propriety, offensive conduct, bunches of keys, asylum walls, and danger. (Pearson, 1975.)

In considering the value of the concept of empowerment in relation to the lives of people with learning disabilities (PWLD) there are at least six different frames of reference which ought to be taken into account:

1. Public/popular perception both shaped and represented by the media and civic institutions such as the education system.
2. The perception and experience of individual members of society in their capacity as neighbours, friends, work and schoolmates, etc. of PWLDs.
3. Professional-academic discourse as represented in articles, books, policy statements, training courses, etc.
4. Perceptions and experience of individual professionals.
5. Perceptions and experience of individual carers.
6. Perceptions and experience of PWLD themselves.

Some of these frames of reference may be accessible to the same person insofar as he or she may be both professional, carer, neighbour, etc. Although PWLDs are not found among the ranks of professionals, a collective voice and experience of citizenship also provide more than one frame of reference. It will be clear that any writer is limited by their own frame of reference. As a professional, parent and consumer I have the advantages and blind spots of having additional and sometimes clashing perspectives in my encounters with other professionals. Dual/multiple perspectives can be a source of fragmented consciousness and inner conflict, or a source of insight and a liberating critical awareness. In the context of the struggle for civil rights for people with disabilities Jane Campbell, Chair of the British Council of Organizations of Disabled People (BCODP), recently discussed the development of her ideas about disability and discrimination:

> I saw disabled people were socially discriminated against in the same way as women. When I worked at the Greater London Council I also saw parallels with black and ethnic minority communities. I found BCODP going in the same direction [as myself] and that, for me, was like finding heaven. They saw my problem in a social context, rather than an impairment one – and that's very liberating. (Crompton, 1994.)

The aim of this chapter is two-fold; firstly to alert providers of human services to be sceptical about 'revolutions in thought and humanization in practice' specifically in relation to claims made for 'consumerism' and 'empowerment'. Secondly, as a parent, professional and human being I write with the aim of rescuing empowerment from the buzz-word collection of the career-minded and the waste paper basket of the cynical. Truly empowering structures, organizations and experiences must still be sought for, preserved and celebrated: cynicism is not a weapon in this struggle, but an excuse for avoiding it.

THE BURDEN OF SYMPATHY

After several changes of mind and heart we decided when Julia was five to have another baby. A midwife covering for my community midwife called: knowing nothing about us she had great difficulty relating to me possibly because I joyfully prattled away while Julia behaved so strangely in the background. Any Christmas carol had a calming effect on Julia's wild uncontrolled behaviour, whether she was shrieking, dancing on a table, climbing bookshelves or whatever. In particular, 'It came upon a midnight clear' brought magical tranquillity.

To relieve this situation, I searched our carols tape for her favourite track, when the midwife said suddenly 'how *do* you cope?' I replied that carols were actually not too bad in summer or autumn, wild behaviour being preferred only in January. As she was leaving, it was clear she had missed the point. 'My dear' she said, 'you have all my sympathy. I just don't know *how* you are going to cope with a baby.'

There is always someone worse off than yourself, isn't there? Imagine going through life with sense of humour difficulties! My dear, allow **me** to offer **you** the burden of my sympathy. I am sure that yours is the greater need.

PRACTICAL SUPPORT

The midwife's sense of humour difficulties notwithstanding, our need for practical support was undoubtedly increasing at this time. However, our history as consumers of care services had begun three years previously. Julia's 'hyperactive' behaviour since her operation at 19 months had led us via our health visitor and home teacher to a family support worker, Claire, who would babysit for us on a regular fortnightly basis so we could go out for a couple of hours. When Claire went to work for the 'Link' foster care scheme she introduced us to a family who she hoped would offer more respite care. Despite much experience, the Link carers lacked all the adaptations we had made to our house for Julia and could only cope for a few hours at a time.

When they eventually pulled out because they were expecting a baby, it was Claire again who introduced us to the newly created outreach scheme, working from a large local respite care centre. This proved to be the service which sustained us until Ali's birth, although it was always poorly resourced and was eventually reduced.

The centre is of the 1960s purpose-built type that is now quite unpopular with many social services departments because of their size, larger staff groups, institutional style kitchens, dormitories and so on. However, these were precisely the aspects which made it much safer than a domestic-scaled establishment with integral kitchen, no space for charging around and fewer staff to support and cover for each other. We were apologetically shown round by a staff member who assumed that we would perceive the horrors of institutionalization and segregation – in fact we saw space, variety, security and opportunity for Julia. As a consequence there was the prospect of a reduction in segregation at home for all of us.

Julia's first outreach worker, Elaine, cared for her for four hours fortnightly 'alongside' ourselves at home, also coming on outings and to hospital appointments. Sometimes she would take Julia out, significantly to numerous cafés. Julia's shrieks, mess, food throwing and general distress had put us off eating out, but Elaine persevered until Julia came to enjoy the experience. This extended the kind of family outings we could then tackle year round, thus widening all our horizons.

The break in care gave me time with my older daughter, then just five and needing to share with her friends the kinds of experiences which they took for granted: boat trips, circus, carefree picnics and library visits. I only really appreciated how restricted Laura's life was when the restrictions were lifted. I also found that working alongside an outreach worker at home was a pleasure, partly because we could do so much more with the help, and also because it reduced the sense of exclusive parental responsibility. No-one had all the answers, and the relationship which I had with Kate (the second worker) was one characterized by a real sense of partnership, mutual support and fun.

Kate and Elaine both admitted to 'burning out' with Julia, who was no less demanding of a paid worker than ourselves, but during the period until Ali was born, this service was a lifeline. It could not be described as 'empowering' in that we were always aware that the help could be withdrawn (we were its principal consumers), funds cut or the worker become ill. Its limited resources meant that staff sickness, family emergencies and school holidays could not be covered, but the help as far as it went was really excellent.

The other 'prop' which I valued highly when Julia was small was the home help service, now superseded by the Home Care Service. The amount of cleaning involved in caring for an incontinent, hyperactive child can scarcely be imagined, and this help gave not only a sense of sharing boring and disliked tasks, but was also a tremendous morale boost. Domestic cleaning is a service from which most social service departments are withdrawing, a state of affairs much regretted by disabled people and their carers as recent research shows (Morris, 1993).

Most patients of children with disabilities whom I know would choose to receive the services of a home help for a couple of hours in preference to the same amount of time with the majority of professionals. A useful tip for consumer surveys which aim to establish the usefulness of doctors, psychologists, social workers, etc. would be to ask of carers:

'Was the time you spent with X more useful or less useful than if an equivalent amount of time had been given by a home help to clean your home?'

If X's time is judged by consumer opinion to be more useful than a home help's time would have been, then he or she deserves a substantial performance related bonus.

If our experience was typical, then the centre's outreach workers would have achieved this bonus every year.

IN AND OUTSIDE A CARING SERVICE

My pregnancy with Ali in the summer of 1990 inevitably led us to consider how to approach the SSD for an increase in support with Julia's care. Managing Julia with only one adult around in any setting was becoming more unsafe at this time, owing to her talents as an opportunist with an eye for danger, mess and escape. If the carer needed to make a meal, answer the phone or go to the lavatory, Julia was likely to make full use of even the briefest lapse in supervision. Denying food and drink and social contact to oneself and Julia while keeping one's legs crossed was one way of keeping her safe. Getting more help at home was our preferred option, but no 'off the peg' solution existed.

Alan's position as an employee and consumer of the SSD had not presented any overt conflicts until this time. Colleagues tended to avoid mentioning Julia, although Alan was happy to talk as freely as anyone else about his home life if it became relevant to a discussion. On the whole it had seemed easier to keep home and work separate, but we were now in a position where this was no longer possible. Alan was very anxious to 'play by the rules', and therefore sounded out a specialist social worker about her willingness to assess Julia's care needs. This she was happy to do, and so with the agreement of her manager she made a home visit.

Unknown to us at the time, however, this arrangement did not suit everyone. Quite out of the blue we received a letter from a hospital team social worker saying that 'a decision had been taken' to allocate our case to herself. Altogether six colleagues who saw Alan daily (including three senior to himself) had been involved in a decision-making process about his family, yet none had felt able to approach Alan to discuss this or even let him know of the proposed change. Although Alan had been carefully 'playing by the rules' in approaching the learning disability social worker, the high handedness of overturning this arrangement left questions which were never answered. Even if Alan had been a 'difficult' person to approach, honesty and courtesy would still have demanded openness in dealing with him as both client and colleague.

The result of this episode was both a powerful sense of humiliation on Alan's part and a loss of confidence in manager-colleagues. On a professional level it begged questions about policies promoting consumerism in the SSD, versus the experience of consumers. If several managers had shown themselves unable to trust another professional (a colleague even!) to identify a way of dealing with the department as a consumer, what chance would less knowledgeable consumers have? The fact that this was not an isolated occurrence was shown earlier this year when a similar scenario began to unfold. Yet another manager began to make arrangements for Julia's care co-ordination without talking first to Alan. His plan (before Alan heard and objected) had been to ask around various social work teams to see if anyone would like to take us on!

At the time of the social worker re-allocation, Alan felt that it was best for him and for us to accept the situation as a *fait accompli* and get on with the urgent business of working on Julia's 'care package' with the new social worker. It was possible to believe at this point that the style of dealing with him as a colleague-consumer was simply the awkwardness of a few individuals in the department. The need for more positive action on our part was not apparent until after the next round in our education as consumers.

MULTIDISCIPLINARY KAFKA

Despite the way she had come into our lives, we were keen to establish a good working relationship with the new social worker, who was known to us both as a colleague. She was knowledgeable about resources and strongly encouraged us to use respite care. It was helpful to have such strong encouragement given our ambivalence about asserting our needs and requesting help as consumers from the SSD for whom Alan worked. This social worker also urged us to use a small residential respite care centre, which turned out to be helpful for unexpected reasons, as described later. Without her encouragement we would not have proceeded, on the grounds that this centre was not safe enough for Julia. Although this turned out to be the case the full extent of Julia's needs and ours would have remained invisible had we not applied.

Julia was still very young (five years) and so our discussions were about the challenge of finding services which would simultaneously ensure her safety, meet our needs for time off, and suit the needs of a younger child. Alan's health had been affected during the previous two years through never being 'off duty' and he was hospitalized with labyrinthitis during my pregnancy, so the need for more support was becoming obvious. Although the new social worker had many ideas about informal arrangements, it was clear to us that a reliable pattern of help was needed, with back-up and support for the staff involved. Julia's needs were such that she had been turned down by the best resourced service in our area, a much publicized children's Haven (hospice) and no further Link family had been found. Although we needed respite care to give us a day 'off duty' a week, we also wanted Julia to be at home for most of the time. However, we were unclear about how this could be achieved or what help to ask for. The only existing service which suited Julia and was safe enough for her was the large respite care centre, but children were not offered places there before the age of seven.

In the circumstances, the social worker suggested that we should put Julia's needs to the newly constituted resources panel, either through herself or by directly representing ourselves. As this seemed to be the only way forward in the circumstances, we agreed to come along to what we understood would be a supportive and informative dialogue with 'resource people'.

Describing our participation in this event is fraught with enduring conflicts. The city we live in is small, the professional world we both work in even smaller. Nevertheless I have chosen to try and describe this meeting because nothing in my experience better illustrates the disastrous consequences to a consumer of ill-thought attempts at 'empowerment'.

We arrived at the venue for the panel meeting in good time with Elaine, our outreach worker. We began to get a flavour of what was to come when the social worker came out and apologetically asked us all to wait while the panel had a preliminary discussion. As we were effectively representing ourselves, we couldn't understand our exclusion from part of the discussion. Elaine knew Julia well, and had worked alongside us at home, but her lower status in relation to a field social worker who had not even met Julia was incidentally illuminated, as she remained outside with ourselves.

We had known that the chair of the panel was a colleague of Alan's, but were not prepared for the fact that virtually everyone else in the room we (eventually) entered was also known to one or other of us as a colleague. In addition to social services staff were staff from agencies with whom Alan liaised as a social work manager, including a member of his own team who was present in her capacity as a representative of a voluntary organization. This situation was difficult enough, but the unfolding of the discussion as led by our social services colleagues was truly Kafkaesque. Firstly, we were offered the opportunity to have our say. Since we had not come with a specific request, this put us in the position of:

1. stressing the difficulty of caring for Julia,
2. pleading our case for more help.

The response to (1) was to pass over this and to (2) to discuss the 'budgetary constraints' of the team which managed outreach and the purpose-built respite care centre. The discussion led around to the only offer of the afternoon, (an idea of the chair's) namely of introducing us to a residential social worker from the centre whom we could then employ privately. Neither the financial costs of this proposal (at least five times the level of Attendance Allowance) nor the ethics were discussed, giving the impression of a casual, off the cuff suggestion. After all, Alan could have been sounded out before the meeting as our needs were known to both Elaine (and through her line manager to the chair) as well as to the field social worker.

We were left with a sense of having devalued our daughter and abased ourselves publicly, only to be met with blanket refusal to help on the grounds of 'budgetary constraints'. The 'introduction service' idea appeared to have the primary value of firmly deterring us from draining anyone's budget. The public arena in which this took place increased our feelings of shame and exposure, and undermined a wider set of Alan's working relationships; it also left us wondering what respect other panel members would feel inclined to offer us if colleagues of Alan's apparently held him in such contempt. This situation could have been avoided in any number of ways. When our requests subsequently became specific it was apparent that they were practical and affordable. This could have been established prior to (or instead of) the panel meeting. Once into the meeting the suggestion that we go away and come up with more specific requests would have spared our dignity and left a way open to negotiate in the event of 'unreasonable demands'.

With the passing of time, the feelings of humiliation and frustration have left us both. Partly this is due to the pragmatic need to get along with people, particularly in a small community. Furthermore, a particular advantage of having an 'insider' perspective is the conscious-ness that there are few mistakes we are not capable of making ourselves. However, we have heard offensive and even brutal opinions about Julia from some doctors and we have left feeling hurt and subsequently angry. We have been frustrated at times by inappropriate advice given by 'experts' who couldn't fathom her. None of these encounters have left us feeling as powerless as attending a meeting whose purpose was ostensibly to inform and **empower** us. The irony was compounded by the fact that it had been organized by theoretically like-minded colleagues. As the following section shows, as 'aggrieved consumers' our difficulties with the department were subsequently resolved, but as disillusioned 'insiders' we can only be satisfied when a better sense of reality enters the culture of social work.

TRANSFORMATIONS: 1

Alan and I recovered from the panel ordeal with a determination to fight for the services we needed, abandoning the pretence of 'partnership'. The Children Act and the National Health Service and Community Care Act created a sense of hope and the SSD was in the process of drafting a complaints procedure. Although Alan wanted to explore all possible avenues of communication first, he and I were in agreement that, if necessary, he would fight his employer as a consumer for the services we needed. We therefore dreamed up our own care package, a 'shopping list' as Alan called it. This was a list of services which would help us to give Julia a normal childhood within a family with a new baby, older sister and two normal mortal parents. The shopping list contained the minimum level of support needed to achieve this; we wanted Julia to be at home, and we preferred not to have paid helpers in and out of our home more than was necessary. Most people's 'shopping lists' would reflect these principles, I believe.

As mentioned previously, Julia's brief stay at the small respite care centre (used for younger children) turned out to be helpful. This was not because she was able to stay regularly (she only had one three-day stay), but because of the clarity of the report about her stay, written by staff who had cared for her. This described Julia's opportunistic escapes, and other incidents such as locking everyone out within hours of arriving, swinging repeatedly on bedroom curtains from a first floor window ledge, and disappearing inside a washing machine, with just one leg sticking out! For the first time, the service providers had a written account of a few days of caring for Julia from people other than ourselves. As Kate, her outreach worker, had made several tea-time visits with Julia beforehand, it was also clear that one-to-one (knowledge-able) supervision made all the difference to her behaviour. Armed with this report and our 'shopping list', Alan met Malcolm, a senior manager, and described the difficulties which his position as employee and client was creating. He was listened to carefully and it was agreed that a meeting would be chaired by Malcolm and attended by Alan's line manager (we lived in Alan's patch) as well as the manager who had chaired the panel. Interestingly, Malcolm told Alan that it had previously been his experience that social services employees often have a worse service as consumers than other people.

By the time the meeting was held, all the services which were asked for had in fact been agreed. These were: outreach or day care at the (purpose-built) centre every Saturday, to give us one work-free day off a week; up to two weeks a year day care at the same centre during school holidays; a further week residential care with extra staff if needed, enabling us to have a holiday, and crucially, after the baby was born, six weeks home care support. The plan was to find someone who would look after the baby with me, freeing me to attend to Julia and maintain her routine while she got used to the change. In addition, our new outreach worker, Kate, had offered to come and stay with Julia day or night, whenever I went into hospital to have the baby. We were finally able to relax and await the arrival of our third child with a sense of optimism.

A BRIEF ENCOUNTER WITH AN ALLY

Ali's arrival in the world could not have been better timed if I had had full control over it. Alan was able to come to hospital in time for the birth, with Kate at home meeting Julia and Laura. Ali's nature and sleeping habits might also have been specially ordered.

This may go some way to explain an attitude to our first family outing after Ali's birth. The unusual thing about this outing was that it was entirely spontaneous, which by 1991 – even pre-baby – was quite unlike us. Most outings were organized like military expeditions with every detail considered, all possible disasters provided for and plenty of bravado to see us through. On this occasion we took baby equipment but completely forgot Julia's normal paraphernalia, i.e. two or three changes of clothing, unbreakable cup, mopping up equipment, etc. We just **went**.

We had discovered that National Trust gardens were reasonably Julia-proofed, being large, traffic-free and reassuringly used by other people with disabilities because of wheelchair accessibility. The plan was to have a walk, followed by lunch in the National Trust café, thus reducing the number of parental tasks that day. As might have been anticipated with a two-week old I spent most of the 'walk' sitting down on the cold March grass, alternately breast feeding and nappy changing. Alan meanwhile attempted to keep Julia and Laura cheerful, while Ali, who had rarely cried before, did nothing else . . .

Our spontaneous outing-ordeal reached a climax when we attempted lunch. We had not thought ahead about the logistics of self-service, which left only one of us to look after Ali and Julia while the other got the food. Alan volunteered to wait, and though stressed by Ali's crying, Laura's irritation and Julia's agitation he had managed to stay on top. Rejoining the others with a full tray was a complicated business as I considered such questions as 'is there anywhere safe for this pot of tea?' and 'do I sit near Julia with Ali in my arms and risk Ali being attacked, or sit further away and risk Julia feeling neglected?' etc. etc. As the tray went down on the table, Julia suddenly saw her chance. Both my arms were in use, and Alan's were too as he managed Ali, chairs, cutlery, etc.

In one movement Julia had seized a bread roll and flung it forcefully into the face of a woman at a nearby table. Julia laughed merrily while Alan, Laura and I shrank with helpless embarrassment.

This is the stuff of everyday nightmares when you live with someone with disinhibited behaviour. This behaviour is not random or immature, but perverse; best described as a strong attraction towards forbidden or dangerous activity. If you choose to live fairly normally, or to 'integrate', to avoid becoming collectively housebound, the price you pay is a constant anxiety about risk taking. There is the risk also of endangering or upsetting unknown others; there is the embarrassment caused to other members of the family, and for the carer, the consequences of always 'living on the edge' because of the constant need to plan, monitor and stay permanently on the alert.

Unable even to look at the victim of Julia's bread roll bowling, I concentrated with Alan on getting through lunch while we all calmed down. As we left, I braced myself to go over, apologise and **explain**. **Explaining** is not the same as explaining if taken to mean 'making a situation clearer'. That kind of explanation would run something like 'I am so sorry about . . . my daughter is autistic and has disinhibited behaviour. Sometimes she is unable to inhibit an impulse to do dangerous or hurtful things'. A truthful explanation of this kind obviously demands too much time, attention and involvement from an injured party. Instead, I **explain**. An **explanation** is something like this: 'I am sorry about . . . my daughter doesn't understand'. This is actually untrue, she is clearly able to spot and make the most of opportunities to cause damage and pain, and strongly inclined to do so when stressed, needing others to protect and 'contain' her. Another **explanation** is 'I am sorry about . . . but my daughter has a mental handicap'. These hated words have the virtue of being plain enough, but they have the consequence of frequently bringing upon us all the burden of sympathy: 'Oh dear, the poor thing'.

Explaining involves a psychological distancing from the words in use, in order to smooth over difficult and distressing situations which arise in brief public encounters. Although it provides a retreat for all the parties involved in such situations, it is at the cost of honesty and real dignity for Julia, myself or, in reality, anyone. The alienating quality of **explaining** has other consequences. To **explain** Julia's behaviour invites the attitude that perfect behaviour in 'normal' children is to be expected, colluding with a very British attitude towards disruptive childish behaviour. Worse, using a 'disability' or 'mental handicap' **explanation** suggests that the association between disability, deviance, disturbance, etc. is a natural one: 'I **see** she is disabled/mentally handicapped, nothing different can be expected.'

Is there an alternative to **explaining** or explaining (or sinking into a deep hole and taking Julia) when she has thrown a bread roll with full force into someone's face? I found one person's answer.

Carrying Ali I went over and started the usual 'I am so sorry . . .' but never managed to get even thus far. Julia's victim was ready with a smile and anticipating my words, repeatedly cut me off. 'I am so glad you came over, we were just saying, how lovely to see a family out together.' (Truly!) After several attempts to **explain** were thwarted, I finally took the point, returned the smile and expressed my heartfelt thanks. 'No, **my** thanks to **you**' came the astonishing reply. 'You will continue to take your lovely family out, won't you? It is so lovely to see.'

Writing as a disabled activist and educator, Micheline Mason advises would-be allies:

> We may . . . need you to remind us of our importance to the world, and to each other, at times of tiredness and discouragement. We can live without patronage, pity and sentimentality, but we cannot live without closeness, respect and co-operation from other people. Above all we need you to refuse to accept any 'segregation' of one group of humans from another as anything else but an unacceptable loss for all concerned. (Mason, 1990.)

Meeting someone who fully understood this was a powerful experience. She refused to accept my thanks at the time. The greatest tribute I can now pay is to include her in our family's roll of honour – our allies. These include Elaine and Kate, Julia's teachers, SSD managers David and Malcolm, friends Anna, Liz, Gina and Mandy, and possibly the greatest ally of all, Mair. Julia's list would have at the top her friend and sister, Laura.

TRANSFORMATIONS: 2

Julia's emotional reactions were so obscure that we had not been able to guess how she would respond to the baby's arrival. While I was in hospital she had smiled briefly when Ali was put on her knee. She also said 'bath' and 'bed' seeing a baby bath and Moses basket respectively. Julia's speech is disordered, making it difficult to assess how much she understands and these words and connections made us hopeful that perhaps like other siblings of new babies she might make a developmental leap.

Although appropriate emotional responses to events are always regarded as a 'good sign' by parents of autistic children, Julia's behaviour after I brought Ali home was so extreme that it was hard to take comfort in this way. I would meet her off the school bus, giving Ali to whichever helper was with me, and try to cope with screams and protests as I brought her into the house. Passers-by might have believed me to be a kidnapper but for her screams of 'bed', the only word she said to me. I dreaded the days when the bus came early or the helper was late. Ali was a baby who recognized when anyone other than myself was taking her, and she was often tearful in the arms of strangers. In desperation I asked for advice from a psychologist who had assessed Julia. She made a home visit, checked through various attempts which I had made to deal systematically with the problem, and could add no further ideas. Julia was very happy at her day school as I found out when I visited her there without Ali, and we decided to end stressful afternoons of 'integration' at our local primary school to give her longer where she was happy.

At home, the only place Julia wanted to be was alone in her bedroom. The previously loved garden seemed to terrify her, and this fear was rapidly generalizing to the living room (which led into the garden), the hall (leading to the living room) and so on. Her screams when the French windows opened were such that we all gave up going out into the garden. When she was not agitated, Julia was liable to be aggressive, especially with Ali.

Our first home carers were employed by the SSD via a nursing agency and their help was essential. It was sometimes difficult even for two people to manage Julia, Ali, dinner and bathing. Although Laura was a very responsible eight year old, she also had needs at the end of a school day. However, different people varied in their ability to find their way into a useful role without causing more disruption, and Laura found some intrusive. Despite the extra help and our vigilance, Ali came close to being injured by Julia several times. Our determination to keep Julia at home as much as before, and to prevent her 'opting out' as a family member seemed questionable to one close friend, who urged me to consider alternatives. Despite the exhaustion of a new baby, an abiding faith in Julia and a sense of the despair that was behind her behaviour drove me on to find a solution. The fact that this became possible was due to the arrival at this time of Mair.

It became obvious that we would need home care for more than the anticipated six weeks, unless Julia was to receive respite care on a daily basis after school. When Ali was two months old, Mair was employed by the SSD Home Care Service to work daily with ourselves. Mair had retired from a hospital-based play worker position, and was looking for a part time job. Her considerable experience with children under stress, her maturity and ability to work alongside parents, and her experience in raising her own family meant that she was able to take initiatives unobtrusively without needing support – on the contrary she supported me. We quickly felt we had always known her and couldn't imagine how we had ever managed before her arrival.

Mair has a great sense of fun and responds to all children with implicit respect and understanding. My 'rescue plan' depended on having a trusted and imaginative helper and I put it into action straight away. It was executed with the help of timetables held by everyone in the house after school, including Laura. This was necessary to achieve my aims of: keeping Julia away from Ali except at prescribed times; keeping Julia away from everyone but myself at dinner time; allowing Julia to have a bath (a favourite activity) only when Ali also had a bath, and allowing Julia into her bedroom no earlier than 6.00 p.m. (when Mair left). The timetables were in 15 minute 'slots' lasting from 4.00 p.m. (when Julia arrived home) until 6.00 p.m. (when Mair left). Laura thought it hilarious and happily showed hers to friends. As Julia came home, I would appear alone at the door and whisk her straight off to the beloved park, before she had time to protest. We varied our walk, and I talked quietly about various landmarks. Her out-of-control behaviour had led us into a pattern of relating that left no room for warmth, laughter or fun, and this short walk provided a chance to restore some of that. We were home within half an hour and Mair, Laura and Ali would be off in a different part of the house, while I prepared dinner as always with Julia by herself, sitting at the table quietly with a puzzle.

After this was bath time, where Mair's other skills came into play. The tension of 'keeping the lid on' with a relaxed air was a considerable challenge for me. Bath time was Mair's creative time, and while helping me to be on the alert for attacks, she came up with wonderful games to help Julia 'play' with Ali, using invented tickling and nursery rhyme games, songs and splashes. Julia was gradually won over, I relaxed and Ali played her part by grinning at Julia whenever she came into view. Just two and a half weeks after Mair started, the need for the timetables faded.

Life is always demanding for and with Julia, but when Mair is around the miraculous thing is that it feels no more so than ordinary family life. Mair's relationship with Ali is a close one, and so when the chance came for me to work part-time, Mair agreed to be her childminder. The difference she has made to all our lives cannot be quantified.

Julia was seen in 1991 by the first professional to have a confident view about the nature of her learning difficulties and a clear sense of the kind of education she would need to develop to her full potential. She recommended schooling in a language unit rather than a SLD school, and a year later our LEA agreed to fund a place for Julia at a residential school for children with communication disorders, where she instantly 'settled'. As school holidays are often longer than local holidays, Mair continues to help when Julia comes home.

For the first time since her first operation, Julia has been able to initiate relationships and to make her own friends. This is the greatest milestone, but there have been others. With the help (sceptically received) of the Light and Sound Therapy Centre in London we discovered that Julia can read and even spell, and a gut feeling that she understood more than she could show us has been confirmed. The school she now attends have staff who are very much on the wavelength of autistic children, and whereas Julia comes home with great enthusiasm, she also returns very happily to school.

Although a residential school place was not what we were looking for in 1991, we feel we would have needed to look for such a place eventually. 'Safety nets' were getting thinner, so Julia depended entirely on our constant good health being maintained under extreme duress. In retrospect, her school place has been good for us all. Nevertheless we remain eternally indebted to Mair, and by implication the SSD managers who made her help possible, for the fact that Julia went to school without any sense of rejection on either side. Her place in the family is assured and she understands this to be so.

CONCLUSION

If empowerment of SSD consumers is to have plausibility as a practice ideal, then both the value of empowering services and strategies, and the difficulties for the profession in handing over power must be acknowledged. I have used our experiences as a paradigm because they illustrate conflicts over the various role aspirations of social work(ers), i.e. between the respective roles of:

- power holder
- carer-enabler
- promoter of social justice.

These conflicts became especially apparent in our dealings with the SSD because in reality we were in a situation of compounded dependency, (Alan being an employee, with a family needing services) which magnified the power imbalance. However, his status as a colleague paradoxically created the illusion of equality, suggesting a reduction in the power imbalance. This may explain Malcolm's observation that SSD employees often fare worse than other consumers.

Social workers' preference for believing in the ideology of professional/ academic discourse rather than facing the effect which power structures have in personal and professional lives is exposed by the muddled and even authoritarian practice which results when the two are brought into conflict with each other. For example, practitioners who deny a 'power holding' role will prefer to present themselves as resistance fighters (promoter of social justice) within a system which he or she presumes the consumer regards as hostile. It will be appreciated from our experience that this is too simplistic, i.e. the SSD provided us with crucial services throughout. Incidentally, the anxiety about an untenable professional persona which lies behind this pose is very apparent to a consumer, and precludes an honest working relationship. Another response to role conflict on the part of practitioners is to flee from the 'carer-enabler' role, which carries obligations to treat consumers as individuals, worthy of respect. It is possible to maintain the 'power holder' and 'promoter of social justice' roles respectively while denying the individual needs of a particular consumer, who may be dismissed as 'manipulative', 'unrepresentative', 'middle class', etc. Activists and campaigners who need services from organizations they are fighting can find themselves deal with in this way as individual consumers. The result is high handedness at best and authoritarianism at worst on the part of the wrong-footed practitioner.

Imbalance of power between consumers and SSD workers does not affect all such relationships. Workers, such as care assistants, residential social workers or 'outreach' staff ('alongsiders') are likely to have the most obvious impact on the self-empowerment of both carers and cared for and they do not have the status or power of other workers such as field social workers, care co-ordinators or managers ('assessors').

The working relationships between consumers, 'alongsiders' and 'assessors' respectively are structurally affected in other ways, and our experience as carers can be summarized in Table 17.1.

It will be apparent that 'assessors' must respond to the demands of their own hierarchy as well as to the needs of various consumers, creating conflicts of interest at several levels. Together with the problems created by the power imbalance between themselves and consumers, it may appear that even the practice ideal of a relationship based on 'partnership' with consumers is unattainable, let alone one

Table 17.1 Relationship between alongsiders and assessors

Alongsiders	Assessors
Have the same status as ourselves	Their power to provide or withhold essential services creates a wide status/power imbalance
Shared reality in that they also look after Julia	Second-hand reality, as their information about Julia comes from other people
The service they provide is their own labour	The service they provide is to recommend or ration the labour of others
Their work reduces the segregation of all family members	Their work may provide information about, or access to, services which reduce segregation of all family members

which could 'empower' consumers. However, our experience did not entirely confirm this. For example, some 'assessors' promoted our take-up of services regardless of service shortfall, giving accurate, comprehensive information and encouragement. Our most recent experience as 'clients' has been with a social worker who is able to manage the power imbalance on a personal level by (briefly) acknowledging potential conflicts on both sides in a non-collusive way, while effectively and humanely helping with the practicalities of Julia's 'care package'. The style of work which is open to 'assessors' and may best promote consumers' self-empowerment might be described as the gate-widening gatekeeper.

On a practical level, the most important help which assessors can provide access to is the service provided by 'alongsiders'. From a carer's point of view, 'alongsiders' meet a basic need for time off from caring insofar as they are both able to establish a relationship with the cared-for person and care competently for them. In this respect they reduce the feeling of exclusive family responsibility which most often affects mothers, wives and daughters. Their work may permanently transform the caring equation by helping the cared-for person find their way in new social situations away from home. Through their direct involvement, 'alongsiders' can be a source of extra physical, emotional and creative energy to carers and cared-for alike.

Unless their health or the cared-for person's safety is an issue, the terms on which carers seek respite usually relate to the need to reduce the oppression which they share with the person with the disability, caused by effective segregation. Few carers will knowingly accept respite care which confirms the oppression of the cared-for person unless they themselves are desperate. Although the main thrust of the struggle against segregation is a collective one, such as the fight for the Civil Rights (Disabled Persons) Bill, segregation permeates private as well as public life. Disabled people living within isolated, struggling families are not 'desegregated' any more than vulnerable people deprived of the care and support they need can be described as 'normalized'. In small practical ways, 'alongsiders' can and do contribute to the breaking down of barriers both by an injection of energy which promotes self-empowerment, and directly, for example in outreach community work. The style of work open to 'alongsiders' which best promotes carers' and cared-for persons' self-empowerment is therefore through a relationship which actively promotes a reduction in segregation.

If professional-academic discourse is to promote these styles of work, it must reflect a sense of optimism, having taken account of the realities of the power structures which govern relationships with SSD service users. I hope to have shown how invaluable good services are, as well as how disempowering high handed practice can be. A principal reason for contributing this chapter has been to answer the question frequently asked within the profession as to whether social work helps anyone. The work itself is hard enough, without identity conflict, the difficulty of managing power, limited resources and lack of autonomy, so the demoralization of students, academics and practitioners is understandable. But as a consumer who could not be writing this article without the help provided by our SSD I would like to offer a heartfelt conclusion, paraphrasing something Kate once said about working with Julia. 'Social work is hard work, but it *is* worth it.'

REFERENCES

Crompton, S. (1994) Civil rights, society's wrongs: disabled people fight discrimination. *Professional Social Work*, May.

Mason, M. (1990) How to be an ally – the role of non-disabled people, *Disability Equality in the Classroom: A Human Rights Issue*, first edn. published by ILEA, second edn. published by Disability Equality in Education (p. 78).

Morris, J. (1993) Achievable goals. *Community Care*.

Pearson, G. (1975) *The Deviant Imagination*, 2nd edn, Macmillan, Basingstoke (p. 16).

Index

Abuse
  corruption of care 260
  in mental health system 209
  organizational 260–2
  see also Elder abuse
Accountability, and levels of hierarchy 266
Administration, see Bureaucracy
ADSS (Association of Directors of Social
  Services) 278, 279–80
Advocacy
  Beth Johnson Foundation 195–8
  element of third age self-help groups 137
  group advocacy 223
  independent living advocates 26–7
  issue or crisis oriented 224
  major roles 126–7
  in mental health care, history 204–5
  Patients' Councils 213–14
  schemes' need for independence 197
  self-advocacy in mental health 213–15
  tasks in, examples of 197
  see also Advocacy training; Citizen
    advocacy; Peer advocacy
Advocacy training
  awareness of sexism and racism 125–6
  Beth Johnson Foundation 196
  Birmingham Citizen Advocacy Project
    124, 125
  objectives 125
  training packs 125
  user experience a prerequisite 124–5
Age Concern 274–5, 276
Age discrimination 273
AGLOW, see Association of Greater
  London Older Women
Alleged Lunatics' Friend Society 204
All Wales Strategy for the Development of
  Services for Mentally Handicapped
  People
  access to hospitals 232, 235
  advocacy partnerships 233–7
  funding 229–30
  implementation problems 228–9
  need for advocacy services 227
  organization and recruitment 231–3
  participation, categories of 228
  and planning 228–9
  principles 228
  see also Citizen advocacy

Alongsiders, v. assessors 305–6
Alzheimer's disease, support groups
  199–200
Appraisal, se Staff appraisal
Assertiveness, in self-help groups 85–6
Assessment
  of individual needs 16–17, 270
  models of 27
Assessors, v. alongsiders 305–6
Association of Directors of Social Services
  (ADSS) 278, 279–80
Association of Grater London Older
  Women (AGLOW)
  address 182
  conference on community care 177–9
  educational programme 179, 180, 181
  source of advice 175
Association of Retired Persons 158, 160
Autonomy
  overriding of 279
  v. protection 278–9

Barclary Report (1982) 259
Beth Johnson Foundation
  advocacy 195–8
  Alzheimer sufferers support groups
    199–200
  Care Line 193–4
  dearth of information 185–6
  health-related activities 194–5
  Leisure Association 195
  peer health counsellors 189, 191–2
  reminiscence 198–9
  self-health care 186–7
  senior centre 194–5
  senior citizens involved in public services
    – health and advocacy (SCIPSHA)
    200–1
  work of 184–5
  see also Senior Health Shop
Beveridge Plan 152
Birmingham Citizen Advocacy Project 120,
  124, 125
Birmingham Community Care Special
  Action Project 23, 26
British Network for Alternatives to
  Psychiatry 204
Bureaucracy
  excess of managerial and administrative

posts? 22
and the internal market 21–2, 32–3
welfare organizations v. self-help groups
    34

CAIT (Citizen Advocacy Information and
    Training) 227
Care, informal 15, 37
Care agencies
    complaints procedure 265
    customer orientated? 262–3
    management role 264, 265
    performance indicators 263–6
    staff relationships 264
    user-first structure 266–7
    user relationships 264, 265
    see also Residential care; Social services
        departments
Care Line (Beth Johnson Foundation)
    193–4
Carers
    informal 15
    untrained 17
Carnegie Inquiry, into third age 134,
    172
Child protection, right to attend meetings
    48, 49
Citizen advocacy
    advocates' comments 235–6
    basic model of need for 234
    befriending 227
    Birmingham Citizen Advocacy Project
        120, 124, 125
    categories of 225
    definition 227
    dilution of principles? 233
    examples of practical help 235
    independence from professional
        interests 226–7, 236
    for individuals and groups 225
    instrumental and expressive dimensions
        227, 234–5
    limited resources 237–8
    v. peer advocacy 116
    the place of 224–8
    see also All Wales Strategy; Peer advocacy
Citizen Advocacy Information and Training
    (CAIT) 227
Club de Jubilados Españoles de Londres
    138
Co-counselling 114–15
    see also Peer counselling
Commerical relationships, not appropriate
    to health services 47
Communication, forms of 61
Communication disorders, residential
    schooling 290, 303–4
Community care
    informal carers 15
    redefinition of responsibility for 12
    untrained carers 17
Community Care Support Forum 19
Competition, and economic independence
    46

Complaints
    redefinition of 50
    reluctance to make 30
    right to make 48
Confidence, from group membership 84
    143, 170, 171
Consultants, *see* Professionals
Consultative bodies, representation on
    86–7
Consumerism
    difference in markets 20–1
    and empowerment 20–2
    empowerment of purchasers 22
    goal of 20
    purchaser–user conflict 20
Consumers
    and complaints 48, 50
    importance of views of 52
    not necessarily purchasers 20–1
    research studies of experiences of
        51–6
    rights of 48
    transfer of power from professionals
        45–6
    see also Users
Corruption of care 260
Counselling, *see* Co-counselling; Peer
    counselling
Customer orientation 262–3
Customers, patients as 47–8

Decision making
    and the elderly 202
    managerial tiers in 266
    rights of users 224
Directness 54
Disability
    professionals' view of 26, 30
    social model of 35–6
Disabled people
    in community care planning 64
    forms of communication 61
    and reseach 70
Discrimination
    on age 273
    and mental health 209–10, 210–12
    mentalism 111–12, 206
    see also Racism; Sexism
Disempowerment, of staff 260–2
Doctors, *see* Professionals
Drugs, psychiatric 208

Education, *see* Training and Education
Elder abuse
    increased campaigning 271–2
    proposal for Emergency Intervention
        Orders 276
    protection for elderly 275–7
Elderly, *see* Older people
Emergency Intervention Orders, proposal
    for 276
Empowerment
    competing ideas 62–4
    definitions 11, 14, 62–3, 282–3

Index

Empowerment *contd*
  a good intent? 3
  models of 63
  see also Enablement; Participation; Power;
    User involvement
Enablement
  v. empowerment 11, 18
  role of the professional 25–9
Ethnic minorities
  pensioners 167
  Self-Help Alliance 246–7
  self-help groups 81, 252, 253
European Community, pensioners'
  parliaments 153–5
European Older Women's Project 180, 182
European Year of the Elder Person and
  Solidarity between Generations 151

Fear
  in asserting rights 261
  in making complaints 30
Feedback from users, collection of 128–9
Funding
  All Wales Strategy 229–30
  in Germany 102, 103
  sources of 181–2
  users' organizations 67
Fundraising, older women's health groups
  175

General practitioners, fundholding leading
  to power 21
Germany, social services
  care insurance 102
  in East Germany 101
  funding 102, 103
  independent welfare organizations 102
  relationship with self-help organizations
    102–4
  Seniorenbüros (senior citizens offices)
    106
  structure, overview of 102
  see also Self-help organizations in
    Germany
Group advocacy 223
Groups, *see* Health groups; Pensioners'
  forums; Retired persons' associations;
  Self-help groups; User groups;
  Women's groups

Health care, needs of elderly likely to be
  met? 185
Health festivals, for older women 173
Health groups, for older women 175
  fundraising 175, 181–2
Health records
  professional reaction to right of access
    49, 50
  right of access to 48
Hearing voices movement 218, 219
Home Care Service 293, 302–4
Home help service 293–4

Independence, of elderly 185

Independent living advocates 26–7
Information, self-help groups as source
  of 83–4
Involvement, *see* Participation; User
  involvement

Ladder of participation 52–3
Language
  of care, an illusion? 43
  as carrier of ideology 45
  in construction of meaning 45
  definition of words 50, 51, 56
  meaning subject to manipulation 44
  metaphor in 45, 47
  not reflection of actual practice 51
  a pivotal concept 44–5
Law Commission reports 273, 276–7
Leisure Association (Beth Johnson
  Foundation) 195
Liberational model of empowerment 63
Light and Sound Therapy Centre 304

McMurphy's (user-controlled project) 215–16
Management
  'bicycle' managers 261
  differences from commercial
    management 47
  implications of user-first organizations
    263–7
  tiers in decision-making 266
Mental Health Act (1983) 223
Mental health services
  abuse in 209
  advocacy movements, history 204–5
  brain damage caused by treatment? 208
  crisis cards 211
  deficiencies in service 110
  diagnosis 207–8
  discouragement of emotion 207
  discrimination in 209–10, 210–12
  drugs 208
  fear in 210
  health promotion units 177
  non-compliant patients' registers 212
  and older women 176–7
  over-protective staff 112
  peer counsellors in 110–11
  power of legal detention 205–6
  professional jargon 112
  professionals in 206–7, 211–12
  psychotherapy 209
  self-help resisted by staff 110
  stigma in 210
  users in no-win situation 112
  users not listened to 206, 210–11
  see also All Wales Strategy; Peer
    advocacy; People with learning
    difficulties; Psychiatric survivor
    movement; Survivors; Survivors Speak
    Out
Mentalism 111–12, 206
Mentor system 109
  professional control 114
  see also Peer counselling

Metaphor 45, 47
Models, of empowerment 63
Mutual aid groups, *see* Self-help groups
Mutuality 53–4

National Citizen Advocacy (NCA) 227
National Council for Voluntary Organiza-
    tions (NCVO) 245–6
National Pensioners' Convention (NPC)
    activities of 150–5, 156
    address 169
    aims of 146, 159–60
    Declaration of Intent 148–9
    educational forums for members 150–1
    in European discussions 153–5
    the future 155–6
    growing influence of 153
    growth in membership 150
    history of 146–7
    non-charitable status 146
    and politics 147–8
    principles of 148–9
    umbrella group for pensioners' organiza-
        tions 145
    see also Pensioners' Forums
National User Involvement Project 67
NCA (National Citizen Advocacy) 227
NCVO (National Council or Voluntary
    Organizations) 245–6
NHS and Community Care Act (1990)
    assessment of needs 177–8
    complaints investigation 265
    and elder abuse 284
    empowerment of purchasers 22
    and user needs 263
Nottingham
    Elderly Voices pensioners' forum 162, 169
    municipal background 79
    Patient's Council 213–14
Nottingham Self-Help Team 244
    enquiries to, types of 79–80
    role 79–80, 82–3
    values 82
    see also Self-help groups in Nottingham
NPC, *see* National Pensioners' Convention

Older peopie
    autonomy v. protection 278–9
    choice in practice 49
    demographic changes 66
    discrimanatory stereotyping 141
    as a distinct group? 272–3, 284
    health care needs met? 185
    limited rsources for 274–5
    need for independence 185
    old age as disability? 273
    professionals' prejudices 30
    see also Beth Johnson Foundation; Elder
        abuse; Older women; Pensioners;
        Third agers
Older women
    as carers 177–9
    confidence building 170, 171
    education and health 175–6

emphasis on health 172–3
    health festivals 173
    health groups 175
    local groups 174–5
    and mental health 176–7
    need for training 181
    needs neglected by professionals 170–1
    numbers and position in society 171
    skills of 180–1
    trivialization of health problems 173, 176
    see also Association of Greater London
        Older Women
Older Women's Groups 174–5
    addresses 182
    funders' addresses 181–2
    see also Association of Greater London
        Older Women
Older Women's Project
    aim of 170
    European Project 180, 182
    mental health users' support groups
        176–7
    reasons for 171–2
Outreach schemes 292–3

Participation
    competing approaches to 61–2
    a dynamic concept 44
    ladder of 52–3
    participative v. participatory practice 53
    theory v. practice 68
    see also User involvement
Participative practice
    conditions for 53–6
    v. participatory practice 53
    professionals' response 56–7
Partnership practice 28
    undermining professionalism? 29
Patient-led services 113
Patients, as customers 47–8
Patients' Councils 213–14
Peer advocacy, in mental health care
    advantages of 123–4
    v. citizen advocacy 116
    crisis advocacy 121–2
    definition 116
    examples of 116–19, 120–2
    features of 122
    need for formal organization 129–30
    obstructionism 119
    professional help 130
    professional objections 120
    systems of 129–30
Peer counselling 109, 110–11, 114–15
    health counselling (Beth Johnson
        Foundation) 189, 191–2
    see also Co-counselling
Peer support
    examples of 108–9
    professional control 114
    see also Peer counselling; Self-help groups
Pensioners
    denial of share in country's wealth 148
    a grey image? 145, 146

Pensioners *contd*
  NPC Declaration of Intent on rights
    of 148–9
  see also National Pensioners' Convention;
    Older people; Pensioners' forums;
    Pensions; Retirement; Third Agers;
    Third age self-help groups
Pensioners's forums
  addresses 168–9
  attracting members 166–7
  development of 157–60
  establishment of 164
  ethnic minorities 167
  future developments 167–8
  information dissemination 163–4
  intergenerational benefit 165–6
  local area based 161–2
  local issues 159–60, 165–6
  matters of interest to 157–8, 158–60
  political independence 158
  purpose of 160–1
  raising the profile 165–6
  relationships with authority 166
  response to militancy 159
  types of 162–4
  umbrella organizations 161
  under-represented groups in 166–7
  ways to success 164–6
  women in 166–7
Pensions
  early retirement 159
  history 155
  loss of value of 150, 152
  not linked to wage rises 148, 150, 152,
    158
  NPC Declaration of Intent on level of
    148–9
People with learning difficulties
  a carer's personal experience 289–307
  empowerment, frames of reference
    290–1
  see also Mental health services
Poverty, definitions 184–5
Power
  client 283
  definition 223
  fundholding GPs 21
  group pressure 223
  inequality between users and providers
    68, 70
  professional 283
  retained by profesionals 11, 39
  taken but not given 16
  transfer from professionals to consumers
    45–6
Practice Guidance for Practitioners and for
  Managers 17–19, 20
Professional imperialism 4
Professional model of empowerment 63
  regulatory and liberatory implications 68
Professionals
  assessing needs 16–17
  interest in empowerment 63
  and the market philosophy 3–4

  in mental health service 206–7, 211–12
  political v. professional viewpoints
    11–12, 13–14, 16
  reactions to legislative changes 49–51
  relationships with self-help groups 35,
    36–8, 88, 111–12
  relationships with service users 13–14
  retention of power 11, 39
  role in enablement 25–9
  tensions of formal v. informal care 35,
    36–8
  transfer of power to consumers 45–6
  unable to empower users? 15, 16–17
  views on self-help groups 84–5
Providers
  conflict of interest with users 60–1, 63–4,
    67–8
  consumerist approach to participation 62
  discourse of 60, 61
  need for constructive partnership 69–70
Psychiatric survivor movement
  avoidance of 'provideritus' 217
  campaigns 215
  creative activities 217–18
  daytime support clubs 216
  reactive survivor action 213–15
  support organizations, addresses 219
  user-controlled systems 215–17
  see also Survivors; Survivors Speak Out
Psychiatry, public perceptions of 290
Psychotherapy 209
Publicity
  elder abuse campaign 271
  self-help groups 88, 89, 90
Purchasers, empowerment of 22

Quality, *see* Standards

Racism
  in mental helath care 117, 125–6, 131,
    209–10
  older women 173
Reciprocity 54
  serial 84
Records, *see* Health records
Reminiscence 198–9
Research
  and disabled people 70
  into user involvement 64–5
  National User Involvement Project 67
  need for changed approach 70
  organizations undertaking 67
Residential care, from independent sector
  15
Resources, redistribution of 69
Resources panels 296–7
Respite care, for younger children 298
Retired persons associations (RPAs) 140
  Association of Retired Persons 158, 160
Retirement, pre-retirement discussions 185
Retirement pensions, *see* Pensions
Rights
  availability v. accessibility 223–4
  consumers' 48

fear in asserting 261
RPAs, *see* Retired persons associations
SCEMSC (Standing Conference on Ethnic
Minority Senior Citizens) 247
Schools, for children with communication
disorders 290, 303–4
SCIPSHA (Senior citizens involved in
public services – health and advocacy)
200–1
Self-advocacy 213–15
Self-health care (Beth Johnson
Foundation) 186–7
Self-Help Alliance (SHA)
appropriate dependency 255–6
criteria for local groups 247
formation of 244–7
'horizontal' support 244, 250, 253
participation of ethnic minorities 246–7
relationship with member groups 252–3
running-in phase 247–9
self-evaluation of projects 250
types of local support 250–1
see also Self-help groups
Self-help groups
assertiveness in 85–6
benefits from membership 34–5, 83–4
challenging nature 85–7
characteristics of 33–4, 34–5
characteristics of self-managing group
254–5
constraints and limitations 84, 92–3
as consumer groups 94
co-operation among 36
definition 33
demanding work 257
differing roles of 87
empowerment of? 92
ethnic minorities 252, 253
group approach 86
growth in number of 31
impact of 94
as information sources 83
local directories of 90
local institutional environment 253
meeting members' needs 254
members' purpose in joining 251–2
members' roles 252
peer support in 109–10
professionals' views of 84–5
publicity for 88, 89, 90
relationship with Self-Help Alliance
252–3
relationships with professionals 35, 36–8,
88, 111–12
representation on consultative bodies
86–7
roles of third agers in 135, 137
schemes of self-empowerment 26
social role 93–4
support and encouragement for 87–92
tensions of informal v. formal care 35,
36–8
types of 33–4
value and importance of 83–6, 94

see also Self Help Alliance; Self-help
groups in Nottingham; Self-help
organizations in Germany; Third age
self-help groups
Self-help groups in Nottingham
definition 82
for ethnic minorities 81
growth in number of 31, 80–1
members' stories 77–8
membership patterns 80–1
see also Nottingham Self-Help Team
Self-help organizations in Germany, for
elderly people
constraints 104–5
definition 96–7
development of 97–100
in East Germany 101–2
fields of activities 99–100
funding of 102–103
future role of 106
growth in numbers of 98–9
increasing independence of elderly 105–6
numbers of 31
political activity and aims 103, 104
reasons for joining 99
relationships with social care system
102–4
social self-help groups, characteristics 97
types of 97
see also Germany, social services
Senior citizens involved in public services –
health and advocacy (SCIPSHA) 200–1
Senior Health Shop (Beth Johnson
Foundation)
cafeteria 187–8
choice of location 187, 188
comparison with formal health services
189
growth in number of users 188
health concerns of visitors 190
recruitment of volunteers 188
user questionnaires 188
Sensitivity 54
Serial reciprocity 84
Service users, *see* Users
Sexism, in mental health care 125–6, 210
SHA, *see* Self-Help Alliance
Sheffield Citizen Advocacy Project 233
Social services departments
conflicts when employee is also user
294–5, 298
customer orientated0 262–3
user involvement policy 64
see also Association of Directors of Social
Services; Care agencies
Social welfare, cultural traditions 32–3
Social work
'in deep trouble' 12
implications for managers 260, 261
limited mandate for empowerment 17–20
organizational abuse in 260–2
a political activity 259
user–services tensions 259
value base 258–60

Staff appraisal 265
Standards, right to services based on 48
Standing Conference on Ethnic Minority
    Senior Citizens (SCEMSC) 247
Stereotyping, of older people 141, 273
Support
    for self-help groups 87–92
    users' limited access to 61, 67
    see also Peer support; Self-Help Alliance;
        Support organizations
Support organizations, addresses
    mental health systems survivor
        movement 219
    pensioners' forums 168–9
    sources of funds 181–2
    women's groups 182
Survivors (from psychiatric system)
    homeless, in USA 216
    peer support for? 115
    personal experiences 203–4, 218
    see also Psychiatric survivor movement
Survivors Speak Out 205, 212, 219
    crisis cards 211
    needs and demands 213
    see also Psychiatric survivor movement
Sympathy, a burden? 292
    or understanding? 299–301

Third age
    Carnegie Inquiry into 172
    definition 134
Third agers
    roles in a multigenerational society 143
    roles in self-help and voluntary groups
        135, 137
    see also Older people; Older women;
        Pensioners
Third age self-help groups
    advocacy element 137
    categories of 135
    changing membership of 135–6
    consciousness-raising groups 140–2
    definition 134
    functions of 135–6
    limited number of key groups 135
    problem-solving groups 137
    responsiveness of 136
    self-development groups 138–40
    types of 136–7
Training and education
    advocacy 196
    AGLOW educational programme 179,
        180, 181
    older women's needs 181
    peer health counsellors 191–2
    see also Advocacy training
Tranquillizers 208
Trust
    demonstrable 53, 54–6
    even-handedness 55

Truth, a flexible concept? 44
Two-tierism 21

Understanding, of an 'ally' 299–301
United Kingdom Advocacy Network 214
University of the Third Age (U3A) 138–40
User groups, funding 67
User involvement
    challenge to traditional relationships 59
    National User Involvement Project 67
    need for new approach to 70–1
    progress of 64–5
    related to broader political issues 65–6
    surveys of 64–5
    in training and assessment of
        professionals 128
    uncertainty in development of 65
    user-led services 113
    see also Participation; Users
User-led services 113
Users
    choice and independence for 284
    conflit of interest with providers 60–1,
        63–4, 67–8
    democratic approach to participation
        62
    disadvantaged compared with providers
        68, 70
    discourse of 60–1
    fearing to complain 30
    finding of organizations 67
    limited access to support 61, 67
    and mainstream services 22, 24–5
    need for constructive partnership 69–70
    personal issues 71
    relationships with professionals 13–14
    see also Consumers; Participation; User
        groups; User involvement

Value systems, and language 45
VC (Volunteer Centre) 245–6
Voluntaryu organizations
    support for self-help groups 90
    user involvement policy 64
Volunteer Centre (VC) 245–6

Wales, *see* All Wales Strategy
Welfare resources, unforeseen demands
    on 151–2
Welfare state, need for change 66–7
WFPU (World Federation of Psychiatric
    Users) 205
Women, *see* Older women; Women's
    groups
Women's groups
    addresses 182
    funders' addresses 181–2
    for older women 174–5
World Federation of Psychiatric Users
    (WFPU) 205